Sports Cardiology

Editor

PETER N. DEAN

CLINICS IN
SPORTS MEDICINE

www.sportsmed.theclinics.com

Consulting Editor
MARK D. MILLER

July 2022 • Volume 41 • Number 3

ELSEVIER

1600 John F. Kennedy Boulevard ● Suite 1800 ● Philadelphia, Pennsylvania, 19103-2899

http://www.theclinics.com

CLINICS IN SPORTS MEDICINE Volume 41, Number 3
July 2022 ISSN 0278-5919, ISBN-13: 978-0-323-84888-6

Editor: Megan Ashdown
Developmental Editor: Diana Grace Ang

Photocopying

Single photocopies of single articles may be made for personal use as allowed by national copyright laws. Permission of the Publisher and payment of a fee is required for all other photocopying, including multiple or systematic copying, copying for advertising or promotional purposes, resale, and all forms of document delivery. Special rates are available for educational institutions that wish to make photocopies for non-profit educational classroom use. For information on how to seek permission visit www.elsevier.com/permissions or call: (+44) 1865 843830 (UK)/(+1) 215 239 3804 (USA).

Derivative Works

Subscribers may reproduce tables of contents or prepare lists of articles including abstracts for internal circulation within their institutions. Permission of the Publisher is required for resale or distribution outside the institution. Permission of the Publisher is required for all other derivative works, including compilations and translations (please consult www.elsevier.com/permissions).

Electronic Storage or Usage

Permission of the Publisher is required to store or use electronically any material contained in this periodical, including any article or part of an article (please consult www.elsevier.com/permissions). Except as outlined above, no part of this publication may be reproduced, stored in a retrieval system or transmitted in any form or by any means, electronic, mechanical, photocopying, recording or otherwise, without prior written permission of the Publisher.

Notice

No responsibility is assumed by the Publisher for any injury and/or damage to persons or property as a matter of products liability, negligence or otherwise, or from any use or operation of any methods, products, instructions or ideas contained in the material herein. Because of rapid advances in the medical sciences, in particular, independent verification of diagnoses and drug dosages should be made.

Although all advertising material is expected to conform to ethical (medical) standards, inclusion in this publication does not constitute a guarantee or endorsement of the quality or value of such product or of the claims made of it by its manufacturer.

Clinics in Sports Medicine (ISSN 0278-5919) is published quarterly by Elsevier Inc., 360 Park Avenue South, New York, NY 10010-1710. Months of issue are January, April, July, and October. Business and Editorial Offices: 1600 John F. Kennedy Blvd., Ste. 1800, Philadelphia, PA 19103-2899. Customer Service Office: 3251 Riverport Lane, Maryland Heights, MO 63043. Periodicals postage paid at New York, NY and additional mailing offices. Subscription prices are $368.00 per year (US individuals), $959.00 per year (US institutions), $100.00 per year (US students), $409.00 per year (Canadian individuals), $988.00 per year (Canadian institutions), $100.00 (Canadian students), $480.00 per year (foreign individuals), $988.00 per year (foreign institutions), and $235.00 per year (foreign students). Foreign air speed delivery is included in all *Clinics* subscription prices. All prices are subject to change without notice. **POSTMASTER:** Send address changes to *Clinics in Sports Medicine*, Elsevier Health Sciences Division, Subscription Customer Service, 3251 Riverport Lane, Maryland Heights, MO 63043. Customer Service (orders, claims, online, change of address): Elsevier Health Sciences Division, Subscription Customer Service, 3251 Riverport Lane, Maryland Heights, MO 63043. **Tel: 1-800-654-2452 (U.S. and Canada); 314-447-8871 (outside U.S. and Canada). Fax: 314-447-8029. E-mail: journalscustomerservice-usa@elsevier.com (for print support); journalsonlinesupport-usa@ elsevier.com (for online support).**

Reprints. For copies of 100 or more of articles in this publication, please contact the Commercial Reprints Department, Elsevier Inc., 360 Park Avenue South, New York, NY 10010-1710. Tel.: 212-633-3874; Fax: 212-633-3820; E-mail: reprints@elsevier.com.

Clinics in Sports Medicine is covered in *MEDLINE/PubMed (Index Medicus) Current Contents/Clinical Medicine*, *Excerpta Medica*, and *ISI/Biomed*.

Contributors

CONSULTING EDITOR

MARK D. MILLER, MD
S. Ward Casscells Professor, Head, Department of Orthopaedic Surgery, Division of
Sports Medicine, University of Virginia, Charlottesville, Virginia; Team Physician, Miller
Review Course, Harrisonburg, Virginia

EDITOR

PETER N. DEAN, MD, FACC
Division of Pediatric Cardiology, Department of Pediatrics, University of Virginia School of
Medicine, UVA Children's Hospital Battle Building, Charlottesville, Virginia

AUTHORS

ERIN S. BARNES, MD
Assistant Professor, Department of Physical Medicine and Rehabilitation and Orthopedic
Surgery, Case Western Reserve University School of Medicine, Cleveland, Ohio

DAVID L. BEAVERS, MD, PhD
Department of Internal Medicine, Division of Cardiac Electrophysiology, University of
Michigan, Ann Arbor, Michigan

ALAN C. BRAVERMAN, MD
Alumni Endowed Professor in Cardiovascular Diseases, Director, Marfan Syndrome and
Aortopathy Clinic, Director, Aortopathy and Master Clinician Fellowship Program,
Cardiovascular Division, John T. Milliken Department of Medicine, Washington University
School of Medicine, St Louis, Missouri

EUGENE H. CHUNG, MD, MSc
Department of Internal Medicine, Division of Cardiac Electrophysiology, University of
Michigan, Ann Arbor, Michigan

JAMIE N. COLOMBO, DO
Assistant Professor, Department of Pediatrics, Division of Cardiology, Washington
University School of Medicine/St. Louis Children's Hospital, St Louis, Missouri

ALFRED DANIELIAN, MD, FACC, FASE
Director of Sports Cardiology and Echocardiography, Las Vegas Heart Associates -
Affiliated with Mountain View Hospital, Las Vegas, Nevada

PETER N. DEAN, MD, FACC
Division of Pediatric Cardiology, Department of Pediatrics, University of Virginia School of
Medicine, UVA Children's Hospital Battle Building, Charlottesville, Virginia

MICHAEL S. EMERY, MD, MS
Sports Cardiology Center, Heart, Vascular, and Thoracic Institute, Cleveland Clinic, Cleveland, Ohio

KIMBERLY G. HARMON, MD
Professor, Departments of Family Medicine and Orthopaedics and Sports Medicine, University of Washington School of Medicine, Sports Medicine Center at Husky Stadium, Seattle, Washington

JONATHAN H. KIM, MD, MSc
Emory University School of Medicine, Emory Clinical Cardiovascular Research Institute, Atlanta, Georgia

JOHN M. MacKNIGHT, MD, FACSM
Professor, Internal Medicine and Orthopaedic Surgery, University of Virginia School of Medicine, University Physicians Clinic, UVA Health System, Charlottesville, Virginia

CHINMAYA MAREDDY, MBBS, MBA
Fellow in Cardiac Electrophysiology, Division of Cardiovascular Medicine, Department of Medicine, University of Virginia, Charlottesville, Virginia

MATTHEW W. MARTINEZ, MD, FACC
Associate Professor of Medicine, Department of Cardiovascular Medicine, Atlantic Health, Morristown Medical Center, Morristown, New Jersey; Sports Cardiology and Hypertrophic Cardiomyopathy

GEORGE MCDANIEL, MD
Associate Professor of Pediatric Cardiology and Electrophysiology, Division of Pediatric Cardiology, University of Virginia, Charlottesville, Virginia

OLIVER MONFREDI, MD, PhD
Assistant Professor of Cardiology and Electrophysiology, Division of Cardiovascular Medicine, University of Virginia, Charlottesville, Virginia

GARY PARIZHER, MD
Sports Cardiology Center, Heart, Vascular, and Thoracic Institute, Cleveland Clinic, Cleveland, Ohio

DERMOT M. PHELAN, MD, PhD
Sanger Heart & Vascular Institute, Atrium Health, Charlotte, North Carolina

KELLI PUGH, MS, ATC, LMT
Associate Athletics Director for Sports Medicine, University of Virginia, McCue Center, Charlottesville, Virginia

CHRISTINE N. SAWDA, MD
Fellow, Department of Pediatrics, Division of Cardiology, Children's National Medical Center, Washington, DC

ANKIT B. SHAH, MD, MPH, FACC
Sports and Performance Cardiology Program, MedStar Health, Baltimore, Maryland

MARY B. SHEPPARD, MD
Assistant Professor, Co-Director, Departments of Family and Community Medicine, Surgery, and Physiology, Saha Aortic Center, University of Kentucky College of Medicine, Lexington, Kentucky

SIOBHAN M. STATUTA, MD, FACSM
Associate Professor, Department of Family Medicine and Physical Medicine and Rehabilitation, University of Virginia School of Medicine, Charlottesville, Virginia

JOHN D. SYMANSKI, MD
Sanger Heart & Vascular Institute, Atrium Health, Charlotte, North Carolina

MATTHEW THOMAS SCM
Pediatric Cardiovascular Genetics Program Director, Division of Pediatric Genetics, University of Virginia, Charlottesville, Virginia

JASON V. TSO, MD
Emory University School of Medicine, Emory Clinical Cardiovascular Research Institute, Atlanta, Georgia

SHELBY C. WHITE, MD
Assistant Professor, Department of Pediatrics, Division of Cardiology, University of Virginia, Charlottesville, Virginia

Contents

Providing medical care for an athlete can be challenging in many aspects. One specific aspect is the athlete's cardiovascular system. Athletic training and physical activity certainly can improve cardiovascular health, but it can also cause cardiac adaptations and place athletes at risk for sudden cardiac arrest. When an athlete has cardiac symptoms, a concerning family history, abnormal cardiac testing, or an underlying cardiac condition, a wide range of professionals are needed to appropriately care for the athlete under evaluation.

Sudden cardiac death (SCD) is the leading cause of medical death in athletes; however, many studies are significantly flawed making an accurate estimation of risk difficult. Incidence studies need to have accurate case ascertainment, a defined study population, and should be stratified by both sex and age. The risk of SCA/d in college-aged males is 1 in 35,000 person-years, black males 1 in 18,000 person-years, and higher-risk sports include men's basketball, men's soccer, and American football. Inherited cardiomyopathies and electrical conditions account for ∼ 2/3 of off SCA/d and can be detected with an ECG. More research is needed to provide more granular estimates.

When considering the variety of complaints an athlete can present with, chest pain is arguably the most concerning given the potential for catastrophic outcomes. Luckily, these do not comprise the majority of cases, and indeed, are quite rare. The bulk of presentations of athletes with chest pain are due to musculoskeletal, gastrointestinal, and pulmonary causes. Each and every healthcare provider who works closely with athletes must have a thorough understanding of contributing conditions that present as chest pain. Here, we explore some of the more prevalent causes of non-cardiac chest pain, classic presentations, and management considerations.

The expanding array and adoption of consumer health wearables is creating a new dynamic to the patient–health-care provider relationship. Providers are increasingly tasked with integrating the biometric data collected from their patients into clinical care. Further, a growing body of evidence is supporting the provider-driven utility of wearables in the screening, diagnosis, and monitoring of cardiovascular disease. Here we highlight existing and emerging wearable health technologies and the potential applications for use within sports cardiology. We additionally highlight how wearables can advance the remote cardiovascular care of patients within the context of the COVID-19 pandemic. Finally, despite these promising advances, we acknowledge some of the significant challenges that remain before wearables can be routinely incorporated into clinical care.

Routine vigorous exercise can lead to electrical, structural, and functional adaptations that can enhance exercise performance. There are several factors that determine the type and magnitude of exercise-induced cardiac remodeling (EICR) in trained athletes. In some athletes with pronounced cardiac remodeling, there can be an overlap in morphologic features with mild forms of cardiomyopathy creating gray zone scenarios whereby distinguishing health from disease can be difficult. An integrated clinical approach that factors athlete-specific characteristics (sex, size, sport, ethnicity, and training history) and findings from multimodality imaging are essential to help make this distinction.

Exercise stress testing (EST) is indicated for diagnostic and prognostic purposes in the general population. In athletes, stress tests can also be useful to inform the risk of high-intensity training and competition, to assess athletic conditioning, and to refine training regimens. Many specific indications for EST are unique to athletes. Treadmill and cycle ergometer protocols each have their strengths and disadvantages; extensive protocol customization may be necessary to answer the clinical question at hand. A comprehensive understanding of the available tools for exercise testing, their strengths, and their limitations is crucial to providing cardiovascular care to athletic individuals.

Myocarditis is a leading cause of sudden death in athletes. Early data demonstrating increased prevalence of cardiac injury in hospitalized patients with COVID-19 raised concerns for athletes recovered from COVID-19 and the possibility of underlying myocarditis. However, subsequent large registries have provided reassuring data affirming low prevalence of myocarditis in athletes convalesced from COVID-19. Although the clinical significance of subclinical myocarditis detected by cardiac MRI remains uncertain, clinical outcomes have not demonstrated an increase in acute cardiac events in athletes throughout the pandemic. Future directions include defining mechanisms underlying "long-haul" COVID-19 and the potential impact of new viral variants.

physical activities are generally prohibited in individuals with aortopathy conditions.

Cardiovascular disease remains the number one cause of death in Americans. It is no secret that exercise mitigates this risk. Exercise and regular physical activity are beneficial for physical health including aerobic conditioning, endurance, strength, mental health, and overall improved quality of life. Unfortunately, today many children and adolescents are sedentary, lacking the recommended daily amount of physical activity, leading to higher rates of obesity, cardiovascular disease, stroke, diabetes, anxiety, and depression. Given this rising concern, the World Health Organization launched a 12-year plan to improve physical activity in children and adolescents by reducing the inactivity rate by 15% in the world. How does this apply to children and adolescents with acquired or congenital heart disease?.

CLINICS IN SPORTS MEDICINE

SERIES OF RELATED INTERESTED

Orthopedic Clinics
https://www.orthopedic.theclinics.com/
Foot and Ankle Clinics
https://www.foot.theclinics.com/
Hand Clinics
https://www.hand.theclinics.com/
Physical Medicine and Rehabilitation Clinics
https://www.pmr.theclinics.com/

THE CLINICS ARE AVAILABLE ONLINE!
Access your subscription at:
www.theclinics.com

Foreword

Sports Cardiology: Put Your Heart into It

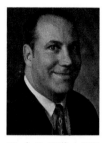

Mark D. Miller, MD
Consulting Editor

I love that Dr Dean, who was gracious enough to accept the job as guest editor for this issue of *Clinics in Sports Medicine*, used a baseball analogy to introduce this topic. I would say that he hit it out of the park! This is a very thorough and comprehensive review of the subject, and I think we can all learn a lot—and not miss a beat. The issue begins with a discussion of the team care of athletes, which is important for all specialists that cover sports. Sudden Cardiac Death is given all the attention it deserves, because none of us want to be on the sidelines when a cardiac emergency occurs. The issue also covers noncardiac mimickers and newer technologies and defines the term "athletic heart." The focus then shifts to stress testing, myocarditis (included that associated with COVID-19), HCM, and genetic arrhythmia syndromes, before concluding with a discussion of aortic disease and pediatric concerns. Thank you to Dr Peter Dean and all of the authors who contributed to this fantastic issue. I think it is safe to say that they all put their heart into it.

Mark D. Miller, MD
Division of Sports Medicine
Department of OrthopaedicSurgery
Surgery University of Virginia, Charlottesville
400 Ray C. Hunt Drive
Suite 330
Charlottesville, VA 22908-0159, USA

E-mail address:
MDM3P@hscmail.mcc.virginia.edu

Clin Sports Med 41 (2022) xiii
https://doi.org/10.1016/j.csm.2022.03.002
0278-5919/22/© 2022 Published by Elsevier Inc.

Preface

The Offense and Defense of Sports Cardiology

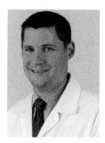

Peter N. Dean, MD
Editor

Just stand out there and stick your glove out in the air. I'll take care of it.
— *Benny "the Jet" Rodriguez, The Sandlot*

Early the movie, *The Sandlot*, Benny "The Jet" Rodriguez recognizes Scotty Smalls has never played baseball and has no hope of catching a fly ball. Instead of shunning him and sending him home, he says the above quote and sends him back to left field. As you may guess, Smalls holds his glove in the air, closes his eyes, and Benny hits a perfect fly ball into the glove.

This is a similar situation for this issue of *Clinics in Sports Medicine*. I, as the guest editor, put my glove in the air and a great group of authors hit perfect fly balls. This group of knowledgeable and experienced authors has written clear, well-researched articles that will help medical providers care for athletes and their hearts.

When I assembled the authors and table of contents, my hope was that readers would gain knowledge in the two major aspects of sports cardiology. The first aspect (the "defense") was preventing adverse events and sudden cardiac arrest (SCA) by appropriate recognition of signs and symptoms of cardiac disease. This incredibly important task can fall into a variety of individuals' fields. Typically, it is in the hands of primary care or sports medicine medical providers and athletic trainers, but other individuals around athletes need to have a solid understanding of the topic (cardiologists, coaches, parents, emergency medical personnel, bystanders, and other subspecialty providers). Typically, preventing SCA is accomplished by performing an appropriate preparticipation evaluation, recognizing and evaluating cardiac symptoms, and carefully performing and interpreting cardiac test results.

The second major aspect of sports cardiology is the appropriate care of athletes with known cardiac disease (the "offense"). This sometimes means restricting an athlete

Clin Sports Med 41 (2022) xv–xvi
https://doi.org/10.1016/j.csm.2022.03.001
0278-5919/22/© 2022 Published by Elsevier Inc.

with a high-risk cardiac condition, and it sometimes means allowing participation when the risk of participation is low. There are significant implications and little data to support either decision, so these decisions and discussions should not be taken lightly. Since the first sign or symptom of cardiac disease can sometimes be an SCA, the "offense" also means responding to emergency situations and SCA with immediate CPR and defibrillation.

Thank you to the authors for your time and important contributions. Thank you also to Mark Miller, Lauren Boyle, Diana Ang, and Megan Ashdown for inviting me to participate and helping put this issue together. Enjoy.

Peter N. Dean, MD
Division of Pediatric Cardiology
Department of Pediatrics
University of Virginia School of Medicine
UVA Children's Hospital Battle Building
1204 West Main Street
Charlottesville, VA, 22903, USA

E-mail address:
pnd8j@virginia.edu

The Importance of Surrounding the Athlete's Heart with a Team

Peter N. Dean, MD, FACC[a],*, Kelli Pugh, MS, ATC, LMT[b],
Siobhan M. Statuta, MD[c], John M. MacKnight, MD[d]

KEYWORDS

- Sports cardiology • Sports participation • Athlete • Sudden cardiac arrest

KEY POINTS

- The care of athletes with cardiac conditions or cardiac symptoms can be challenging and requires a variety of specialized professionals.
- It is important to differentiate between exercise-induced cardiac remodeling and cardiac pathologic conditions.
- Knowing of the causes of sudden cardiac arrest (SCA) in athletes as well as red flags that suggest an underlying cardiac condition is vital to caring for athletes.
- Preparticipation evaluation will never diagnose every cause of SCA, so onsite providers need to quickly recognize SCA and provide appropriate emergency treatment.

INTRODUCTION

The importance of a team surrounding and caring for an athlete's heart can be illustrated in a recent case (**Fig. 1**).

> A 20-year-old collegiate athlete called his athletic trainer one evening after he felt the abrupt onset of palpitations at rest. The palpitations lasted approximately 1 hour and resolved spontaneously. The athletic trainer discussed the symptoms with the athlete and appropriately thought he did not require urgent medical care.

[a] Division of Pediatric Cardiology, Department of Pediatrics, University of Virginia School of Medicine, UVA Children's Hospital Battle Building, 1204 West Main Street, Charlottesville, VA 22903, USA; [b] University of Virginia, McCue Center, Room 112, 290 Massie Road, Charlottesville, VA 22904, USA; [c] Department of Family Medicine and Physical Medicine and Rehabilitation, University of Virginia School of Medicine, PO Box 800729, 1415 Jefferson Park Avenue-McKim Hall 3152, Charlottesville, VA 22908, USA; [d] Internal Medicine & Orthopaedic Surgery, University of Virginia School of Medicine, University Physicians Clinic, UVA Health System, Box 800671, Charlottesville, VA 22908, USA
* Corresponding author.
E-mail address: pnd8j@virginia.edu

Clin Sports Med 41 (2022) 357–368
https://doi.org/10.1016/j.csm.2022.02.001
0278-5919/22/© 2022 Elsevier Inc. All rights reserved.

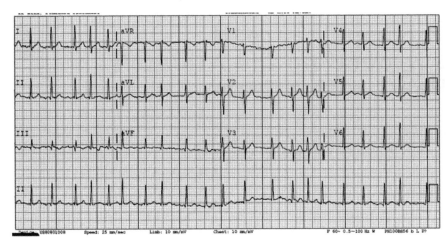

Fig. 1. ECG demonstrating atrial fibrillation in the 20-year-old collegiate athlete in the introduction.

The following morning he had recurrence of symptoms and saw his primary sports medicine physician. Examination and electrocardiogram (ECG) in the office diagnosed atrial fibrillation. The athlete was directed to the emergency department where his other workup was reassuring, and he underwent a successful cardioversion. Because this event occurred 2 to 3 weeks after a novel coronavirus-19 (COVID-19) infection, he also underwent additional cardiac evaluation. His echocardiogram and cardiac magnetic resonance imaging (MRI) showed slight abnormalities, but his cardiologist and radiology team believed these findings were consistent with athletic cardiac remodeling and not cardiac pathologic conditions. There was no late gadolinium enhancement or other evidence of myocardial scar or myocarditis.

This athlete was then evaluated by an electrophysiologist who specializes in sports cardiology. At that visit, they discussed the risks and benefits of nonintervention, medical management, and catheter ablation. His risk for embolic stroke was deemed low, so he was not started on anticoagulation. The electrophysiologist also walked him through a shared decision-making process regarding whether or not he should continue playing football.

He subsequently experienced significant anxiety surrounding his new diagnosis of atrial fibrillation and his future in sports, thus he met with his primary sports medicine physician several times. Eventually, he was referred for psychological counseling and initiated an anxiolytic medication.

Given that he was at a low risk for complications related to the atrial fibrillation and displayed no other risk factors, he and his electrophysiologist opted for nonintervention and no cardiac medications. Once his anxiety was also addressed, he was then able to resume sport participation with gradual reconditioning guided by his athletic trainer.

This case shows the complexity in caring for athletes with cardiac symptoms or cardiac conditions and the multispecialty providers that are often required.

THE CHALLENGE OF SPORTS CARDIOLOGY

Before 2020, the challenges surrounding caring for athletes with cardiac conditions or cardiac symptoms were recognized by a fairly limited number of individuals. With the advent of the novel coronavirus-19 (COVID-19) pandemic, however, these challenges were quickly recognized by many in the general population. The international media outlets and general medical community caught onto the concern for the complication of myocarditis from viral infections, and the apprehension encompassing return-to-exercise and sports participation. The media also discovered the concerning initial findings of abnormal cardiac MRIs in athletes following a COVID-19 infection[1,2] and reports of high-level athletes with myocarditis.[3,4] Fortunately, large follow-up registries in young athletes eventually demonstrated a low prevalence of myocardial injury after COVID-19,[5,6] thus allaying some of the fears associated with returning to sports and exercise participation.

The COVID-19 pandemic has also added a huge stress on the workload of medical professionals, highlighting the importance of a team approach to caring for athletes. Preparticipation clearance has never been a simple process, and COVID-19 adds yet another layer of complexity for the primary care providers. In addition to their typical full workload, athletic trainers and primary care physicians are now responsible for COVID-testing athletes, following up results, mandating appropriate quarantining and isolating practices, and supervising return-to-play. Once athletes are cleared to resume sports, this new history of a previous COVID-19 infection requires heightened vigilance by all parties to survey for cardiac symptoms.

In brief, the specific challenges in caring for athletes' hearts are as follows:

1. Athletic training causes adaptations in the heart.[7,8] These changes alter the typical diagnostic cardiac testing (ECGs, echocardiograms, MRIs, and so forth) and can make it seem the athlete has pathologic conditions when there is no true pathologic condition present. Sometimes, as may have happened in the above case, the adaptations can cause atrial fibrillation or worsen other preexisting cardiac disease.
2. In the setting of preexisting cardiac disease, there is very little scientific data and no randomized controlled trials exploring the safety and impact of athletic training and sports participation. Most guidelines come from suboptimal evidence or expert recommendations.
3. Athletes, despite a cardiac diagnosis or concerning cardiac symptoms, typically desire to continue their sport and training and therefore will continue to add both acute and chronic stress to their heart.
4. There are significant negative implications when an athlete is restricted from sports. Although the diagnosis of heart disease is traumatic and difficult for any patient, an athlete potentially feels a greater loss given that so much of their identity is intertwined with sport and exercise. Restriction from sport thus strips them from an action or lifestyle that adds to their general well-being and quality of life.[9-11]
5. A missed diagnosis of cardiac disease can be catastrophic in an athlete. Sometimes, the first symptom or sign of cardiac disease can be a malignant arrhythmia or lethal aortic dissection. Not all athletes will have symptoms of their cardiac condition before their sudden cardiac arrest (SCA).
6. Even with extensive and appropriate preparticipation cardiac testing, SCAs still occur.[12,13] This is an unsatisfying and anxiety-provoking realization for those caring for athletes.

PREPARTICIPATION EVALUATION

With those particular challenges and more, team physicians and primary care providers do their best to mitigate risk to each individual athlete. Sudden cardiac death (SCD) is the devastating outcome each medical team endeavors to prevent. Athlete screening protocols exist with the goal to identify at-risk individuals and take appropriate precautions. Many clues to the examining physician will come from past personal history or family history, yet even before delving into those, there are broad considerations to help determine risk. These can be particularly helpful when contemplating the varied population involved in sports activities today. The first factor to note is athletes' age, as the causes of SCD vary. Occurrences of SCA in athletes aged less than 35 years are mostly the outcomes of congenital heart disease (CHD), cardiomyopathies, or inherited arrhythmia syndromes. However, coronary heart disease is more commonly the cause for athletes aged more than 35 years. Another element to understand is the specific sport and intensity that the athlete desires. The environment of competitive sports places an individual under greater pressures to excel, and potentially higher training levels with exertional extremes. However, recreational athletes, although still training hard, are likely not experiencing these same physical and thus cardiac stresses.[14] These generalities can serve as influencers toward assessment, but careful exploration of personal and family history remains essential because each athlete carries his/her own unique set of risk factors.

When completing the preparticipation assessment, the history provides an invaluable insight into possible harbingers of bad outcomes. There exists no standard screening form, as questionnaires vary depending on sport, state/country, and athletic agency. In the United States, however, consensus statements by the American Heart Association and European Society of Cardiology[15] as well as the 2019 release of the *Preparticipation Physical Evaluation*, 5th Edition (PPE)[16] guide much of the current practice.

The personal history aims to identify clinical warning signs noted on thoughtful and systematic review. Previous episodes of lightheadedness, syncope or near syncope during exercise, chest pains, seizures, shortness of breath beyond normal degrees, excessive fatigue, any cardiac testing completed or known cardiac diagnoses including murmur are vital questions to review carefully (**Box 1**).

Family history is essential to raise red flags to potential inherited conditions to which the athlete may be predisposed. A history of genetic heart problems in relatives or placement of a defibrillator/pacemaker at younger ages in relatives should raise suspicion. An occurrence of nontraumatic sudden death, especially younger than 50 year old, ought to be considered cardiac related. Similarly, any history of unexplained syncope, motor vehicle collision, seizure activity, drowning/near drowning, or sudden infant death syndrome may similarly indicate the existence of a familial cardiac pathologic condition.

Cardiovascular systematic screening programs vary greatly worldwide. Standard practice in the United States is to complete a personal history, family history, and physical examination (without ECGs). Italy and Israel are 2 countries well known for their inclusion of 12-lead ECGs with all preparticipation encounters.[15] Much debate and controversy surround these particular approaches as well as other countries' rejection of any systemic cardiovascular screening programs altogether.

CARE DURING SPORTS PARTICIPATION AND EMERGENCY ACTION PLANS

Even with extensive preparticipation testing, SCA can still occur in athletes.[12,17] Due to this, professionals at sporting venues need to be prepared for SCA and other cardiac symptom presentations.

Athletic trainers are medical professionals with comprehensive education in injury prevention, clinical evaluation and diagnosis, immediate and emergency care, and the treatment and rehabilitation of injuries. The athletic trainer is often the most consistent medical provider available to an athlete in the high school or collegiate setting, as well as the first responder to a traumatic or nontraumatic injury. SCD and exertional

> **Box 1**
> **Abnormal cardiac history follow-up questions recommended by the PPE 5th Edition**
>
> Abnormal History Follow-up Questions
>   Personal History
>   Have you ever experienced chest pain or chest discomfort with exercise?
>   Have you ever nearly lost or actually lost consciousness?
>   Have you ever had excessive shortness of breath or fatigue with exercise beyond what is expected for your level of fitness?
>   Have you ever been told that you have a heart murmur?
>   Do you experience the skipped, irregular, or racing heartbeats (palpitations) with exercise?
>   Family History
>   Has anyone in your family aged less than 35 years died suddenly or died unexpectedly of heart disease?
>   Has anyone in your family aged less than 35 years been disabled from heart disease or had cardiac treatments including surgery?
>   Are there any cardiac conditions in your extended family members such as hypertrophic or dilated cardiomyopathy, long QT syndrome or other ion channelopathies, Marfan syndrome, or arrhythmias?
>
> Additional, further in-depth follow-up questions may be found in the original resource.[15]
>
> *Data from* Preparticipation Physical Evaluation (PPE) Monograph, 5th Edition, https://www.acsm.org/education-resources/books/preparticipation-physical-evaluation-monograph.

conditions (ie, exertional sickling collapse, exertional heat stroke) are the 2 leading nontraumatic causes of death in athletes.[18,19]

The athletic trainer's familiarity with an athlete's medical history, sport training history, and observation of his/her typical recovery patterns during exertion provides a great advantage during the on-field differential diagnosis. An athlete with shortness of breath, pale clammy skin, or holding their chest who does not recover quickly during interval rest periods warrants further medical attention. A history should identify acute symptoms and address pertinent medical/lifestyle questions, such as the following:

- What did you eat before exercise?
- Did you hydrate well yesterday, and/or before this workout?
- Did you sleep well last night?
- Have you had any recent symptoms of illness?
- Have you performed physical training of this exercise and intensity recently?
- Has your recent exercise been indoors or outdoors?

These and similar questions can help provide reassurance that the athlete's symptoms may be attributed to lack of appropriate preparation before exercise, deconditioning, or lack of environmental acclimatization, as opposed to an emergent medical condition. In the conscious, responsive athlete, a period of observation with rest, hydration, fueling with easily digestible carbohydrates, and cooling measures should provide relief of symptoms rapidly.

The athletic trainer should also use a variety of vital signs to help quantify the athlete's status and potentially determine the cause of symptoms. Pulse oximetry is helpful in ruling out exertional sickling conditions, as well as providing an accurate heart rate when the athlete's pulse is too fast to count. Obtaining a rectal temperature is the only way to accurately assess for exertional heat stroke versus heat exhaustion. There are also devices that can be paired with smart phones to capture a medical-grade single lead ECG in the field. The corresponding phone application typically can provide a quick analysis of "sinus rhythm," "abnormal rhythm," or "atrial fibrillation." The ECG can be emailed immediately to the team physician, allowing for real-time determination of whether transport to the emergency department is necessary versus routine clinical follow-up.

Nontraumatic sudden collapse of an athlete requires a coordinated emergency response by the athletic trainer and any available support personnel such as coaches or other athletes. The athletic trainer should initially assess level of consciousness, breathing, and pulse. Early activation of emergency medical services (EMS), prompt administration of cardiopulmonary resuscitation (CPR), and rapid application of an automatic external defibrillator (AED) are critical to the athlete's survival.[20]

Every athletic venue should have a unique emergency action plan (EAP) rehearsed annually by relevant sports medicine and coaching staff members. Per the National Collegiate Athletic Association (NCAA) Sport Science Institute "Interassociation Recommendations: Preventing Catastrophic Injury and Death in Collegiate Athletes"[21] best practices document, EAPs should provide responses for the following nontraumatic catastrophic events:

1. Cardiac arrest.
2. Exertional heatstroke.
3. Asthma.
4. Exertional collapse associated with sickle cell trait.
5. Any exertional or nonexertional collapse.
6. Mental health emergency.

The EAP should ideally be posted in an easily accessible location and include the facility address as well as EMS access points. Once EMS is activated by calling 911, coaches or other support staff should station at specific points along the route to help guide EMS to the location of the athlete. EAPs are revised any time there is facility construction, with the pertinent changes communicated to local EMS providers. Emergency equipment ought to be easily accessible and well maintained. AEDs must be visible and their locations noted prominently throughout the venue, with a goal of a collapse-to-shock in less than 3 minutes.[22.]

Athletic trainers are required to submit proof of current certification for CPR and AED use every 2 years when they recertify through their national organization. To emphasize the role of coaches in the emergency response, in 2014, the NCAA mandated all full time coaching staff—including strength and conditioning coaches—must remain certified in first aid, CPR, and AED use.[23] Regular education and annual rehearsal of the EAP promotes a culture of readiness and reinforces the expectation that coaches are participants in the execution of the EAP.

Emergency preparedness by athletic trainers and coaches can help an athlete survive an SCA. Once an acute intervention is provided and the athlete has stabilized or recovered, primary care physicians and sports cardiologists are left with the challenging determination of whether resumption of sport participation is safe.

OFFICE EVALUATION WHEN CARDIAC SYMPTOMS OR CONCERNS ARE PRESENT

Athletes presenting with chest pain or other potential cardiac symptoms always warrant prompt and thorough assessment. Because even mild symptoms arising with exertion may have serious implications, up to and including SCA, a cardiac cause should always be assumed until proven otherwise. In the office setting, it is preferable for these evaluations to be performed by a dedicated primary care or sports medicine practitioner whose comfort level with sport training and exercise physiology ensures an appropriate evaluation.

A detailed history will often rapidly narrow the differential diagnosis at the time of presentation. For chest pain, it is vital to determine severity, location, and quality of pain as well as any pattern of radiation and factors that either provoke or relieve. For dyspnea, it is important to determine whether this is present with exertion or at rest, and whether there are associated features such as wheezing, cough, or inspiratory obstructive symptoms. Syncope or presyncope should always suggest a potentially serious underlying cardiac cause; distinguishing events that are postexertional from those that occur during exercise helps to differentiate benign from more serious causes. It is also important to review underlying medical history and medication use. Substance use/abuse history should always be obtained with particular attention to stimulant products or illicit drugs. The nature of the athlete's sport, present level of training and fitness, and the relation of symptoms to specific training activities should also be obtained.

Following the history, a focused physical examination is performed with attention to the cardiopulmonary systems and then broadened to other areas as suggested by the history. Vital signs are reviewed for hypertension or hypotension, abnormal or irregular pulse, elevated respiratory rate, and presence or absence of fever. A thoughtful cardiac assessment includes auscultation with attention to rate, rhythm, murmurs, gallops, and ectopy as well as quality and symmetry of peripheral pulses. Pulmonary examination should focus on the presence of full breath sounds bilaterally, rales, wheezes or other signs of obstruction, inspiratory stridor, or evidence of focal consolidation. Remaining physical examination components may focus on other organ systems including gastrointenstinal, musculoskeletal, and neurologic.

History and physical examination alone have a low sensitivity for detecting many causes of occult cardiac disease, but the addition of an ECG can improve the diagnostic ability. A truly normal ECG gives the practitioner reassurance at the time of the initial assessment; however, it should always be remembered that a normal ECG does not completely exclude the potential for significant cardiac pathologic condition in a symptomatic athlete.

Useful ancillary data may include selective laboratory testing with complete blood count/profile, comprehensive chemistry profile with blood glucose, troponin, thyroid testing, and urinalysis. These basic parameters may be useful tools to evaluate for metabolic or hormonal abnormalities. Chest radiographs should be obtained in any patient with cardiac symptoms or dyspnea.

The final step in the office evaluation of an athlete with potential cardiac symptoms is a disposition. Those with ominous historical features, significant physical exam findings, or clearly abnormal ECGs should be held from physical activity until their diagnosis is clearly defined. For individuals who do not have findings that are definitive, a return to modified exercise with gradual progression and close follow-up is generally appropriate. Having a care provider with practical experience in return to play determinations helps to avoid unnecessary sport limitation in those whose medical status allows it.

CARDIAC TESTING FOR ATHLETES WHEN CONCERN FOR CARDIAC PATHOLOGIC CONDITION

In the setting of an athlete who is presenting with a potential cardiac concern, the list of potential cardiac testing modalities is extensive. The exact test depends on the athlete and the specific situation.

- *ECG:* When responding to cardiac symptoms or other abnormalities, the ECG is typically the first step. ECGs are fairly sensitive and specific for diagnosing electrical abnormalities that predispose athletes to SCA (Wolff-Parkinson-White, long QT syndrome, Brugada syndrome, and short QT syndrome). The ECG is reasonable, but certainly not perfect, at suggesting other structural or anatomic conditions (hypertrophic cardiomyopathy (HCM), dilated cardiomyopathy, CHD, pulmonary hypertension, myocarditis, and arrhythmogenic right ventricular cardiomyopathy). As noted in the clinical assessment, unfortunately there are times when an athlete will have a normal ECG and still have a condition that predisposes them to SCA (anomalous coronary artery origin, catecholaminergic polymorphic ventricular tachycardia, and some variants of cardiomyopathies).

- *Echocardiogram:* Echocardiograms are excellent at evaluating cardiac structure, ventricular size and wall thickness, ventricular function, and valve function. Echocardiograms can be diagnostic or raise suspicion for pathologic condition in the most common causes of SCA (HCM, dilated cardiomyopathy, anomalous coronary artery origins, pulmonary hypertension, myocarditis, and CHD). A key limitation of an echocardiogram assessment is the inability to detail myocardial tissue characteristics. Furthermore, the ultrasound technology can sometimes make it difficult to evaluate all aspects of the cardiac anatomy (atrial septum, coronary arteries and/or pulmonary venous drainage).

- *CT and MRI:* Cross-sectional and three-dimensional imaging, such as cardiac MRI and cardiac CT angiograms (CTAs), can also be used for confirming or diagnosing cardiac conditions. Although grossly simplified (and there is certainly overlap), MRI typically excels at evaluating the myocardium and ventricular function, whereas CTAs are better at assessing artery and vein course and size. Due to this, MRIs are very helpful to evaluate conditions such as HCM, arrhythmogenic right ventricular cardiomyopathy, or myocarditis. CTAs are excellent at appraising thoracic vessels (aorta size, pulmonary venous drainage, and so forth) as well as coronary artery origins and their course. Therefore, CTAs are helpful for diagnosing aortopathies, coarctation of the aorta, anomalous pulmonary venous drainage, anomalous coronary artery origins, myocardial bridging, and acquired coronary artery disease.

- *Cardiac Monitors:* Cardiac event monitors, either continuous or looping event-type, can be helpful to observe the athlete's cardiac rhythm while at home or performing activities. They can also demonstrate the exact heart rate and rhythm at the time of cardiac symptoms.

- *Exercise Stress Testing:* Provocative or stress testing is also an important component to cardiac testing. The basic form is an exercise stress test in which the athlete rides a stationary bike or runs on a treadmill while a 12-lead ECG monitors the athlete. With this particular modality, it is important to customize the stress test protocol to simulate the athlete's sport or activity they were doing at the time of cardiac symptoms.
  - Other more advanced types of stress testing also exist. For example, a cardiopulmonary exercise test is an option that measures gas exchange during participation. This information can be used to determine effort and overall exercise capacity as well as assess cardiac, respiratory, and skeletal muscle function. Additional imaging modalities that combine imaging with exercise/stress testing (stress echo, stress MRI, nuclear perfusion, and so forth) can be considered for even greater detailing.

IMPORTANCE OF OTHER MEDICAL SUBSPECIALISTS

Access to—and communication with—supporting subspecialists is vital because it is impossible for a cardiologist to be an expert across every cardiac field. This is especially important when there are abnormal or borderline results. Although not an exhaustive list, some of these subspecialists are as follows:

1. *Sports cardiologist:* Although general cardiologists and pediatric cardiologists certainly have experience with athletes and other active patients, there is clearly a role for a dedicated sports cardiologist. A sports cardiologist is a resource to primary care providers and general cardiologists due to their experience caring for athletes with known heart disease or symptoms with exercise, their knowledge of the cardiovascular response to exercise, and their understanding of "gray zone" cardiac testing results. Sports cardiologists can also be helpful with shared decision-making with athletes, particularly at the elite end of the athletic spectrum.

2. *Electrophysiologist:* Typically, a primary care provider and general cardiologist will be able to perform noninvasive testing and diagnose arrhythmias, but an electrophysiologist is vital when abnormal or borderline results are found. The electrophysiologist is needed to discuss the risks and benefits of nonintervention, medications, invasive testing, and/or cardiac device placement. They are typically the most appropriate person to perform shared decision-making with the athletes found to have an inherited condition (long QT syndrome, Wolff-Parkinson-White syndrome, and so forth) or when an arrhythmia is diagnosed. The electrophysiologist is likely the best to determine the risk status of exercise and whether medications and/or procedures can modulate the risk.

3. *HCM specialist:* Similar to the electrophysiologist, the HCM specialist is critical in confirming the diagnosis of HCM, assessing the need for adjunct testing, and determination of risks associated with sports participation. Although recent guidelines suggest that patients with HCM may be able to participate in exercise and sports,[24] there continues to be some controversy in this area.[25] An HCM specialist should be the medical specialist participating in the shared decision-making with the athlete under these unique circumstances given their experience and expertise.

4. *CHD specialist:* Outcomes for patients with CHD have dramatically improved during the past several decades. Due to this trend, there will continue to be an increase in the number of CHD patients wanting to participate in sports. CHD encompasses a vast range of cardiac disease with countless implications for exercise and sports participation. A thorough understanding of the impact of exercise on specific forms of CHD (as well as degree of residual disease following varying degrees of repair) is essential in determining the risk of sports participation. Similar to electrophysiology and HCM, the shared decision-making process for athletes with CHD should be performed by these subspecialists.

5. *Cardiovascular genetic counselors:* Because many of the cardiac conditions that have implications for exercise and sports are genetic in origin, genetic counselors are important to help diagnose and manage these conditions. These counselors evaluate whether genetic testing is indicated, determine the exact testing required, navigate the implications of the results, and provide subsequent counseling to the athlete. With the increase of genetic testing options as well as results that are not clearly black or white, genetic counselors' roles will continue to increase.

6. *Psychologists/psychiatrists:* Cardiac symptoms or diagnoses are inherently unsettling for anyone, including athletes. Involvement of a psychologist or psychiatrist is desirable because these specialists greatly aid in providing emotional support and coping strategies in the face of a new cardiac diagnosis. This may help to allay fears and anxiety while building a positive outlook for the future. In situations in which the future cardiac status is unknown, mental health providers can assist with the shared decision-making process for a return to sport or to manage the intense disappointment of retirement. These specialists are also critical to the treatment of the more pervasive underlying mental health conditions such as anxiety and depression, which may manifest as chest pain, palpitations, or other cardiac symptoms.

SUMMARY

Although there will be other articles in this issue that go in to further detail of the above subjects, one can begin to appreciate the complexities of caring for athletes' hearts. A wide range of medical professionals is therefore indispensable to provide the highest quality care for athletes. This care ranges from ensuring athletes are safe to initiate participation, responding to events or symptoms during sport, thoughtfully evaluating athletes when questions or concerns arise, and proper management once a condition has been diagnosed.

CLINICS CARE POINTS

- Emergency action plans should be created and practiced for each individual athletic venue.In the section "Cardiac testing for athletes when concern for cardiac pathologic condition.
- Cardiac testing should be largely guided by athlete's history and bystander's history.
- Many times an athlete with cardiac symptoms can be cleared after a history, examination, ECG, and echocardiogram. A normal ECG and echocardiogram will identifiy the majority of causes of sudden cardiac death but not all causes. If the history is concerning for cardiac pathology more extensive or directed cardiac testing is required (stress testing, ambulatory monitors, cross sectional imaging, etc).In the section "Importance of other medical subspecialists.
- No provider or cardiologist can be the expert for every cardiac diagnosis. Providers and cardiologists must know when to ask for help from other specialists.

DISCLOSURE

The authors have nothing to disclose.

REFERENCES

1. Rajpal S, Tong MS, Borchers J, et al. Cardiovascular Magnetic Resonance Findings in Competitive Athletes Recovering from COVID-19 Infection. JAMA Cardiol 2020. https://doi.org/10.1001/jamacardio.2020.4916.
2. Brito D, Meester S, Yanamala N, et al. High Prevalence of Pericardial Involvement in College Student Athletes Recovering From COVID-19. JACC Cardiovasc Imaging 2021. https://doi.org/10.1016/j.jcmg.2020.10.023.
3. Boston Red Sox pitcher Eduardo Rodriguez done for season due to heart issue. ESPN.com. 2020. https://www.espn.com/mlb/story/_/id/29579222/boston-red-sox-pitcher-eduardo-rodriguez-done-season-due-heart-issue.
4. Streeter K. For This College Athlete, Covid-19 Was Just the Start of a Nightmare. New York Times. 2021. https://www.nytimes.com/2021/02/12/sports/ncaabasketball/college-sports-myocarditis.html.
5. Martinez MW, Tucker AM, Bloom OJ, et al. Prevalence of Inflammatory Heart Disease Among Professional Athletes With Prior COVID-19 Infection Who Received Systematic Return-to-Play Cardiac Screening. JAMA Cardiol 2021. https://doi.org/10.1001/jamacardio.2021.0565.
6. Moulson N, Petek BJ, Drezner JA, et al. SARS-CoV-2 Cardiac Involvement in Young Competitive Athletes. Circulation 2021. https://doi.org/10.1161/circulationaha.121.054824.
7. Arbab-Zadeh A, Perhonen M, Howden E, et al. Cardiac remodeling in response to 1 year of intensive endurance training. Circulation 2014. https://doi.org/10.1161/CIRCULATIONAHA.114.010775.

8. Wasfy MM, Weiner RB, Wang F, et al. Endurance Exercise-Induced Cardiac Remodeling: Not All Sports Are Created Equal. J Am Soc Echocardiogr 2015. https://doi.org/10.1016/j.echo.2015.08.002.

9. Dean PN, Gillespie CW, Greene EA, et al. Sports participation and quality of life in adolescents and young adults with congenital heart disease. Congenit Heart Dis 2015. https://doi.org/10.1111/chd.12221.

10. Berg AE, Meyers LL, Dent KM, et al. Psychological impact of sports restriction in asymptomatic adolescents with hypertrophic cardiomyopathy, dilated cardiomyopathy, and long QT syndrome. Prog Pediatr Cardiol 2018. https://doi.org/10.1016/j.ppedcard.2018.05.001.

11. Luiten RC, Ormond K, Post L, et al. Exercise restrictions trigger psychological difficulty in active and athletic adults with hypertrophic cardiomyopathy. Open Hear 2016. https://doi.org/10.1136/openhrt-2016-000488.

12. Malhotra A, Dhutia H, Finocchiaro G, et al. Outcomes of Cardiac Screening in Adolescent Soccer Players. N Engl J Med 2018. https://doi.org/10.1056/nejmoa1714719.

13. Berge HM, Andersen TE, Bahr R. Cardiovascular incidents in male professional football players with negative preparticipation cardiac screening results: An 8-year follow-up. Br J Sports Med 2018. https://doi.org/10.1136/bjsports-2018-099845.

14. Riebe D, Franklin BA, Thompson PD, et al. Updating ACSM's recommendations for exercise preparticipation health screening. Med Sci Sports Exerc 2015. https://doi.org/10.1249/MSS.0000000000000664.

15. Maron BJ, Levine BD, Washington RL, et al. Eligibility and Disqualification Recommendations for Competitive Athletes With Cardiovascular Abnormalities: Task Force 2: Preparticipation Screening for Cardiovascular Disease in Competitive Athletes. J Am Coll Cardiol 2015. https://doi.org/10.1016/j.jacc.2015.09.034.

16. American Academy of Pediatrics, American Academy of Family Physicians, American College of Sports Medicine, American Medical Society for Sports Medicine, American Medical Society for Sports Medicine, American Orthopaedic Society for Sports Medicine and AOA of SM. Preparticipation physical evaluation. 5th edition. Elk Grove Village, IL: American Academy of Pediatrics; 2019. Available at: https://ebooks.aappublications.org/content/9781610023023/978161 0023023.

17. Eriksen had cardiac arrest but test results are normal, Danish team doctor says. Reuters. Available at: https://www.reuters.com/lifestyle/sports/denmarks-eriksen-still-hospital-condition-is-stable-2021-06-13/.

18. Camp SPV, Bloor CM, Mueller FO, et al. Nontraumatic sports death in high school and college athletes. Med Sci Sports Exerc 1995. https://doi.org/10.1249/00005768-199505000-00005.

19. Yau R, Kucera KL, Thomas LC, et al. Catastrophic sports injury research: Thirty-fifth annual report Fall 1982-Spring 2017. In: National Center for Catastrophic Sport Injury Research at the University of North Carolina at Chapel Hill. 2018.

20. Casa DJ, Guskiewica KM, Anderson SA, et al. National athletic trainers' association position statement: preventing sudden death in sports. J Athl Train 2012; 47(1):96–118.

21. Parsons JT, Anderson SA, Casa DJ, et al. Preventing catastrophic injury and death in collegiate athletes: Interassociation recommendations endorsed by 13 medical and sports medicine organisations. J Athl Train 2019. https://doi.org/10.4085/1062-6050-54.085.

22. Hainline B, Drezner JA, Baggish A, et al. Interassociation Consensus Statement on Cardiovascular Care of College Student-Athletes. J Am Coll Cardiol 2016. https://doi.org/10.1016/j.jacc.2016.03.527.

23. Association NCA. Division I Proposal – 2013-17. Athletics Personnel – Conduct of Athletics Personnel – First Aid, CPR, and AED Certification. 2014. Available at: https://web3.ncaa.org/lsdbi/search/proposalView?id=3044. Accessed August 3, 2021.

24. Ommen SR, Mital S, Burke MA, et al. 2020 AHA/ACC Guideline for the Diagnosis and Treatment of Patients with Hypertrophic Cardiomyopathy: Executive Summary: A Report of the American College of Cardiology/American Heart Association Joint Committee on Clinical Practice Guidelines. Circulation 2020. https://doi.org/10.1161/CIR.0000000000000938.

25. Drezner JA, Malhotra A, Prutkin JM, et al. Return to play with hypertrophic cardiomyopathy: Are we moving too fast? A critical review. Br J Sports Med 2021. https://doi.org/10.1136/bjsports-2020-102921.

Incidence and Causes of Sudden Cardiac Death in Athletes

Kimberly G. Harmon, MD[a,b,c,]*

KEYWORDS

- Sudden cardiac death • Athlete • Incidence • Sudden cardiac arrest

KEY POINTS

- Most studies on the incidence of SCA/d are flawed producing inaccurate assessments of the rate of SCA/d in different populations.
- Risk should be stratified by age group, as the risk and underlying etiology of SCA/d varies significantly with age.
- Incidence studies with more robust design indicate the presence of higher risk groups for SCA/d. These include male athletes, black athletes, and athletes playing men's basketball, men's soccer, and American football.
- Cardiomyopathies and electrical disease are common causes of SCA/d in athletes.

INTRODUCTION

Sudden cardiac death (SCD) is the leading medical cause of death in athletes; however, attempts to define risk have been challenged by imprecise epidemiologic methods that may not convey helpful information.[1] Accurate information is important to make decisions about screening and prevention strategies. In this article we will explore basic epidemiologic concepts and how they apply to our understanding of SCD and sudden cardiac arrest (SCA) in athletes and identify current knowledge gaps. The causes of sudden cardiac arrest and death (SCA/d) are also important when considering screening and prevention strategies and existing studies will be reviewed.

---

[a] Department of Family Medicine, University of Washington School of Medicine, Seattle, WA, USA; [b] Department of Orthopaedics and Sports Medicine, University of Washington School of Medicine, Seattle, WA, USA; [c] Sports Medicine Center at Husky Stadium, 3800 Montlake Boulevard, Seattle, WA 98195, USA
* Sports Medicine Center at Husky Stadium, 3800 Montlake Boulevard, Seattle, WA 98195.
E-mail address: kharmon@uw.edu
Twitter: @DrKimHarmon (K.G.H.)

Clin Sports Med 41 (2022) 369–388
https://doi.org/10.1016/j.csm.2022.02.002

EPIDEMIOLOGY
The Basics – Numerator and Denominator

Risk or incidence is a measure of disease prevalence in a population over a defined period of time.[2] The cases identified, or the numerator, needs to be accurate for a precise estimation of incidence. Most studies of SCA/d in athletes rely on media reports, registries, or reviews of diagnoses on autopsy reports to identify cases for inclusion; therefore, it is likely that cases will be missed, and the incidence will appear artificially low. There are few studies whereby there is required reporting to a central database of SCD in athletes. When evaluating the quality of an incidence study, the accuracy of the numerator should be considered.

The denominator of an incidence proportion is the number of persons at the start of an observation period.[2] Studies of SCA/d should clearly define what is meant by an athlete and how the group is determined. Many studies estimate participation (ie, "there are about 8,000,000 high school athletes") which can result in either over or under-estimation of risk. Perhaps more importantly is grouping populations with widely varying risks. For example, when determining the risk of breast cancer in a population one would not include men, who are at significantly less risk for breast cancer, in that calculation. To do so would provide a distorted picture of the risk in a female. Similarly, when trying to understand the risk of SCD in a population, age and sex stratification are critical.

Risk of Sudden Cardiac Arrest and Death by Sex

Studies of SCD in athletes and nonathletes alike have consistently shown that men have a much higher rate of SCD than women.[2–8] A recent meta-analysis found that the incidence of SCA/d in men was 3 times that of women.[4] They found a median incidence was 2.7 SCD per 100,000 person-years (1 in 37,000) (IQR 1.8–4.4, range 1.3–36) in men, compared with a median incidence in women of 0.9 cases per 100,000 person-years (1 in 111,111) (IQR 0.6–1.4, range 0–7).[4] Therefore, for an accurate understanding of the incidence rate of SCA/d, male and female events should be analyzed and reported separately (**Table 1**).

Risk of Sudden Cardiac Arrest and Death by Age

Grouping wide ranges of ages together can lead to inaccurate estimates of the incidence of SCA/d. Population-based studies demonstrate a peak in SCD in those less than 1 year of age followed by a relatively low rate of SCD that increases again around age 15 before rising precipitously at age 25 due to the increasing contribution of coronary artery disease.[9–12] (**Fig. 1A**). In those under 25 years old, the primary causes of SCA/d are congenital.[9,12,13] (see **Fig. 1B**). Many studies of SCA/d group wide swaths of ages (12–40 years old) with widely varying incidence rates together. For an accurate estimation of incidence rate, it is important that age grouping reflects a similar prevalence of SCA/d **Table 1** includes low risk of bias studies that stratify groups by age. Similar to population-based studies, high school age athletes appear to have a slightly lower risk of SCA/d than those that are college aged although this could also be the result of less robust case reporting. High school athletes still represent a higher number of SCA/d as there are roughly 8,000,000 high school athletes compared with roughly 500,000 college athletes.

Exercise-Associated Sudden Cardiac Death

Perhaps one of the biggest issues when considering SCA/d in athletes is the differentiation between exercise-associated (sometimes called sports related) SCA/d and

Table 1
Incidence of sudden cardiac arrest and death in athletes in low risk of bias studies with sex, race, and sport rates

Study	SCD or SCA/d?	Age Range; Number of Cases	Overall Incidence of SCA/d	Male SCA/d Incidence	Female SCA/d Incidence	Black SCA/d Incidence	White SCA/d Incidence	Sex/Sport Specific Incidence
Wide Age Range (12–35)								
Corrado et al,[42] 2003	SCD	12–35 N = 51	1:47,000	1:41,000	1:93,000	-	-	
High School Age (~14–18)								
Toresdahl et al,[5] 2014	SCA/d	14–18 N = 44	1:88,000	1:58,000	1:323,000	-	-	
Drezner et al,[43] 2014	SCA/d	14–18 N = 13	1:71,000		-			Male, basketball 1:21,000
Malhotra et al,[20] 2018	SCD	15–17 N = 8						Male, soccer 1:14,794
Peterson et al,[8] 2021	SCA/d	14–18 N = 204	1:66,000	1:44,000	1:204,000			Male Ice Hockey 1:24,000 Male Basketball 1:40,000 White Football 1:20,000
College/University Age (~18–25)								
Harmon et al,[6] 2015	SCD	17–26 N = 79	1:53,000	1:38,000	1:122,000	1:21,000	1:68,000	Football 1:36,000 Male, soccer 1:24,000 Male, basketball 1:9000 Male, black, basketball 1:5300 Male, Div. I basketball 1:5200
Peterson et al,[8] 2021	SCA/d	18–24 N = 39	1:51,000	1:35,000	1:123,000	Black male 1:18,000	White Male 1:39,000	Black Male Basketball 1:4800 White Male Basketball 1:15,000 Black Football 1:28,000 White Football 1:20,000

A

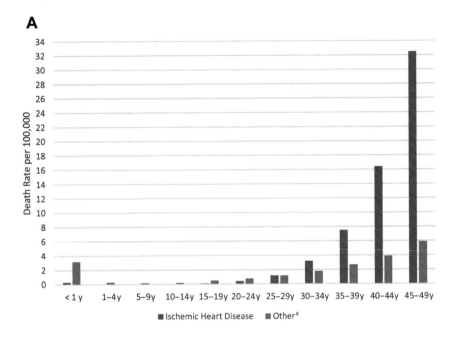

B

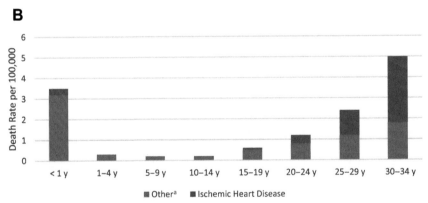

Fig. 1. Cardiac Causes of Death by Age. (*A*) The increasing Contribution of Ischemic Heart Disease Cardiac Causes of Death with Age (2011–2020). (*B*) Relative Contributions of Ischemic and other[a] causes of SCD by Age (2011–2020). [a]ICD-10 Codes I40.0 (Infective myocarditis); I40.1 (Isolated myocarditis); I40.8 (Other acute myocarditis); I40.9 (Acute myocarditis, unspecified); I42.0 (Dilated cardiomyopathy); I42.1 (Obstructive hypertrophic cardiomyopathy); I42.2 (Other hypertrophic cardiomyopathy); I42.3 (Endomyocardial (eosinophilic) disease); I42.4 (Endocardial fibroelastosis); I42.5 (Other restrictive cardiomyopathy); I42.8 (Other cardiomyopathies); I42.9 (Cardiomyopathy, unspecified); I45.6 (Pre-excitation syndrome); I46.1 (Sudden cardiac death, so described); I46.9 (Cardiac arrest, unspecified); Q24.5 (Malformation of coronary vessels).[12]

SCA/d that occurs in an athlete with any activity or during any time. Exercise-associated SCA/d is typically defined as death that occurs during or within an hour of death and is a subset of SCD in athletes. Estimates for exercise-associated SCA/d will underestimate the total number of SCA/d in athletes. While some studies suggest that up to 90% of deaths in athletes occur during exercise,[14] other suggests that number is closer to 50%.[6,15] In a recent systematic review on the incidence of SCA/d in young athletes and military members 25/40 (62.5%) identified studies included only exercise-associated deaths in their collection or did not state if included SCA/d were exercise associated.[16] Another systematic review excluded studies that only included exercise-associated deaths as not truly representative of the incidence of SCD.[4] If incidence rates of SCA/d are being used to calculate resources needed for events, then estimates occurring associated with exercise activity may be appropriate. If incidence rates are being used to inform screening practices, then the incidence SCA/d occurring at any time is needed.

Sudden cardiac arrest and death and sudden cardiac death

Most studies only include SCD in their analyses; however, some also include athletes who had cardiac arrests, were resuscitated, and survived. The inclusion of SCA is important to understand the scope of the problem; however, there are less reliable ways to track SCA compared with SCD. One study prospectively followed high school students more than 2 years while they were on campus and reported 26 SCAs, of which only 4 suffered SCD. Thus, 85% of those that had an SCA, while on school grounds were resuscitated.[17] If only SCDs had been included this would significantly underestimate the problem of SCA. The high rate of resuscitation found in this study may be because all but one school whereby arrests occurred had an automated external defibrillator (AED) program in place and the study did not include SCA/d that occurred at home or while away from campus whereby access to a defibrillator would be less reliable making resuscitation less likely. Another study examined SCA and SCD in athletes 11 to 29 which occurred at any time (exercise associated, at rest or while sleeping) and found 48% of athletes were resuscitated.[8] (**Table 2**) Finally, in the Fédération Internationale de Football Association (FIFA) Sudden Death Registry, a world-wide endeavor studying SCA/d in soccer, an overall survival rate of 23% was noted which varied drastically if CPR and an AED were used by trained staff immediately (85% survival).[18] The discrepancy in reported survival between studies is likely explained by the availability of AEDs in different settings and whether or not the arrest

Table 2
Percent of sudden cardiac arrests resuscitated by age[8]

Athlete Level	Number of SCAs	Number of SCDs	% Resuscitated
Middle School	22	29	43%
High School	108	96	53%
College	21	23	48%
Semi-professional/professional	4	7	36%
Recent/former athlete (within a year)	3	18	14%

Data from Peterson DF, Kucera K, Thomas LC, Maleszewski J, Siebert D, Lopez-Anderson M, Zigman M, Schattenkerk J, Harmon KG and Drezner JA. Aetiology and incidence of sudden cardiac arrest and death in young competitive athletes in the USA: a 4-year prospective study. *Br J Sports Med.* 2021;55:1196-1203.

was witnessed. This data suggests that studies that only include SCD may miss a significant amount of cardiac arrest events.

Sport Specificity

More recent studies which include sport as a potential variable have shown differential risks between sports.[6–8,19,20] Specifically, men's basketball, men's soccer, and American football consistently seem to be higher risk. It is hypothesized that this may be related to the physiologic demands of these sports; however, more research is needed to better understand this phenomenon.

INCIDENCE

There have been 2 recent systematic reviews on the incidence of SCA/d in the young.[4,16] The first looked at the incidence of SCD in a general population aged 12 to 39 and included 26 studies (9 in athletes) of SCA/d that occurred at any time; studies that examined only exercise-related SCD were excluded.[4] They reported an incidence of 1 in 58,000 person-years (1.7 per 100,000 person-years (IQR 1.3–2.6)) which did not differ between athletes and nonathletes.[4] A meta-analysis was not performed because of study heterogeneity. This estimate is limited by the inclusion of both men in women in the same group and the wide age range. Similarly, the second systematic review reported an incidence of 1 in 52,000 person-years (1.91 (95%CI: 0.71–5.14)) in competitive athletes.[16] Thirty-four studies in athletes were included in the analysis but only 8 that were considered low risk of bias and included in the meta-analysis.[16] This analysis included studies of SCA/d that occurred at any time and studies that reported on exercise-related SCA/d only. A specific rate for men or women was not calculated due to a paucity of included studies reporting. While the calculated incidence of SCA/d from both these systematic reviews, around 1 in 50,000 person-years, is concerning, evolving understanding based on more granular data points to the existence of high-risk groups and calls for more focused analysis.

Table 3 includes a list of studies on SCA/SCD along with a risk of bias assessment using a risk of bias tool addressing study design, accuracy of numerator and denominator, type of SCD (SCA, SCD, exercise-associated SCA), and age and sex specificity. There were 26 studies of athletes in total. In studies that used the same data set the most recent, complete, or lowest risk of bias was included in the table leaving 20 total studies (10 studies at high risk of bias, 4 intermediate, and 6 low). Low risk of bias studies was the only included studies from which a sufficiently granular assessment of SCA/d could be obtained and are included in **Table 1**. This table highlights the existence of groups that are at much higher risk of SCA/d including males, black athletes, and athletes playing men's basketball, men's soccer, and American football.

CAUSES OF SUDDEN CARDIAC DEATH IN ATHLETES

Like incidence, there are problems with currently available studies which report on causes of SCD. In the United States, there is no coordinated system for postmortem evaluation relying instead on a patchwork of medical examiners and coroners which result in variable quality and specificity of autopsies. In other parts of the world, specialized referral centers exist but data from these centers may reflect ascertainment bias as cases with more obvious causes may remain at local sites. In addition, our current understanding of pathology is evolving, and things once diagnosed as one entity, may today be diagnosed as another. Despite these issues, there are consistent findings in many studies with sudden arrhythmic death syndrome (SADS)/electrical issues,

Table 3
Incidence of sudden cardiac arrest and death in athletes

Study	Study Design and Population	Case Identification (Numerator)	Population Definition (Denominator)	Sports-Related SCD or all SCD?	SCD or all SCA/d?	Study Years	Age Range; Number of Cases	Annual Incidence	Risk of Bias
Van Camp et al,[44] 1996	Retrospective cohort; high school and college athletes	National Center for Catastrophic Sports Injury Research and media reports	Data from NCAA, NFHS, NAIA, and NJCAA, added together with conversion factor (1.9 for high school and 1.2 for college) used to account for multisport athletes "based on discussions with representatives from the national organizations."	Sports-related	SCD	1983–1993	13–24 N = 160	*College + High School* Overall 1:188,000 Male 1:134,000 Female 1:752,000 *High School* Overall 1:213,000 Male 1:152,000 Female 1:861,000 *College* Overall 1:94,000 Male 1:69,000 Female 1:356,000	High
Corrado et al,[42] 2003	Prospective cohort; athletes and nonathletes in the Veneto Region of Italy	Mandatory reporting of sudden death	Registered athletes in the Sports Medicine Database of the Veneto Region of Italy and the Italian Census Bureau	All	SCD	1979–1999	12–35 N = 51 12–35 N = 208	*Athletes* Overall 1:47,000 Male 1:41,000 Female 1:93,000 *Non-Athletes* Overall 1:143,000	Low
Drezner et al,[45] 2005	Retrospective survey; college athletes	Survey of NCAA Division I institutions (244/326 responded)	Reported number of athletes	All	SCD	—	N = 5	*College* Overall 1:67,000	Intermediate
Maron et al,[21] 2009	Retrospective cohort; amateur and competitive athletes	US Registry for Sudden Death in Athletes	An estimated 10.7 million participants per year ≤ 39 y of age in all organized amateur and competitive sports	All	SCA + SCD	1980–2006	8–39 N = 1046	*Athletes* 1:164,000	High

(continued on next page)

Table 3
(continued)

Study	Study Design and Population	Case Identification (Numerator)	Population Definition (Denominator)	Sports-Related SCD or all SCD?	SCD or all SCA/d?	Study Years	Age Range; Number of Cases	Annual Incidence	Risk of Bias
Drezner et al,[46] 2009	Cross-sectional survey; high school athletes	Survey of 1710 high schools with AEDs	Reported number of student athletes	All cases occurring on campus	SCA + SCD	2006–2007	14–17 N = 14	*High School* 1:23,000 (SCA + SCD) 1:64,000 (SCD)	Intermediate
Holst et al,[47] 2010	Retrospective cohort; athletes and general population in Denmark	Review of death certificates, Cause of Death Registry, and National Patient Registry in Denmark	Interview data of people age 16–35 y from the National Danish Health and Morbidity Study	Sports-related SCD in athletes vs all SCD in the general population	SCD	2000–2006	12–35 N = 15; 12–35 N = 428	*Athletes* 1:83,000; *General Population* 1:27,000	High
Marijon et al,[48] 2011	Prospective cohort; general population in France	Data from emergency medical system	General population statistics, data from the Minister of Health and Sport to estimate young competitive athlete population	Sports-related SCA or SCD with moderate or vigorous exercise	SCA + SCD	2005–2010	10–75 N = 820; 10–35 N = 50	*General Population* 1:217,000; *Young Competitive Athlete* 1:102,000; *Young Non-competitive Athlete* 1:455,000	High
Steinvil et al,[49] 2011	Retrospective cohort; athletes in Israel	Retrospective review of 2 Israeli newspapers	Competitive athletes registered in the Israel Sport Authority in 2009; extrapolated this data for prior 24 y based on the growth of the Israeli population (age 10–40) from the Central Bureau of Statistics; allowed for a presumed doubling of the sporting population over 24 y	All	SCD	1985–2009	12–44 N = 24	*Athletes* 1:38,000	High

Maron et al,[50] 2013	Retrospective cohort; Minnesota high school athletes	US Registry for Sudden Death in Athletes	Minnesota State High School statistics (Estimated using conversion factor of 2.3 to account for multisport athletes)	All	SCD	1986–2011	12–18 N = 13	High School Overall 1:150,000 Male 1:83,000 Female 0	Intermediate
Toresdahl et al,[5] 2014	Prospective observational; high school students and student-athletes	2149 high schools monitored for SCA events on school campus	Reported number of students and student-athletes	All cases occurring on school campus	SCA + SCD	2009–2011	14–18 N = 44	Student-athlete Overall 1:88,000 Male 1:58,000 Female 1:323,000 Student Non-athlete Overall 1:326,000 Male 1:286,000 Female 1:357,000	Low
Drezner et al,[43] 2014	Retrospective cohort; Minnesota high school athletes	Public media reports	Minnesota State High School statistics (Sum of unduplicated athletes 2003–04 through 2011–12 school years)	All	SCA + SCD	2003–2012	14–18 N = 13	High School Overall 1:71,000 Female 0 Male, basketball 1:21,000	Low
Risgaard et al,[51] 2014	Retrospective cohort; competitive and noncompetitive athletes in Denmark	Review of death certificates and the Danish National Patient Registry	Competitive and noncompetitive athlete populations in Denmark estimated based on survey data from the Danish National Institute of Public Health	Sports-related SCD in competitive vs noncompetitive athletes	SCD	2007–2009	12–35 N = 44	Competitive Athlete 1:213,000 Non-competitive Athlete 1:233,000	High

(continued on next page)

Table 3
(continued)

Study	Study Design and Population	Case Identification (Numerator)	Population Definition (Denominator)	Sports-Related SCD or all SCD?	SCD or all SCA/d?	Study Years	Age Range; Number of Cases	Annual Incidence	Risk of Bias
Harmon et al,[6] 2015	Retrospective cohort; college athletes	Parent Heart Watch database, NCAA Resolutions list, catastrophic insurance claims	Participation data from the NCAA	All	SCD	2003–2013	17–26 N = 79	*College* Overall 1:53,000 Male 1:38,000 Female 1:122,000 Black 1:21,000 White 1:68,000 Football 1:36,000 Male, soccer 1:24,000 Male, black 1:16,000 Male, basketball 1:9000 Male, black, basketball 1:5300 Male, Div. I basketball 1:5200	Low
Bohm et al,[52] 2016	Prospective cohort; sports-related SCD in all persons in Germany	Voluntary reporting to German National Registry, web-based media search, regional institutes	Physical activity estimated from the German Health Update study and extrapolated to population data from the German Federal Statistical Office	Sports-related SCD	SCD	2012–2014	10–79 N = 144	*Sports Participants* 1:1,200,000	High
Grani,[53] 2016	Retrospective; sports-related SCD in all persons in German-speaking Switzerland	Forensic reports	Physical activity estimated from survey on sports participation by the Swiss Federal Office of Sports	Sports-related SCD	SCD	1999–2010	10–39 N = 69	*Sports Participants* Competitive: 1:90,000 Recreational: 1:192,000	High

Study	Design	Source	Population	Data	Outcome	Years	Age	N	Incidence	Quality
Maron et al,[54] 2016	Retrospective cohort	Records of the Medical Examiner	All	Data from the Minnesota Department of Education, National Center for Education Statistics, and the Minnesota State High School League for Hennepin County, Minnesota	SCD	2000–2014	14–23	N = 27	Non-athlete 1:39,000 Athlete 1:121,000	High
Harmon et al,[7] 2016	Retrospective cohort, US high school athletes	Media reports	All	NFHS participation statistics	SCA/SCD	2007 = 2013	14–18	N = 104	High School Overall 1:67,000 Male 1:45,00 Female 1:237,000 Male, basketball 1:37,000	Intermediate
Chatard, et al,[27] 2018	Prospective, Pacific Island athletes who were screened	Prospectively followed	All	Defined cohort of 1450 athletes	SCD	2012–2015	10–40	N = 3	Pacific Island Athletes 1:2416	High
Malhotra, et al,[20] 2018	Prospective,	Followed from time of screen to 2016	All	Defined cohort of 11,168 elite soccer athletes	SCD	1996–2016	15–17	N = 8	Elite Male Soccer Athletes 1:14,794	Low
Peterson et al,[8] 2021	Prospective	National Center for Catastrophic Sports Injury Research	All	Has defined cohort for high school and college athletes	SCA/SCD	2014–	14–18 18–24	20,181: N = 204 N = 39	High School Overall 1:66,000 Male 1:44,00 Female 1:204,000 Male Ice Hockey 1:24,000 Male Basketball 1:40,000 College Overall 1:51,000 Male 1:35,000 Female 1:123,000 Black Male 1:18,000 White Male 1:39,000 Black Male Basketball 1:4800 White Male Basketball 1:15,000 Black Football 1:28,000 White Football 1:20,000	Low

cardiomyopathies, coronary artery abnormalities, myocarditis-related pathology, and aortic dissection all important causes of SCA/d **Table 4** includes studies of SCA/d in young people and the relative contributions in each study. Atherosclerotic coronary artery disease represents an average of 5% of the cases represented (range 0% - 27%), which is largely reflective of the age range of the athletes/sportsmen included in each study and possibly their smoking status.

Sudden Arrhythmic Death Syndrome

SADS is a diagnosis of exclusion when there is a presumed SCA, a morphologically normal heart with normal histopathology, and a negative toxicology screen. SADS is cited as a cause of death in 2%–44% of cases (see **Table 4**). Diagnoses that are represented in this category include channelopathies including long QT syndrome (LQTS) and Brugada syndrome, catecholaminergic polymorphic ventricular tachycardia (CPVT), and conduction abnormalities such as Wolff–Parkinson–White Syndrome which may not be diagnosed premortem. SADS may have been underrepresented in earlier pathologic studies that relied on autopsy diagnosis as morphologically normal hearts were sometimes excluded.[21]

Cardiomyopathies

Cardiomyopathies are myocardial disorders in the heart muscle and can be primary (genetic), secondary (due to other conditions such as hypertension), or acquired (postinfectious).

Hypertrophic cardiomyopathy

Hypertrophic cardiomyopathy (HCM) is an important cause of SCD with a prevalence in the general population of 1 in 500, and in athletes 1 in 2,000.[22] Studies cite HCM as a cause of SCD in athletes in 0% - 36% of cases (see **Table 4**). HCM is characterized by left ventricular hypertrophy (LVH) and histologic analysis shows disorganized cellular architecture or myocyte disarray. HCM is inherited in an autosomal dominant fashion although there is variable penetrance of the gene with some never developing phenotypic HCM. These individuals are considered low risk for SCA. Morphologic features may appear in childhood but often develop in adolescence or young adulthood; therefore, screening for HCM needs to continue into young adulthood to be effective.[23] The presenting symptoms of HCM is SCA 80% of the time. Exertional syncope or chest pain, light-headedness, or dyspnea may also occur. ECG will detect 93% of HCM[24] if suspected, a cardiac MRI is indicated as echocardiogram may miss apical hypertrophy, the most common variant in athletes.[25] Late gadolinium enhancement on cardiac MRI may predict future risk.[26] Exercise increases the risk of ventricular tachycardia/fibrillation and is a modifiable risk factor. Shared-decision making for return-to-play is becoming more common; however, it should be noted that there are multiple cases of SCD after returning to play with HCM.[23,27] An in-depth discussion of risks, including death, should be part of the decision-making process.

Arrhythmogenic cardiomyopathy

The prevalence of AC in population is reported as 1 in 5000.[28] It is estimated to cause 2% – 36% of athlete SCDs (see **Table 4**). It was formerly characterized as arrhythmogenic right ventricular cardiomyopathy; however, there is increasing recognition as a biventricular entity.[28] AC is an inherited muscle disorder characterized by myocardial fibro-fatty replacement. Exercise causes progression of disease and should generally be avoided after diagnosis.[29,30]

Table 4
Studies of the causes of sudden cardiac arrest and death in young people

Study	Years of Study	Methods	Autopsy	Country	"Sports-Related" or all Deaths	Age Range	Cases	HCM	Idiopathic LVH/Fibrosis	Coronary Artery Anomalies	ARVC	DCM	AN-SUD/SADS	CAD	Myocarditis Related	Aortic Dissection	LQTS	WPW	Other
Corrado et al,[55] 2001	1979–1999	Prospective, mandatory reporting, all deaths in Veneto region	standard procedure at referral center	Italy	All	12–35	46	2%	0%	13%	26%	2%	2%	22%	11%	2%	2%	0%	17%
De Noronha et al,[56] 2009	1996–2008	All cases SCD referred to CRY	standard procedure at referral center	UK	All	6–34	88	13%	32%	7%	10%	0%	30%	0%	3%	0%	0%	0%	6%
Maron, et al,[21] 2009	1980–2006	Retrospective, registry, media reports	review of available autopsy,	US	All - includes SCA	8–39	1049	24%	5%	11%	3%	1%	34%	2%	4%	2%	2%	1%	10%
Holst et al,[47] 2010	2000–2006	retrospective, death certificates	autopsy reports, hospital records	Denmark	Sports-related	12–35	14	0%	7%	7%	29%	0%	29%	14%	7%	0%	0%	0%	7%
Suarez-Mier et al,[57] 2013	1995–2010	SCD referred to National Institute of Forensic Sciences of Madrid	standard procedure at referral center	Spain	Sports-related	9–35	81	10%	9%	6%	15%	0%	23%	14%	5%	0%	0%	0%	19%
Harmon et al,[6] 2015	2003–2013	NCAA data base	autopsy reports	US	All	18–26	64	8%	17%	11%	5%	3%	25%	9%	9%	5%	2%	3%	3%
Finochiaro et al,[15] 2016	1994–2014	All cases SCD referred to CRY	standard procedure	UK	All	18–35	179	8%	14%	4%	14%	1%	44%	0%	2%	0%	0%	0%	13%

(continued on next page)

Table 4
(continued)

Study	Years of Study	Methods	Autopsy	Country	"Sports-Related" or all Deaths	Age Range	Cases	HCM	Idiopathic LVH/Fibrosis	Coronary Artery Anomalies	ARVC	DCM	AN-SUD/SADS	CAD	Myocarditis Related	Aortic Dissection	LQTS	WPW	Other
Bohm et al,[52] 2016	2012–2014	retrospective	media reports, registry	Germany	Sports-related	10-34	29	7%	3%	10%	3%	3%	17%	21%	31%	0%	0%	0%	3%
Harmon et al,[7] 2016	2007–2013	retrospective, media reports	autopsy reports	US	All	14-18	50	14%	28%	8%	2%	0%	18%	6%	14%	0%	0%	0%	12%
Morentin et al,[58] 2021	2010–2017	Retrospective	standard procedure at referral center	Spain	Sports-related	15-24	14	14%	21%	0%	36%	0%	0%	0%	21%	0%	0%	0%	7%
Thiene et al,[59] 2019	1980–2015	Prospective	Standard procedure at referral center	Italy	All	< 40	75	5%	0%	16%	27%	0%	11%	23%	4%	0%	0%	0%	15%
Wisten et al,[60] 2019	2000–2010	Retrospective	death certificates, autopsy and medical records	Sweden	EA-SCA/d	<35	62	16%	10%	0%	13%	6%	24%	11%	11%	0%	0%	0%	8%
Egger et al,[18] 2022	2014–2018	media reports, registry	autopsy reports and interviews	many	SCA/d	<35	104	11%	9%	13%	4%	1%		14%	13%	0%	0%	0%	42%
Peterson et al,[8] 2021	2014–2018	media reports, reports to NCCSIR	autopsy reports	US	SCA/d	11-29	209	21%	13%	12%	6%	3%	10%	2%	4%	3%	5%	4%	16%
Total							2050	18%	9%	10%	7%	1%	27%	5%	5%	1%	2%	1%	256

Dilated cardiomyopathy

The prevalence in population is 1 in 2500. Dilated cardiomyopathy can be the end stage of other cardiomyopathies such as HCM or arrhythmogenic cardiomyopathy (AC). It is less commonly diagnosed in athletes (0%–5%) than other cardiomyopathies but is still an important cause of SCA/d (see **Table 4**).

Idiopathic left ventricular hypertrophy/left ventricular hypertrophy with fibrosis/ cardiomyopathy not otherwise specified (NOS)

An increasing number of SCDs are being characterized as caused by Idiopathic LVH, LVH with Fibrosis, or Cardiomyopathy NOS. **Table 4** demonstrates 0%–32% of athletes in postmortem studies may carry this diagnosis. These are hearts that may not meet the defined pathologic criteria to be categorized as HCM. It is unknown whether some of these cases represent an early expression of HCM, another entity, or are an acquired response to exercise.

Coronary Artery Abnormalities

Coronary artery abnormalities cause between 0% and 16% of SCD in athletes (see **Table 4**). Abnormal origin of the left coronary artery arising from the right sinus of Valsalva is most common. Other features that may contribute to ischemia during exercise include an acute angled take-off, hypoplastic ostium, or impingement of the anomalous artery as it traverses between the expanding great vessels during exercise. Coronary artery abnormalities may cause chest pain or exertional syncope and are not detectable with ECG. Transthoracic echocardiogram can visualize the coronary ostia greater than 90% of the time in athletes; however, a recent study reported that less than 20% of echo laboratories routinely report the coronary origins in athletes.[31] Depending on abnormality surgical repair may be indicated. Return to play after surgical repair is reasonable.

Aortic Dissection

Aortic rupture accounts for 0%–5% of SCD in athletes (see **Table 4**) and is usually associated with Marfan syndrome or other connective tissue abnormalities. Marfan syndrome can cause progressive dilatation and weakness (cystic medial necrosis) of proximal aorta and myxomatous degeneration of mitral and aortic valves. An echocardiogram to assess aortic diameter should be obtained in those with typical Marfanoid features. Return to play should be guided by a specialist familiar with aortic root pathology and is based on aortic dimensions and pathologic features of the disease.

Myocarditis

Myocarditis is an acute inflammatory process involving the myocardium which has historically been reported as a cause of death in 2%–31% of SCD in athletes (see **Table 4**). Previously Coxsackie B virus was implicated in more than 50% of cases, but echovirus, adenovirus, influenza, and *Chlamydia pneumoniae* have also been associated with myocarditis. Pathologic features noted at postmortem examination include lymphocytic infiltrate of myocardium with necrosis or degeneration of adjacent myocytes. With the advent of the SARS-CoV-2 virus, there has been increasing concern for post–COVID-19 myocarditis. Early studies of hospitalized patient[32] and later single-center studies in athletes[33,34] suggested a high rate of post–COVID-19 cardiac involvement and prompted recommendations for wide-spread screening in athletes.[35] Larger registry studies suggested a much lower prevalence of 0.5%-0.6% of myocarditis accompanied by clinical symptoms and 1.5%-1.7% prevalence inclusive of only imaging findings of unclear clinical significance.[36–38] A recent study in college athletes with over a year of follow-up had no adverse cardiovascular outcomes related to COVID-19 (submitted for publication). Future studies will be needed to understand if COVID-19 increases the amount of SCA/d due to myocarditis.

PREVENTION

Prevention can be considered from 2 view points; primary or identifying the cardiac conditions associated with SCA/d with screening or secondary or treated the SCA/d once it has occurred. SCA/D is the leading cause of medical death in athletes and causes more death than heat stroke, sickle cell trait and head injury combined.[6] Current recommendations from the American Heart Association recommend a 14-point history and physical examination for screening,[39] although the sensitivity for detecting conditions associated with SCA/d is low and the false positive rate is high.[22] The European Society for Cardiology and most American professional leagues add an ECG to their screening protocols increasing the ability to detect cardiovascular conditions associated with SCA/d[40] Of the conditions listed above many cardiomyopathies are detectable with screening ECG. In particular, ECG changes are often the first manifestation of HCM before phenotypic changes occur. Channelopathies and conduction disorders such as WPW can also be detected on ECG. It is estimated around 2/3 of cardiovascular conditions associated with SCA/d are present on an ECG.[41] Coronary artery abnormalities and aortopathies are not typically associated with an abnormal ECG. In high-risk populations, if adequate resources are available, consideration of adding a screening ECG to the preparticipation evaluation should be considered.

AED programs and emergency action plans should also be developed at sites whereby SCA/d might occur. Basketball arenas, soccer and football fields, and along marathon routes can all be considered. Access to an AED is important but also a maintenance plan for the AED and education to coaches and administrators.

SUMMARY

The incidence of SCA/d is important for understanding the need for prevention strategies such as primary screening and presence of AEDs and emergency action plans. Studies are difficult given the relatively low prevalence of the condition and a lack of mandatory, centralized reporting. Many studies have imprecise case ascertainment (numerators), inexactly defined study populations (denominators), groups with widely varying risks that give inaccurate assessments of individual risk. These studies suggest a risk of SCA/d of 1 in 50,000 person-years but this represents a regression to the mean with the existence of high-risk groups. Studies addressing these issues indicate the presence of higher risk groups including men (1 in 35,000 person-years) black athletes (1 in 18,000 person-years), and sports including men's basketball (1 in 9000 person-years), men's soccer (1 in 24,000 person-years), and American football (1 in 36,000 person-years). As we move to individualized medicine concepts, consideration should be given toward targeting more aggressive screening to higher risk groups and placing AEDs whereby arrests are more likely to occur. Ongoing studies of incidence should focus on addressing the issues outlined above and include both SCA and SCD.

CLINICS CARE POINTS

- Studies on the incidence of sudden cardiac arrest and death must be interpreted with attention to the methodology. They should differentiate between sex and age groups.

- Approximately 2/3 of conditions that can lead to SCA/D can be detected with the use of a screening ECG.

- 1/3 of conditions will still go undetected. Athletes that play men's basketball, men's soccer or American football appear to be at higher risk for SCA/D than other athletes.

DISCLOSURE

The author has no relevant disclosures.

REFERENCES

1. Harmon K, Asif IM, Maleszewski JJ, et al. Incidence, cause, and comparative frequency of sudden cardiac death in National Collegiate Athletic Association Athletes: a decade in review. Circulation 2015;132:10–9.
2. Lesson 3: Measures of Risk Principles of Epidemiology in Public Health Practice, An Introduction to Applied Epidemiology and Biostatistics. 2012.
3. Harmon KG, Drezner JA, Wilson MG, et al. Incidence of sudden cardiac death in athletes: a state-of-the-art review. Br J Sports Med 2014;48:1185–92.
4. Couper K, Putt O, Field R, et al. Incidence of sudden cardiac death in the young: a systematic review. BMJ Open 2020;10:e040815.
5. Toresdahl BG, Rao AL, Harmon KG, et al. Incidence of sudden cardiac arrest in high school student athletes on school campus. Heart Rhythm 2014;11(7): 1190–4.
6. Harmon KG, Asif IM, Maleszewski JJ, et al. Incidence, Cause, and Comparative Frequency of Sudden Cardiac Death in National Collegiate Athletic Association Athletes: A Decade in Review. Circulation 2015;132:10–9.
7. Harmon KG, Asif IM, Maleszewski JJ, et al. Incidence and etiology of sudden cardiac arrest and death in high school athletes in the United States. Mayo Clin Proc 2016;91:1493–502.
8. Peterson DF, Kucera K, Thomas LC, et al. Aetiology and incidence of sudden cardiac arrest and death in young competitive athletes in the USA: a 4-year prospective study. Br J Sports Med 2021;55:1196–203.
9. Winkel BG, Holst AG, Theilade J, et al. Nationwide study of sudden cardiac death in persons aged 1-35 years. Eur Heart J 2011;32:983–90.
10. Pilmer CM, Kirsh JA, Hildebrandt D, et al. Sudden cardiac death in children and adolescents between 1 and 19 years of age. Heart Rhythm 2014;11:239–45.
11. Virani SS, Alonso A, Benjamin EJ, et al. American Heart Association Council on E, Prevention Statistics C and Stroke Statistics S. Heart Disease and Stroke Statistics-2020 Update: A Report From the American Heart Association. Circulation 2020;141:e139–596.
12. Centers for Disease Control and Prevention, National Center for Health Statistics. Underlying Cause of Death 1999-2020 on CDC WONDER Online Database, released in 2021. Data are from the Multiple Cause of Death Files, 1999-2020, as compiled from data provided by the 57 vital statistics jurisdictions through

the Vital Statistics Cooperative Program. Available at: http://wonder.cdc.gov/ucd-icd10.html. Accessed January 16, 2022.

13. Pilmer CM, Porter B, Kirsh JA, et al. Scope and nature of sudden cardiac death before age 40 in Ontario: a report from the cardiac death advisory committee of the office of the chief coroner. Heart Rhythm 2013;10:517–23.

14. Corrado D, Basso C, Pavei A, et al. Trends in sudden cardiovascular death in young competitive athletes after implementation of a preparticipation screening program. JAMA 2006;296:1593–601.

15. Finocchiaro G, Papadakis M, Robertus JL, et al. Etiology of Sudden Death in Sports: Insights From a United Kingdom Regional Registry. J Am Coll Cardiol 2016;67:2108–15.

16. Lear A, Patel N, Mullen C, et al. Incidence of sudden cardiac arrest and death in young athletes and military members: a systematic review and meta-analysis. J Athl Train 2021.

17. Toresdahl B, Courson R, Borjesson M, et al. Emergency cardiac care in the athletic setting: from schools to the Olympics. Br J Sports Med 2012;46(Suppl 1): i85–9.

18. Egger F, Scharhag J, Kastner A, et al. FIFA Sudden Death Registry (FIFA-SDR): a prospective, observational study of sudden death in worldwide football from 2014 to 2018. Br J Sports Med 2022;56:80–7.

19. Peterson DF, Siebert DM, Kucera KL, et al. Etiology of Sudden Cardiac Arrest and Death in US Competitive Athletes: A 2-Year Prospective Surveillance Study. Clin J Sport Med 2018;30(4):305–14.

20. Malhotra A, Dhutia H, Finocchiaro G, et al. Outcomes of cardiac screening in adolescent soccer players. N Engl J Med 2018;379:524–34.

21. Maron BJ, Doerer JJ, Haas TS, et al. Sudden deaths in young competitive athletes. Analysis of 1866 Deaths in the United States, 1980-2006. Circulation 2009;119:1085–92.

22. Harmon KG, Zigman M, Drezner JA. The effectiveness of screening history, physical exam, and ECG to detect potentially lethal cardiac disorders in athletes: a systematic review/meta-analysis. J Electrocardiol 2015;48:329–38.

23. Malhotra R, West JJ, Dent J, et al. Cost and yield of adding electrocardiography to history and physical in screening Division I intercollegiate athletes: a 5-year experience. Heart Rhythm 2011;8:721–7.

24. Zorzi A, Calore C, Vio R, et al. Accuracy of the ECG for differential diagnosis between hypertrophic cardiomyopathy and athlete's heart: comparison between the European Society of Cardiology (2010) and International (2017) criteria. Br J Sports Med 2018;52:667–73.

25. Drezner JA, Sharma S, Baggish A, et al. International criteria for electrocardiographic interpretation in athletes: Consensus statement. Br J Sports Med 2017; 51:704–31.

26. Finocchiaro G, Sheikh N, Leone O, et al. Arrhythmogenic potential of myocardial disarray in hypertrophic cardiomyopathy: genetic basis, functional consequences and relation to sudden cardiac death. Europace 2021;23:985–95.

27. Chatard JC, Espinosa F, Donnadieu R, et al. Pre-participation cardiovascular evaluation in Pacific Island athletes. Int J Cardiol 2019;278:273–9.

28. Miles C, Finocchiaro G, Papadakis M, et al. Sudden death and left ventricular involvement in arrhythmogenic cardiomyopathy. Circulation 2019;139(15): 1786–97.

29. James CA, Bhonsale A, Tichnell C, et al. Exercise increases age-related penetrance and arrhythmic risk in arrhythmogenic right ventricular dysplasia/

cardiomyopathy-associated desmosomal mutation carriers. J Am Coll Cardiol 2013;62:1290–7.

30. Sawant AC, Bhonsale A, te Riele AS, et al. Exercise has a disproportionate role in the pathogenesis of arrhythmogenic right ventricular dysplasia/cardiomyopathy in patients without desmosomal mutations. J Am Heart Assoc 2014;3:e001471.

31. Petek BJ, Moulson N, Drezner JA, et al. Echocardiographic reporting of proximal coronary artery origins in young competitive athletes. JACC Cardiovasc Imaging 2022;15(3):544–6. S1936-878X(21)00892-00895.

32. Shi S, Qin M, Shen B, et al. Association of cardiac injury with mortality in hospitalized patients with COVID-19 in Wuhan, China. JAMA Cardiol 2020;5:802–10.

33. Rajpal S, Tong MS, Borchers J, et al. Cardiovascular Magnetic resonance findings in competitive athletes recovering from COVID-19 Infection. JAMA Cardiol 2021;6:116–8.

34. Brito D, Meester S, Yanamala N, et al. High Prevalence of Pericardial Involvement in College Student Athletes Recovering From COVID-19. JACC Cardiovasc Imaging 2021;14:541–55.

35. Phelan D, Kim JH, Chung EH. A Game Plan for the Resumption of Sport and Exercise After Coronavirus Disease 2019 (COVID-19) Infection. JAMA Cardiol 2020; 5:1085–6.

36. Moulson N, Petek BJ, Drezner JA, et al. Baggish AL and Outcomes Registry for Cardiac Conditions in Athletes I. SARS-CoV-2 cardiac involvement in young competitive athletes. Circulation 2021;144:256–66.

37. Daniels CJ, Rajpal S, Greenshields JT, et al. Prevalence of clinical and subclinical myocarditis in competitive athletes with recent SARS-CoV-2 Infection: Results From the Big Ten COVID-19 Cardiac Registry. JAMA Cardiol 2021;6:1078–87.

38. Martinez MW, Tucker AM, Bloom OJ, et al. Prevalence of inflammatory heart disease among professional athletes with prior COVID-19 infection who received systematic return-to-play cardiac screening. JAMA Cardiol 2021;6:745–52.

39. Maron BJ, Friedman RA, Kligfield P, et al. Assessment of the 12-lead electrocardiogram as a screening test for detection of cardiovascular disease in healthy general populations of young people (12-25 years of age): a scientific statement from the American Heart Association and the American College of Cardiology. J Am Coll Cardiol 2014;64:1479–514.

40. Pelliccia A, Sharma S, Gati S, et al. 2020 ESC guidelines on sports cardiology and exercise in patients with cardiovascular disease. Rev Esp Cardiol (Engl Ed) 2021;74:545.

41. Drezner JA, O'Connor FG, Harmon KG, et al. AMSSM Position Statement on cardiovascular preparticipation screening in athletes: current evidence, knowledge gaps, recommendations and future directions. Br J Sports Med 2016;15(5): 359–75.

42. Corrado D, Basso C, Rizzoli G, et al. Does sports activity enhance the risk of sudden death in adolescents and young adults? J Am Coll Cardiol 2003;42:1959–63.

43. Drezner JA, Harmon KG, Marek JC. Incidence of sudden cardiac arrest in Minnesota high school student athletes: the limitations of catastrophic insurance claims. J Am Coll Cardiol 2014;63:1455–6.

44. Van Camp SP, Bloor CM, Mueller FO, et al. Nontraumatic sports death in high school and college athletes. Med Sci Sports Exerc 1995;27:641–7.

45. Drezner JA, Rogers KJ, Zimmer RR, et al. Use of Automated External Defibrillators at NCAA Division I Universities. Med Sci Sports Exerc 2005;37:1487–92.

46. Drezner JA, Rao AL, Heistand J, et al. Effectiveness of emergency response planning for sudden cardiac arrest in United States high schools with automated external defibrillators. Circulation 2009;120:518–25.

47. Holst AG, Winkel BG, Theilade J, et al. Incidence and etiology of sports-related sudden cardiac death in Denmark–implications for preparticipation screening. Heart Rhythm 2010;7:1365–71.

48. Marijon E, Tafflet M, Celermajer DS, et al. Sports-related sudden death in the general population. Circulation 2011;124:672–81.

49. Steinvil A, Chundadze T, Zeltser D, et al. Mandatory electrocardiographic screening of athletes to reduce their risk for sudden death proven fact or wishful thinking? J Am Coll Cardiol 2011;57:1291–6.

50. Maron BJ, Haas TS, Ahluwalia A, et al. Incidence of cardiovascular sudden deaths in Minnesota high school athletes. Heart Rhythm 2013;10:374–7.

51. Risgaard B, Winkel BG, Jabbari R, et al. Sports-related sudden cardiac death in a competitive and a noncompetitive athlete population aged 12 to 49 years: data from an unselected nationwide study in Denmark. Heart Rhythm 2014;11: 1673–81.

52. Bohm P, Scharhag J, Meyer T. Data from a nationwide registry on sports-related sudden cardiac deaths in Germany. Eur J Prev Cardiol 2016;23:649–56.

53. Grani C, Chappex N, Fracasso T, et al. Sports-related sudden cardiac death in Switzerland classified by static and dynamic components of exercise. Eur J Prev Cardiol 2016;23:1228–36.

54. Maron BJ, Haas TS, Duncanson ER, et al. Comparison of the frequency of sudden cardiovascular deaths in young competitive athletes versus nonathletes: should we really screen only athletes? Am J Cardiol 2016;117:1339–41.

55. Corrado D, Basso C, Thiene G. Sudden cardiac death in young people with apparently normal heart. Cardiovasc Res 2001;50:399–408.

56. de Noronha SV, Sharma S, Papadakis M, et al. Aetiology of sudden cardiac death in athletes in the United Kingdom: a pathological study. Heart 2009;95:1409–14.

57. Suarez-Mier MP, Aguilera B, Mosquera RM, et al. Pathology of sudden death during recreational sports in Spain. Forensic Sci Int 2013;226:188–96.

58. Morentin B, Suarez-Mier MP, Monzo A, et al. Sports-related sudden cardiac death in Spain. A multicenter, population-based, forensic study of 288 cases. Rev Esp Cardiol (Engl Ed) 2021;74:225–32.

59. Thiene G, Rizzo S, Schiavon M, et al. Structurally normal hearts are uncommonly associated with sudden deaths in athletes and young people. J Am Coll Cardiol 2019;73:3031–2.

60. Wisten A, Borjesson M, Krantz P, et al. Exercise related sudden cardiac death (SCD) in the young - Pre-mortal characterization of a Swedish nationwide cohort, showing a decline in SCD among athletes. Resuscitation 2019;144:99–105.

Non-Cardiac Conditions that Mimic Cardiac Symptoms in Athletes

Siobhan M. Statuta, MD[a],*, Erin S. Barnes, MD[b],
John M. MacKnight, MD[c]

KEYWORDS

- Non-cardiac chest pain • Athlete • Musculoskeletal (MSK)
- Gastroesophageal reflux (GER) • Asthma

KEY POINTS

- Any team physician or healthcare provider caring for an athlete with chest pain must be able to quickly and efficiently assess for life-threatening conditions.
- The majority of athletes presenting with chest pain have non-cardiac etiologies such as musculoskeletal, pulmonary, gastrointestinal, or from other sources.
- A deliberate and thoughtful approach to these athletes is crucial in uncovering essential historical and examination clues to assist with an efficient diagnosis and treatment plan.

INTRODUCTION

Chest pain is one of the most serious and worrisome complaints encountered in the field of sports medicine due to its potential for catastrophic outcomes. Part of the challenge is that chest pain can indicate a wide variation of etiologies spread across an expansive continuum (**Table 1**), ranging from the simple musculoskeletal strain, to the acute and life-threatening arrhythmia. In active or athletic populations who withstand high levels of physiologic exertion, an acute presentation of chest pain requires the treating physician and medical staff to be skilled at a thorough yet appropriate assessment. They must expeditiously rule out urgent scenarios using sound clinical judgment while providing appropriate and thoughtful evaluation and management

[a] Department of Family Medicine and Physical Medicine and Rehabilitation, University of Virginia School of Medicine, Box 800729, 1415 Jefferson Park Avenue- McKim Hall 3152, Charlottesville, VA 22908, USA; [b] Department of Physical Medicine and Rehabilitation and Orthopedic Surgery, Case Western Reserve University School of Medicine, Cleveland, OH, USA; [c] Internal Medicine & Orthopaedic Surgery, University of Virginia School of Medicine, University Physicians Clinic, UVA Health System, Box 800671, Charlottesville, VA 22908, USA
* Corresponding author.
E-mail address: sms5bb@virginia.edu

Clin Sports Med 41 (2022) 389–404
https://doi.org/10.1016/j.csm.2022.02.003
0278-5919/22/© 2022 Elsevier Inc. All rights reserved.
sportsmed.theclinics.com

Table 1
Non-cardiac causes of chest pain in athletes

Musculoskeletal	Pulmonary	Gastrointestinal	Psychiatric	Miscellaneous
• Costochondritis	• Exercise-induced bronchospasm (EIB)	• Biliary colic	• Hyperventilation syndrome	• Eating disorder
• Intercostal myalgia	• Pleurisy	• Boerhaave's syndrome	• Psychogenic	• Drug abuse
• Muscular strain	• Pneumomediastinum	• Delayed gastric emptying		• Herpes zoster
• Myofascial pain syndrome	• Pneumonia	• Esophagitis		• Malignancy
• Osteomyelitis (thoracic spine, sternum, rib)	• Pneumothorax	• Gastritis		• Medications/ supplements
• Radiculopathy (cervical, thoracic)	• Pulmonary contusion	• Gastroesophageal reflux		• Mondor disease
• Rib fracture (traumatic, stress)	• Pulmonary embolus	• Gastric ulcer		• Precordial catch syndrome
• SAPHO syndrome	• Vocal cord dysfunction	• Hiatal hernia		• Pregnancy
• Slipping rib syndrome		• Pancreatitis		• Puberty
• Sternalis syndrome				
• Sternoclavicular joint injury				
• Tietze Syndrome				
• Trigger points				
• Xiphodynia				

(Fig. 1).[1] If not completed in a deliberate and methodical fashion, a work-up can prove to be inappropriately excessive, costly, and anxiety provoking for patients.

Chest pain accounts for 1% of all ambulatory primary care visits, prompting millions of physician encounters annually.[2] Of these, up to 50% are related to chest wall pain, 20% from reflux esophagitis, and 13% due to costochondritis, with additional contributors including pulmonary and psychiatric causes.[2] Specifically for athletes, the most common cause of chest pain in those under 35 year old is gastroesophageal reflux followed by exercise-induced bronchospasm. Despite these trends, the initial differential in the case of chest pain in an athlete should remain broad with particular consideration toward the unique nuances of the individual sporting event at hand. Here, we explore some of the non-cardiac contributors that should be considered in evaluating any athlete with chest discomfort.

Musculoskeletal

Once life-threatening causes of chest pain have been ruled out, more common etiologies can be considered. Musculoskeletal chest pain accounts for at least 20% of chest pain presentations in all athletes.[3] Pathology can arise from issues with the bone, joint, muscle, fascia, and peripheral nerve. Diagnosis is often clinical, with key

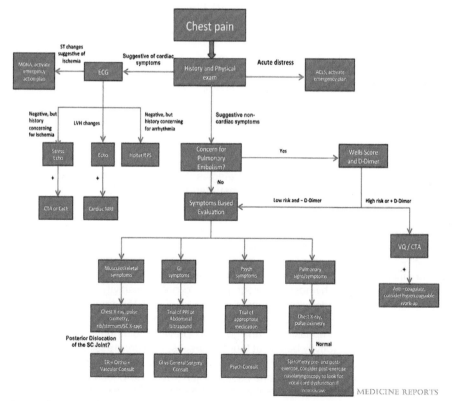

Fig. 1. Algorithm for assessment diagnostic evaluation of chest pain in the athletes. (*From* Moran B, Bryan S, Farrar T, Salud C, Visser G, Decuba R, Renelus D, Buckley T, Dressing M, Peterkin N, Coris E. Diagnostic Evaluation of Nontraumatic Chest Pain in Athletes. Curr Sports Med Rep. 2017 Mar/Apr;16(2):84-94. https://doi.org/10.1249/JSR.0000000000000342. PMID: 28282354., with permission.)

history components including trauma history, aggravating activities, and associated neurologic symptoms, followed by a focused examination. While the majority of cases of musculoskeletal thoracic pain are focal in nature, presentations involving radicular symptoms should prompt consideration of cervical or thoracic segmental dysfunction and concomitant multi-joint complaints may suggest an underlying rheumatologic disorder.[4]

Costochondritis

Costochondritis, costosternal syndrome, and anterior chest wall syndrome are terms used to describe a condition characterized by local pain and tenderness at the costochondral and/or costosternal junctions, most frequently at the second through fifth articulations. Cited to account for up to one-third of emergency room visits for chest pain, it is the most common diagnosis of musculoskeletal chest pain, though its pathophysiology is not well understood.[5] It is thought to be related to functional overload and microtrauma from repetitive physical activity as emphasized by its high prevalence in volleyball players, rowers, and weightlifters.[6] Symptoms are often unilateral and elicited by deep inspiration and upper extremity movement. Diagnosis is made by identification of multiple chest wall tender points reproducible upon palpation and exclusion of other causes. It is differentiated from Tietze's syndrome (see below) by an absence of swelling or inflammation. Treatment is symptomatic and the course is usually self-limiting with the majority of cases resolving within 1 year.[7] In refractory cases, rib manipulation, soft tissue mobilization, and corticosteroid or sulfasalazine injections can improve outcomes.[8]

Tietze syndrome

Tietze syndrome manifests similarly to costochondritis, however non-suppurative inflammation at the costochondral junction is the key distinguishing feature of this rare idiopathic condition. Unlike the more diffuse nature of costochondritis, the majority of patients are affected at a single site, most commonly at the second and third costal cartilage articulations.[9] Findings of elevated erythrocyte sedimentation rate, increased uptake on bone scintigraphy, and inflammatory findings on ultrasonography support the diagnosis.[10,11] Treatment strategies that reduce inflammation including local corticosteroid injections have demonstrated favorable results.[12]

Traumatic rib fracture

These injuries result from blunt thoracic trauma and most commonly occur at the posterolateral angle of ribs four through nine. Clinically, pleuritic pain is often present and patients may demonstrate respiratory splinting. Exam findings suggestive of rib fracture include point tenderness, focal tenderness elicited by rib cage compression, bony crepitus, and ecchymosis. Radiographs yield poor sensitivity and generally do not influence the management of uncomplicated injuries.[13] Rib fractures in isolation have limited clinical significance beyond the acute pain and dysfunction. Management is conservative with emphasis on analgesia to prevent pulmonary complications. Gradual return to the activity begins at four to 6 weeks, with progression to full activity as tolerated at eight to 10 weeks.[6] In the setting of a traumatic thoracic injury, more concerning concomitant or resultant visceral injury, such as pneumothorax, hemothorax, and splenic or liver lacerations, should be ruled out if suspected.

Chest wall stress fractures

This type of injury should be considered in the athlete who presents with atraumatic chest wall pain associated with repetitive activity. Stress fractures at the anterolateral fourth through ninth ribs are seen predominantly in rowers, but have also been reported in golfers and swimmers. The underlying mechanism is thought to be from repetitive tensile loading from the inserting serratus anterior and abdominal muscles.[14,15] First rib stress fractures are found in throwing and overhead sports, such as tennis, baseball, javelin, and basketball, with the anterior scalenes implicated in their development.[16] Less common are stress fractures of the manubriosternum, which have been described in wrestlers and golfers.[6] Patients with these conditions typically present with insidious onset of vague chest pain, which can progress to more localized, pleuritic pain made worse with provocative activities. As with other stress injuries, bone scan and magnetic resonance imaging are the preferred imaging modalities due to their superior specificity over radiographs. More recently, however, ultrasound has been increasingly utilized for diagnosis.[17] Management includes relative rest, activity modification, and rehabilitation focused on scapular stabilization and serratus anterior strengthening.[18]

Slipping rib syndrome
Additionally known as 'twelfth rib', 'clicking rib', and 'rib-tip syndrome', this condition is characterized by pain in the lower ribs with associated clicking, popping, or slipping sensation. It is seen in sports with repetitive trunk motion such as running, rowing, and lacrosse. The large female predominance (70%) suggests a possible correlation with hyperlaxity phenotype.[19] These risk factors may contribute to the incompetence of the fibrous attachments of the floating ribs that allow superior slippage of the cartilage resulting in intercostal nerve irritation, intercostal muscle strain, or costal cartilage sprain.[20] The "hooking maneuver," in which the examiner places curled fingers under the ribs at the costal margin and applies an anterior force, is considered positive if reproducible of pain or popping sensation and can aid in diagnosis. Ultrasound can identify abnormalities in the rib and cartilage anatomy, as well as soft tissue swelling. The mainstays of treatment remain conservative, though there are roles for prolotherapy, botulinum toxin injections, and surgical treatments in refractory cases.[21]

Sternoclavicular (SC) joint injury
Sternoclavicular sprains, subluxations, and dislocations are rare traumatic injuries that result from high-velocity forces directly on the diarthrodial joint or indirectly via medial compression from the shoulder. In athletes, this is most commonly seen in collision sports like football, hockey, and rugby, but is also observed in cycling. The direction of the dislocation is important to identify as it dictates management. The majority of SC joint injuries are anterior, and while a true dislocation should be reduced within 24 hours, they are generally uncomplicated and treated symptomatically. Contrastingly, posterior dislocations are medical emergencies due to potential compression of vital mediastinal structures by the clavicular head. These patients may present with dysphagia, dyspnea, hoarseness, venous congestion in the neck, and upper extremity paresthesias, with any of these findings prompting urgent reduction using a traction-abduction maneuver or a sterile towel clip. Further treatment options include open or closed reduction under anesthesia, the latter of which confers lower risk with demonstrated success up to 1-week post-injury.[22] In stable patients, serendipity view on x-ray is best for evaluating the SC joint, though CT is the diagnostic modality of choice for definitive diagnosis.[23]

Precordial catch syndrome
Also known as "Texidor's twinge," precordial catch is a benign cause of chest pain in adolescents and children of unclear etiology. Sudden episodes of well-localized pain are characterized as sharp and stabbing, but last seconds to minutes and are not

associated with other symptoms.[24] Symptoms usually occur at rest and are made worse with inspiration. Management is reassurance.

Pulmonary Chest Pain

Exercise-induced bronchospasm

Exercise-induced bronchospasm (EIB) is defined as transient airway narrowing that occurs during or after exercise. EIB is the most common cause of exercise-related chest pain and has been reported in 10% to 20% of athletes and up to 90% of asthmatic patients.[3,25] EIB is also commonly seen in those without underlying asthma, particularly in children where it may account for up to 75% of chest pain diagnoses,[26] in those with atopy or rhinitis, and following respiratory infections. Intensity, duration, and type of exercise have been associated with the occurrence of EIB with higher prevalence rates in high-level athletes competing in endurance sports, winter disciplines, and swimming.[3,25]

Airway hyper-reactivity, bronchospasm, wheezing, and mucus hypersecretion occur via a number of environmental mechanisms and result in progressive airway narrowing. Clinical features of EIB include burning substernal chest pain, chest tightness, wheezing, dry cough, shortness of breath, increased sputum production, and unusual fatigue.[25–27] Patients often complain of difficulty with inspiration and a hyper-expanded, "full" chest because of air-trapping and inefficient exhalation.

Current guidelines recommend distinguishing EIB in those with underlying asthma from exercise-induced bronchial obstruction in those without other symptoms or signs of asthma.[27,28] Many other conditions may mimic the "wheezing" of asthma (**Box 1**); as such, it is essential to obtain a definitive diagnosis via spirometry.[29] Post-exercise pulmonary function tests (PFTs) and peak expiratory flow (PEF) rate are typically utilized to make the diagnosis. An exercise-induced decrease in FEV_1 by 10% to 15% or a decrease in peak flow by 15% to 20% should be considered diagnostic of EIB. In athletes, provocative testing via methacholine challenge, eucapneic voluntary

---

Box 1
Non-Asthmatic conditions which May Be associated with a complaint of "wheezing"

- Allergic rhinitis
- Laryngotracheobronchitis
- Foreign body
- Vocal cord dysfunction (VCD)
- Laryngeal webs, tracheal stenosis, enlarged lymph nodes, tumors
- Cystic fibrosis
- Bronchiectasis
- Bronchopulmonary dysplasia
- Congestive heart failure
- α-1 antitrypsin deficiency
- Aspiration
- Gastroesophageal reflux disease (GERD)
- Laryngeal reflux disease

hyperpnea, mannitol, or hypertonic saline may be required to discern a decline in pulmonary function with exercise.

EIB management varies from inhaled pre-exercise β-2 agonist therapy (albuterol) to long-acting β-2 agonist therapy (salmeterol) with or without inhaled corticosteroids (eg, fluticasone, betamethasone). Oral leukotriene antagonists (eg, montelukast) may be helpful as well.

Pneumothorax

A pneumothorax is a collapse of the lung due to loss of negative intrathoracic pressure from air entering the chest cavity. The primary mechanism is a tear in the protective pleural surface of the lung, often due to a rupture of pleural blebs or bullae in tall, slender males, usually under 40 years old.[30] On the playing field, rib fractures and significant direct blows to the chest wall may also predispose to pneumothorax. A pneumothorax is one of a small number of potential on-field emergencies and, as such, should always be considered high in the differential of any athlete presenting with new-onset chest pain or shortness of breath, even without trauma.

Chest pain occurs in 80% to 90% of patients with a pneumothorax, making it the most common clinical feature. In addition, shortness of breath, hypotension, and tachycardia[31] may be observed as well. Physical exam is notable for decreased or absent breath sounds in the affected lung field with associated hyper-resonance to percussion. Progressive accumulation of air and rise in positive pressure within the chest may create a tension pneumothorax which may be life-threatening as it shifts mediastinal structures away from the pneumothorax and compromises venous return to the heart. These athletes present as critically ill with tracheal deviation away from the pneumothorax, cyanosis, tachypnea, and impending circulatory collapse.

Chest radiographs are the initial diagnostic study of choice for a suspected pneumothorax. If a standard chest x-ray fails to demonstrate a pneumothorax in a patient with high clinical suspicion, further investigation is best accomplished with a chest CT scan.

Small pneumothoraces (15%–25% collapse) may be safely monitored via serial x-rays if the patient is clinically stable and without evidence of cardiopulmonary compromise. Moderate/large, progressive, or bilateral pneumothoraces should be treated with urgent chest tube decompression.[32–34] A tension pneumothorax requires immediate needle decompression and emergent transport for definitive management.

Pulmonary contusion

Bruising of the lung parenchyma in sport results from high force blunt trauma as seen in bicycle racing or motor sports. Focal lung damage and inflammation may progress to alveolar edema, hemorrhage, and significant respiratory compromise.

Onset of symptoms is insidious and includes chest pain, dyspnea, tachypnea, cyanosis, and tachycardia; approximately 50% of patients will develop hemoptysis.[33] Pulmonary exam may reveal rales or diminished breath sounds in the area of injury. It is important to note that the most severe pulmonary contusions are often found without concomitant rib fracture; the lack of force dissipation when the rib does not break conveys a more severe blow to the underlying lung.

Classic radiographic findings include patchy irregular alveolar infiltrates. When the diagnosis remains in question, CT scanning should be utilized because of its high sensitivity for detection of early lung injury.[35] Patients should be observed in the hospital setting to monitor for progressive respiratory failure. Guidelines for return to play after pulmonary contusion are largely based on case reporting. Athletes should not return to sports in the presence of continued hemoptysis, dyspnea, or exercise intolerance. In the absence of respiratory symptoms, if the athlete is able to tolerate strenuous exercise for 48 hours and able to perform at an appropriate level, return to sports participation may be allowed.[36]

Pneumomediastinum

Pneumomediastinum (PM) is characterized by free air in the mediastinum due to injury to the alveolar space or to the communicating bronchial tree. Spontaneous PM is an uncommon condition accounting for 0.3% of patients with chest pain, most of whom are male adolescents with a history of preexisting asthma.[37] In athletes, an exertional increase in airway pressure induced by heavy weightlifting or similar high intensity activity may cause alveolar rupture with resultant PM, even in the absence of underlying lung disease.

Clinically, chest pain is typically retrosternal, worsened by inspiration, and present in 50% to 90% of cases. Pain may radiate to the shoulders or back and may mimic myocardial infarction or pericarditis. The classic physical exam finding is palpable subcutaneous crepitus. Auscultation may reveal the "Hamman sign," precordial systolic crepitations and diminution of heart sounds. Pneumothorax may be a concomitant finding.

Chest radiographs typically demonstrate air outlining mediastinal structures, producing the "double bronchial wall" sign. Spontaneous resolution is the rule, and management is directed toward possible co-morbidities, particularly pneumothorax or musculoskeletal injuries. There are no reported cases of athletes requiring intervention for PM.

Pulmonary embolism

Pulmonary embolism (PE) is a potentially life-threatening complication of deep venous thrombosis (DVT) which occurs uncommonly in athletes.[38–42] Nonetheless, PE should always be included in the differential diagnosis of chest pain because thromboembolic risks in athletes are common. Venous stasis with immobilization from injury or surgery, venous trauma, hypercoagulability from dehydration, genetic clotting syndromes (Factor V Leiden mutation, Prothrombin/Factor II mutation, Protein S and Protein C deficiencies) and oral contraceptive use may all predispose to DVT and PE.[43]

Presentations vary considerably and are often subtle. Although chest pain, dyspnea, and/or tachycardia are present in 97% of those diagnosed with PE, no single clinical feature effectively supports or rules out its diagnosis.[44] Chest pain is typically pleuritic and may be associated with hemoptysis. Physical exam may reveal an uncomfortable, tachypneic patient with tachycardia, fever, focal rales, and increased S2 heart sound, though the exam may be largely normal. The classic electrocardiogram reveals sinus tachycardia and an S wave in Lead I, and a Q wave and T wave inversion in Lead III ("$S_1Q_3T_3$" pattern).

The Wells clinical prediction rule (**Table 2**) is a validated tool that can be used to accurately predict a low, moderate, or high likelihood of PE.[45] ELISA D-dimer assay, pulmonary CT angiography, V/Q scanning, and lower extremity venous Doppler may be helpful in making the diagnosis.[45,46]

Low clinical suspicion for PE (Wells score < 2) and a normal quantitative ELISA D-dimer assay have a negative predictive value for PE of greater than 99.5%.[47–49] Although largely replaced by non-invasive CT scanning, selective pulmonary angiography is still considered the gold standard for diagnosis of PE.

Pulmonary emboli are treated with warfarin or direct oral anticoagulants (DOACs) such as apixaban, dabigatran, or rivaroxaban for 6 months. Athletic participation during that time may be considered in low impact sports without contact risk. Future participation will depend on PE etiology and long-term anticoagulation status.

Table 2
Wells prediction rule for pulmonary embolus

Clinical Feature	Points
Clinical symptoms of DVT	3
Other diagnosis less likely than PE	3
Heart rate >100 beats per minute	1.5
Immobilization or surgery within past 4 wk	1.5
Previous DVT or PE	1.5
Hemoptysis	1
Malignancy	1
Total points	

Probability of pulmonary embolus: HIGH RISK: score of greater than 6 points (78.4%); MODERATE RISK: score of 2 to 6 points (27.8%); LOW RISK: score less than 2 points (3.4%).

Pneumonia

Pneumonia is an uncommon cause of chest pain in athletes. Typically resulting from viral, atypical bacterial (eg, mycoplasma), or community-acquired bacterial (eg, *Strep. pneumoniae, H. influenzae*) pathogens, pneumonia may produce chest pain as a result of pleural inflammation. In addition, patients present with a broad constellation of symptoms including fever, chills, rigors, cough with purulent sputum, malaise, and shortness of breath. The presence of cough, fever, and focal inspiratory rales on examination are the most useful clinical tools.[50] Egophony, dullness to percussion of the posterior thorax, and respiratory rate greater than 20 breaths per minute are also highly suggestive of pneumonia.[51]

Chest radiographs classically demonstrate focal areas of lobar consolidation or diffuse interstitial infiltrates, but may be normal. Atypical pneumonias often demonstrate bilateral patchy infiltrates which appear more impressive than the clinical presentation of the patient. Management is either supportive or with broad-spectrum antibiotics depending on the causative organism.

Pleurisy

Inflammation of the pleura with resultant chest pain may arise from a variety of conditions. In athletes, the majority of pleuritic pain results from viral respiratory infections due to adenovirus, Coxsackie virus, cytomegalovirus (CMV), Epstein-Barr virus (EBV), influenza, parainfluenza, and respiratory syncytial virus (RSV). Pneumonia may produce pleuritic pain by direct involvement of the pleura or via parapneumonic effusion. Pulmonary embolism commonly presents with pleuritic pain and is the most frequently observed life-threatening cause of pleuritic chest pain. Management focuses on accurate diagnosis of the underlying cause, and therapies are condition-specific.

Gastrointestinal

When assessing an athlete with complaints of chest pain, one must keep gastrointestinal (GI) etiologies in consideration. Up to 50% of recreational athletes report having experienced GI complaints at some point during sport.[52] This prevalence increases to 70% in the endurance athlete.[53] Due to the nature of the abdomen and its close proximity to the thorax, various conditions can present as chest pain or precipitate other issues such as esophageal spasm or pulmonary complaints, making diagnosis challenging. Several GI conditions have a predilection for active persons compared to the general population, with factors such as mechanical forces from sporting activity, alterations in GI perfusion during exercise, and neuroendocrine changes placing them at greater risk of GI irritation.[54]

Gastrointestinal reflux

Gastrointestinal reflux (GER) is a pervasive condition worldwide, yet has no universally accepted definition. Typically thought of as the *problematic* result of the reflux of stomach contents, the classic presentation is of burning epigastric discomfort, dyspepsia, and regurgitation with diagnosis via testing or symptom description alone. However, GER can alternatively manifest with a constellation of atypical symptoms including sore throat, hoarseness, cough, bronchitis, asthma, recurrent pneumonia, choking, or chest pain/angina. While, the incidence of GER is high across the general population, exertional activities further induce symptoms and place athlete populations at greater risk. The physiologic mechanisms of exercise promote GER in multifaceted fashion. Sympathetic relaxation of the lower esophageal sphincter, increased jostling of epigastric contents, slowed GI clearance and decreased splanchnic perfusion all contribute. Symptoms increase in frequency postprandially or with increased activity intensity or endurance, and dehydration further exacerbates symptoms. Other causes of gastric distress common in athletes such as nonsteroidal anti-inflammatory drug (NSAID) use, protein and/or caffeine supplementation, and consumption of certain sports drinks can intensify discomfort. Sports such as weightlifting or cycling that involve increased abdominal pressures have greater propensity toward symptomatic reflux.

The shared sensory pathway of the esophagus and heart presents a challenge for clinicians, at times confounding simple gastric causes as chest pain. In athletes complaining of chest pain, even those with known GER, it can be difficult to differentiate between benign and more nefarious etiologies. In addition to obtaining a careful history and thorough cardiovascular/abdominal exams, additional testing with electrocardiogram, chest x-ray, endoscopy, or esophageal pH monitoring will assist with the proper diagnosis. Laboratory studies including hemoglobin, hematocrit, transaminases, and amylase can be helpful in ruling out other less common causes of GI pathology such as peptic ulcer disease, hepatitis and pancreatitis. Moreover, GER can simultaneously worsen true angina-a consideration that should not be dismissed.[55]

Once GER is determined as the underlying cause, a four to 6 week trial of lifestyle modifications is a reasonable initial treatment option.[55] Adjusting training and eating times to allow for three or 4 hours between consumption and exercise may alone be enough to alleviate symptoms. Incorporating a more prolonged warmup and cool down, improving hydration, limiting unnecessary NSAID use, and modifying size and composition of meals can also help. If symptoms persist despite these attempts, a 2 week trial of a twice-daily H2 blocker or a once-daily proton pump inhibitor (PPI) taken prior the first meal of the day should be initiated. If effective, the medication can be extended to an 8 week course followed by efforts to eventually wean off.

Substance Abuse

Abuse of any of a variety of legal and illicit substances may result in chest pain either directly or indirectly and thus should be part of the differential in the assessment of chest pain in an athlete.

Energy drinks/weight loss products

In the hypercompetitive climate of sport today, immense pressure is placed on athletes to succeed; to win. It is no wonder, then, that the market for energy drinks has skyrocketed with promises to provide the desired added edge to sports performance. Despite their allure to some, current evidence regarding efficacy and safety of energy drinks is lacking. These drinks are categorized as 'dietary supplements' within the U.S. Food and Drug Administration (FDA), allowing for minimal regulation and failure to warn consumers of potential side-effects. While over-the-counter foods/beverage products are limited in how much caffeine their products contain, there exists no maximum dosage restriction for energy drinks. Consequently, their higher caffeine levels have been linked to disrupted sleep, anxiety, and even seizures. Acute cardio-vascular effects are widespread and include impaired arterial endothelial function, blood pressure spikes, coronary artery spasm, changes on electrocardiograms (increased QTc interval), arrhythmias, aortic dissection, and even sudden cardiac death.

Similarly, weight-loss supplements are not subject to the strict federal product reg-ulations either. They target those vulnerable to fit a societal mold of the ideal body type, while avoiding full disclosure of potential harmful ingredients.[56] These pills and powders are commonplace in athlete settings particularly for those in aesthetic sports or weight-derived classifications for competition such as wrestling or gymnastics.

These products must be considered by the medical staff in the setting of a partici-pant chest pain. If the athlete acknowledges consumption, obtaining a chemistry panel and EKG will assist with ruling out the more dangerous effects. Immediate cessation and education regarding these products should follow.

Stimulants

As of 2016, there were 6.1 million children under age seventeen diagnosed with attention-deficit/hyperactivity disorder (ADHD) with nearly two-thirds (62%) on medica-tion for treatment.[57] Specific to young athletes, prevalence rates of ADHD range from 4% to 14.3% thus commonplace.[58] Concerns regarding safety profiles of the medica-tions are compounded when considering use in the athletic population. The collegiate level of play comes with even more pressures to practice, hone skills, and earn playing time while juggling rigorous academic workloads. Psychostimulant medications in-crease levels of neurotransmitters within the central nervous system, allowing the brain to focus and function at a greater capacity. Studies have demonstrated that stimulants, if taken near competition, can provide athletic advantages (improved strength, acceler-ation, anaerobic capacity, time to exhaustion, fine motor skills and balance, atten-tion).[59,60] Other less desirable effects of these drugs are frequently encountered include an elevated pulse rate and blood pressure—both of which have serious conse-quences in the athletic population already pushing their bodies to physical extremes. In addition to chest pain, stimulant use can result in abdominal pain, cause decreased appetite/weight loss, headaches, constipation, and sleep disturbance.

Beyond caffeine products and stimulant medications, there exists a plethora of products that are misused for performance benefits or simply for recreational pur-poses. The more notorious substances such as cocaine, marijuana, and anabolic ste-roids are well identified, however misuse of legitimate medications such as diuretics or beta-blockers can also be used for competitive advantages yet can result in adverse health consequences. It is important to keep these products in mind while evaluating an individual presenting with chest pain.

Psychogenic

An assortment of psychosocial stressors including generalized anxiety disorder, panic disorder, depression, and somatization can result in chest pain.[61] Anxiety in particular can manifest itself as fear, apprehension, worry or tension in response to an actual or perceived threat.[62] Within athletic cohorts, these 'threats' go beyond an obvious high-stakes competition and into the daily struggle of maintaining life/training balance, po-sition on the desired team, playing time, or securing future financial security. Rice and colleagues found that the rates of combined anxiety disorders in the elite athlete are similar to that of the general population,[63] yet it is speculated that in the world of athletics, symptoms are frequently underreported due to stigma and unsupportive environments regarding mental health. Such settings preclude proper identification of mental health symptoms and can lead to unanticipated symptom escalation manifesting as chest pain, panic attacks and hyperventilation syndrome.

In the acute setting, if an athlete presents with chest pain and is hyperventilating, it is important to move the athlete to a quiet environment. Members of the healthcare team should assist with slowing the respiration rate and pulse through a variety of techniques such a breathing into a paper bag or mindfully focusing on specific sensations of the outside world ("feel your hand touching the ground"). Once the event has passed and safety confirmed, appropriate in-office follow-up should be arranged to assess the underlying conditions.

In the non-acute setting, open and direct discussion is recommended, addressing personal and family history mental health as well as current safety status. Referral to psychological/psychiatric services should strongly be considered for additional diagnosis and treatment of symptoms, as cognitive behavioral and mindfulness-based therapies have been proven effective.[64] If symptoms remain problematic, the addition of a serotonin-specific reuptake inhibitor may be warranted such as escitalopram, sertraline, and fluoxetine.[65]

SUMMARY

The evaluation of chest pain in active individuals is an essential skill for all who practice in the sports medicine realm. A systematic assessment is crucial because the differential diagnosis for an athlete suffering from chest pain is extensive, complicated, and frequently convoluted. True life-threatening emergencies must be expeditiously ruled out with particular attention paid to worrisome cardiac etiologies. A thorough history coupled with an understanding of the baseline fitness and physical demands of the athlete are generally sufficient to direct a focused physical exam and judicious use of ancillary testing. Once concerning cardiac pathologies are excluded, the practitioner should methodically assess for a wide range of non-cardiac conditions as detailed in this chapter. A meticulous and attentive approach by the healthcare team is the key to keeping the athlete safe, active, and performing at the highest level.

CLINICS CARE POINTS

- Chest pain accounts for 1% of all ambulatory primary care visits with 50% of these related to chest wall pain. If a workup is not completed in a deliberate and methodical fashion, it can prove to be inappropriately excessive, costly and anxiety provoking for patients.

- Traumatic rib fractures result from blunt thoracic trauma, most commonly occuring at the posterolateral angle of ribs four through nine. In the acute traumatic setting, concomitatnt or other resultant visceral injuries such as pneumothorax, hemothorax, or other organ lacerations (splenic, liver) should be ruled out.

- In the setting of high clinical suspicion for a pneumothorax, if a standard chest x-ray is negative, a chest CT scan is reasonable for definitive diagnosis.

- When considering a pulmonary embolus, the Wells clinical predicition rule is a validated tool to assess the likelihood. Classic electrocardiogram (EKG) findings associated with a pulmonary embolism is sinus tachycardia, an S wave in Lead I, and a Q wave and T wave inversion in Lead III ("S1Q3T3" pattern).

DISCLOSURE

The authors have nothing to disclose.

REFERENCES

1. Moran B, Bryan S, Farrar T, et al. Diagnostic evaluation of nontraumatic chest pain in athletes. Curr Sports Med Rep 2017;16(2):84–94.
2. McConaghy JR, Sharma M, Patel H. Acute chest pain in adults: outpatient evaluation. Am Fam Physician 2020;102(12):721–7.
3. Sik EC, Batt ME, Heslop LM. Atypical chest pain in athletes. Curr Sports Med Rep 2009;8(2):52–8.
4. Ayloo A, Cvengros T, Marella S. Evaluation and treatment of musculoskeletal chest pain. Prim Care 2013;40(4):863–87.
5. Disla E, Rhim HR, Reddy A, et al. Costochondritis. a prospective analysis in an emergency department setting. Arch Intern Med 1994;154(21):2466–9.
6. Gregory PL, Biswas AC, Batt ME. Musculoskeletal problems of the chest wall in athletes. Sports Med 2002;32(4):235–50.
7. Aspegren D, Hyde T, Miller M. Conservative treatment of a female collegiate volleyball player with costochondritis. J Manipulative Physiol Ther 2007;30(4):321–5.
8. Barranco-Trabi J, Mank V, Roberts J, et al. Atypical costochondritis: complete resolution of symptoms after rib manipulation and soft tissue mobilization. Cureus 2021;13(4):e14369. Published 2021 Apr 8.
9. Fam AG, Smythe HA. Musculoskeletal chest wall pain. CMAJ 1985;133(5): 379–89.
10. Oh JH, Park SB, Oh HC. 18F-FDG PET/CT and bone scintigraphy findings in tietze syndrome. Clin Nucl Med 2018;43(11):832–4.
11. Kamel M, Kotob H. Ultrasonographic assessment of local steroid injection in Tietze's syndrome. Br J Rheumatol 1997;36(5):547–50.
12. Yıldız ÖÖ, İnan K, Ağababaoğlu İ, et al. Local treatment of pain in Tietze syndrome: a single-center experience. Turk Gogus Kalp Damar Cerrahisi Derg 2021;29(2):239–47. Published 2021 Apr 26.
13. Chapman BC, Overbey DM, Tesfalidet F, et al. Clinical utility of chest computed tomography in patients with rib fractures CT chest and rib fractures. Arch Trauma Res 2016;5(4):e37070. Published 2016 Sep 13.
14. Dragoni S, Giombini A, Di Cesare A, et al. Stress fractures of the ribs in elite competitive rowers: a report of nine cases. Skeletal Radiol 2007;36(10):951–4.
15. Karlson KA. Thoracic region pain in athletes. Curr Sports Med Rep 2004; 3(1):53–7.
16. Coris EE, Higgins HW 2nd. First rib stress fractures in throwing athletes. Am J Sports Med 2005;33(9):1400–4.
17. Roston AT, Wilkinson M, Forster BB. Imaging of rib stress fractures in elite rowers: the promise of ultrasound? Br J Sports Med 2017;51(14):1093–7.
18. Warden SJ, Gutschlag FR, Wajswelner H, et al. Aetiology of rib stress fractures in rowers. Sports Med 2002;32(13):819–36.
19. Foley CM, Sugimoto D, Mooney DP, et al. Diagnosis and treatment of slipping rib syndrome. Clin J Sport Med 2019;29(1):18–23.
20. Udermann BE, Cavanaugh DG, Gibson MH, et al. Slipping rib syndrome in a collegiate swimmer: a case report. J Athl Train 2005;40(2):120–2.
21. Foley Davelaar CM. A clinical review of slipping rib syndrome. Curr Sports Med Rep 2021;20(3):164–8.

22. Deren ME, Behrens SB, Vopat BG, et al. Posterior sternoclavicular dislocations: a brief review and technique for closed management of a rare but serious injury. Orthop Rev (Pavia) 2014;6(1):5245. Published 2014 Mar 12.

23. Ferrera PC, Wheeling HM. Sternoclavicular joint injuries. Am J Emerg Med 2000; 18(1):58–61.

24. Gumbiner CH. Precordial catch syndrome. South Med J 2003;96(1):38–41.

25. Rowland TW. Evaluating cardiac symptoms in the athlete. Clin J Sport Med 2005; 15(6):417–20.

26. Carlsen KH, Anderson SD, Bjermer L, et al. Exercise-induce asthma, respiratory and allergic disorders in elite athletes: epidemiology, mechanisms and diagnosis: part I of the report from the joint task force of the european respiratory society (ERS) and the european academy of allergy and clinical immunology (EACCI) in cooperation with GA2LEN. Allergy 2008;63:387–403.

27. Wiens L, Sabath R, Ewing L, et al. Chest pain in otherwise healthy children and adolescents is frequently caused by exercise-induced asthma. Pediatrics 1992; 90:350–3.

28. Allen TW. Return to play following exercise-induced bronchoconstriction. Clin J Sport Med 2005;15:421–5.

29. Bonini M, Silvers W. Exercise-induced bronchoconstriction: background, prevalence, and sport considerations. Immunol Allergy Clin North Am 2018;38(2):205–14.

30. Orenstein D. Asthma and sports. In: BO O, editor. The child and adolescent athlete. Oxford: Blackwell Science; 1996. p. 433–54.

31. Sahn SA, Heffner JE. Spontaneous pneumothorax. N Engl J Med 2000;342: 868–74.

32. Cvengros R, Lazor J, Pneumothorax- a medical emergency. J Ath Train 1996; 31(2):167–8.

33. Collins JC, Levine G, Waxman K. Occult traumatic pneumothorax. Am Surg 1992; 58:743–6.

34. Eckstein M, Henderson S, Markochick V. In: Marx JA HR, Walls RM, editors. Thoracic trauma. Rosen's emergency medicine. St. Louis: Mosby; 2002. p. 381–414.

35. Sherwood DH, Gill BD, Schuessler BA, et al. Posttraumatic Pneumothorax in sport: a case report and management algorithm. Curr Sports Med Rep 2021; 20(3):133–6.

36. Brooks AP, Olson LK. Computed tomography of the chest in the trauma patient. Clin Radiol 1989;40:127–32.

37. Chan JS, Wee JC, Ponampalam R, et al. Pulmonary contusion and traumatic pneumatoceles in a platform diver with hemoptysis. J Emerg Med 2017;52(2): 205–7.

38. Tobushi T, Hosokawa K, Matsumoto K, et al. Exercise-induced pneumomediastinum. Int J Emerg Med 2015;8(1):43.

39. Moffatt K, Silberberg PJ, Gnarra DJ. Pulmonary embolism in an adolescent soccer player: a case report. Med Sci Sports Exerc 2007;39(6):899–902.

40. Freeman L. Pulmonary embolism in a 13-year-old boy. Pediatr Emerg Care 1999; 15:422–4.

41. Melanson SW, Silver B, Heller MB. Deep vein thrombosis, pulmonary embolism, and white clot syndrome. Am J Emerg Med 1996;14:558–60.

42. Rossdale M, Harvey JE. Diagnosing pulmonary embolism in primary care. BMJ 2003;327:393.

43. Van Ommen CH, Heyboer H, Groothoff JW, et al. Persistent tachypnea in children: keep pulmonary embolism in mind. J Pediatr Hematol Oncol 1998;20: 570–3.

44. Croyle PH, Place RA, Hilgenberg AD. Massive pulmonary embolism in a high school wrestler. JAMA 1979;241:827–8.

45. West J, Goodacre S, Sampson F. The value of clinical features in the diagnosis of acute pulmonary embolism: systematic review and meta-analysis. QJM 2007; 100(12):763–9.

46. Wells PS, Anderson DR, Rodger M, et al. Excluding pulmonary embolism at the bedside without diagnostic imaging: management of patients with suspected pulmonary embolism presenting to the emergency department by using a simple clinical model and d-dimer. Ann Intern Med 2001;135:98–107.

47. Stein PD, Sostman HD, Bounameaux H, et al. Challenges in the diagnosis of acute pulmonary embolism. Am J Med 2008;121:565–71.

48. Wells PS, Anderson DR, Rodger M, et al. Derivation of a simple clinical model to categorize patients probability of pulmonary embolism: increasing the models utility with the SimpliRED D-dimer. Thromb Haemost 2000;83:416–20.

49. Stein PD, Hull RD, Patel KC, et al. D-dimer for the exclusion of acute venous thrombosis and pulmonary embolism: a systematic review. Ann Intern Med 2004;140:589–602.

50. Perrier A, Roy PM, Aujesky D, et al. Diagnosing pulmonary embolism in outpatients with clinical assessment, D-dimer measurement, venous ultrasound, and helical computed tomography: a multicenter management study. Am J Med 2004;116:291–9.

51. Metlay JP, Kapoor WN, Fine MJ. Does this patient have community-acquired pneumonia? Diagnosing pneumonia by history and physical examination. JAMA 1997;278:1440–5.

52. Htun TP, Sun Y, Chua HL, et al. Clinical features for diagnosis of pneumonia among adults in primary care setting: a systematic and meta-review. Sci Rep 2019;9(1):7600.

53. Waterman JJ, Kapur R. Upper gastrointestinal issues in athletes. Curr Sports Med Rep 2012;11(2):99–104.

54. Rehrer NJ, Janssen GM, Brouns F, et al. Fluid intake and gastrointestinal problems in runners competing in a 25-km race and a marathon. Int J Sports Med 1989;10(Suppl 1):S22–5.

55. Peters HP, Bos M, Seebregts L, et al. Gastrointestinal symptoms in long-distance runners, cyclists, and triathletes: prevalence, medication, and etiology. Am J Gastroenterol 1999;94(6):1570–81.

56. Higgins JP, Babu K, Deuster PA, et al. Energy drinks: a contemporary issues paper. Curr Sports Med Rep 2018;17(2):65–72.

57. Cappelletti S, Piacentino D, Fineschi V, et al. Caffeine-related deaths: manner of deaths and categories at risk. Nutrients 2018;10(5):611.

58. Danielson ML, Bitsko RH, Ghandour RM, et al. Prevalence of parent-reported ADHD diagnosis and associated treatment among U.S. children and adolescents, 2016. J Clin Child Adolesc Psychol 2018;47(2):199–212.

59. Poysophon P, Rao AL. Neurocognitive deficits associated with ADHD in athletes: a systematic review. Sports Health 2018;10(4):317–26.

60. Chandler JV, Blair SN. The effect of amphetamines on selected physiological components related to athletic success. Med Sci Sports Exerc 1980;12(1):65–9.

61. Hickey G, Fricker P. Attention deficit hyperactivity disorder, CNS stimulants and sport. Sports Med 1999;27(1):11–21.

62. MacKnight J, Mistry D. Chest pain in the athlete: differential diagnosis, evaluation, and treatment. In: Lawless C, editor. Sports card ess. New York, NY: Springer; 2011.

63. American Psychiatric Association. Diagnostic and statistical manual of mental disorders (DSM-5®). Washington: American Psychiatric Pub; 2013.

64. Rice SM, Gwyther K, Santesteban-Echarri O, et al. Determinants of anxiety in elite athletes: a systematic review and meta-analysis. Br J Sports Med 2019;53(11): 722–30.

65. Reardon CL, Creado S. Psychiatric medication preferences of sports psychiatrists. Phys Sportsmed 2016;44(4):397–402.

Wearables in Sports Cardiology

David L. Beavers, MD, PhD*, Eugene H. Chung, MD, MSc

KEYWORDS

- Wearables • Digital health • Electrocardiogram • Smartphone • Athletes
- Sports cardiology

KEY POINTS

- With the rapid expansion and adoption of consumer health wearables, health-care providers are challenged with interpreting and incorporating patient-generated biometric data into daily clinical care.
- A growing body of research acknowledges the potential utility of wearables in the screening, diagnosis, and monitoring of cardiovascular health.
- The COVID-19 pandemic has necessitated the expansion of virtual health care, and wearables can provide a useful adjunct to providing effective remote clinical care.

INTRODUCTION

Over the last decade, there has been a meteoric increase in the availability and adoption of direct-to-consumer health-related wearable devices. Rapid advances in device processing speed and miniaturization of components have contributed to a proliferation of commercial biosensors. These advances coupled with the near-ubiquitous presence of smartphones and associated mobile wireless technology has empowered consumer's unparalleled access to biometric data. Cardiovascular-related health monitoring has been one of the fields most directly impacted by the proliferation of wearables. Medical providers are now challenged with not only how to respond to the data collected independently from their patient population but also how they might harness this technology to advance the care for their patients. In this article, we highlight emerging wearable technologies and their potential applications to the practice of sports cardiology.

The History of Cardiovascular Health Wearables

Perhaps the earliest origins of a health-related wearable can be traced back to the first pedometer developed in the 1700s. Although the exact origins are unclear, Thomas

Department of Internal Medicine, Division of Cardiac Electrophysiology, University of Michigan, 1500 East Medical Center Drive, SPC 5853, Ann Arbor, MI 48109-5853, USA
* Corresponding author.
E-mail address: dbea@med.umich.edu

Clin Sports Med 41 (2022) 405–423
https://doi.org/10.1016/j.csm.2022.02.004
0278-5919/22/© 2022 Elsevier Inc. All rights reserved.

Jefferson is often attributed with introducing the United States to a rudimentary mechanical device based on horological technology that could be used for counting steps. Norman Holter pioneered the use of backpack-based radio for the transmission of electrocardiographs in the 1940s. Oximetry was also developed in the 1940s and used to monitor the safety of pilots in World War II. However, commercial fingertip oximeters did not reach market until the 1990s.

The origins of the more modern concept of cardiovascular fitness and health trackers began with the development of microelectromechanical systems, or MEMS, in the 1960s. This technology allowed for the miniaturization of technology into self-contained devices. The Manpo-kei was an early modern wearable pedometer developed by Dr. Yoshiro Hatano in the 1960s centered on his concept of maintaining health with 10,000 steps per day.[1] The 1970s saw the initial development of wearable heart rate monitors with the first commercial wireless monitor released by Polar in 1982.

The subsequent significant strides in personal computing power including the invention of smartphones and Bluetooth technology brought exponential growth to the wearables sector in the late 1990s and early 2000s. Popular technology and apparel companies began to commercialize health-tracking devices. In 2006, Nike and Apple partnered to release a fitness tracking system that consisted of a wireless chip, a compatible Nike shoe, an iPod, and an iTunes and Nike + membership. FitBit successfully pioneered this emerging market sector with the release of their first fitness tracker in 2009. It clipped onto clothing and was capable of tracking steps, activity, sleep quality, and predict calorie expenditure. AliveCor, Inc, released the US Food and Drug Administration (FDA)-approved, smartphone-connected single-lead electrocardiogram (EKG) device in 2012. Many analysts declared 2013 "the year of the smartwatch" with new releases from companies such as Pebble, Samsung, Sony, and Qualcomm while many other large tech companies disclosed active development.[2] The Apple watch, currently the top-selling smartwatch, was released in 2015.

The most prevalent incorporated technologies include an accelerometer, gyroscope, and/or global positioning system (GPS) for activity tracking and photoplethysmography (PPG) or electrodes for the measurement of vitals including advanced heart rate monitoring, EKG, and pulse-oximetry. In addition to dedicated health wearable devices, multifunctional smart devices are also beginning to incorporate biosensors. There has been an expansion in the available form factors of wearables including smart rings, earrings, necklaces, eyewear, clothing, tattoos, and patches. Additionally, these devices have begun incorporating novel biosensors using technologies such as microfluidics, bioresponsive polymers, reverse iontophoresis, and various types of spectroscopy. Today, wearable technology is a multibillion-dollar industry with 1 in 5 Americans owning a health-tracking device.[3]

CLINICAL APPLICATIONS OF WEARABLES IN CARDIOLOGY

With wearable-generated health data becoming more prevalent, clinicians need to consider the scenarios where these data may prove useful in patient care.

Assessing Paroxysmal Symptoms

Cardiologists are often tasked with elucidating the cause of paroxysmal symptoms that do not manifest during routine clinical visits, resting diagnostics, or supervised stress testing. There has been a growth in the availability of prescribed ambulatory EKG and blood pressure monitors. However, these are generally limited to monitoring for several hours to a few weeks and may have a form factor that limits their use during everyday activities. Loop recorders are the gold standard for providing longer term ambulatory rhythm monitoring but are costly and can face delays in data transmission. So at present are largely reserved for use within high risk populations such as patients with cryptogenic stroke rather than routine screening, but there may a role for them in cases of infrequent but potentially concerning symptoms not easily captured on a routine EKG monitor.[4] Consumer health wearables provide the potential for longer term monitoring and correlation of symptoms with biometric data.

Palpitations and Cardiac Arrhythmia Screening

Palpitations are a common symptom often secondary to a noncardiac cause such as stress, anxiety, strenuous exercise, stimulant medications or substances including alcohol, or underlying endocrinopathy. However, they may also be attributable to cardiac arrhythmias including premature atrial or ventricular contractions, atrial fibrillation or flutter, supraventricular tachycardia, or ventricular tachycardia. Further, these arrhythmias may be a manifestation of underlying structural heart disease. Wearable devices offer a potentially useful screening tool to identify patients who have an undiagnosed cardiac arrhythmia and have been reported to be an acceptable or preferable approach compared with conventional cardiac monitoring even among older populations.[5–7] EKG-based devices typically provide a single-lead tracing congruent to lead I, although several studies have described techniques to serially acquire additional vectors to simulate multiple leads.[8,9] PPG-based devices do not measure cardiac electrical activity directly. They use light to detect volumetric changes in microvasculature, and extrapolate peaks in volume change to correlate with R waves, or ventricular contraction (**Fig. 1**).

Arrhythmia detection and discrimination by wearables has been the focus of numerous studies, resulting in recent guidelines acknowledging the potential utility of these devices in arrhythmia management.[10] To date, the use of wearables in the screening for arrhythmias has largely focused on the detection of atrial fibrillation given its prevalence and associated morbidity. Within higher risk, asymptomatic, older populations, several prospective studies have shown an increased incidence of atrial fibrillation detection using smart phone-based single-lead EKG compared with routine care.[5,11] The Apple Heart study included a larger, more diverse asymptomatic population and detected a 0.5% prevalence of suspected atrial fibrillation. Again, the highest incidence of irregular pulse notification was within participants aged more than 65 years (3.1%), whereas only 0.16% of those aged 22 to 40 years received an irregular pulse alert. Adherence to confirmatory follow-up protocols was limited, but the positive predictive value of an individual irregular tachogram was 71% and 84% for irregular pulse notification triggered by the detection of 4 additional serial irregular tachograms.[12] The Huawei Heart Study was a similar, large-scale PPG-based wristband screening study within a younger population in China demonstrating a 0.2% prevalence of suspected atrial fibrillation. Among those that provided follow-up, PPG signals demonstrated a positive predictive value of 91.6%.[13] A meta-analysis of smartphone PPG-based applications showed a high sensitivity (94.2%) and specificity (95.8%) for the detection of asymptomatic atrial fibrillation. Modeling within the higher risk, older subgroup showed a negative predictive value of 99.9% but only a 19.3% positive predictive value.[14] Mobile EKG devices have demonstrated similarly high levels of sensitivity and specificity in patients with known atrial fibrillation admitted for antiarrhythmic drug loading or postablation monitoring.[15,16] Advances in software-based diagnostic algorithms including the incorporation of machine learning techniques offer the promise of improved sensitivity and specificity for rhythm discrimination.[17,18]

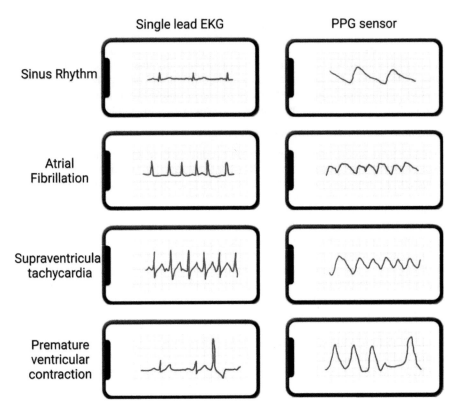

Fig. 1. Heart rhythm waveforms obtained from mobile electrode-based EKG and PPG-based sensors. Images not drawn to scale.

Although the utility of wearables as a screening and monitoring tool has been more thoroughly investigated, fewer studies have assessed their use as an ambulatory diagnostic device in symptomatic patients. Additionally, there is limited data on the use of wearables to detect arrhythmias aside from atrial fibrillation. Small studies have demonstrated the ability of PPG-based sensors to identify episodes of tachycardia and bradycardia, and distinguish atrial fibrillation from other arrhythmias including atrial flutter, atrial tachycardia, and premature contractions although with lower degrees of accuracy.[19–22] The AliveCor Kardia device was found to be noninferior to an external loop recorder in the diagnostic evaluation of patients with palpitations.[23] Common wearables demonstrate variable accuracy in the detection of sudden heart rate increases in paroxysmal supraventricular tachycardia (SVT), particularly if it is short-lived.[24] Given that rhythm-tracking devices often incorporate an accelerometer, algorithms exist to detect heart rates that are incongruent to the level of activity as a potential marker of arrhythmia. One prospective, randomized controlled trial compared the use of a smartphone-based EKG device to standard care in the 90-day follow-up of patients who presented to the emergency department with palpitations and no obvious cause at the initial evaluation. The use of the smartphone device resulted in the symptomatic rhythm detection in 55.6% of patients within an average of 9.5 days. Standard care resulted in the symptomatic rhythm detection in only 9.5% of patients within an average of 42.9 days. Although the most symptomatic events correlated with benign causes such as sinus rhythm, sinus tachycardia, or infrequent ectopy, a symptomatic arrhythmia was detected in 8.9% of patients in the intervention group compared with just 0.9% in the control group.[25] A small case series used mobile single-lead EKG tracings to confirm the absence of dangerous arrhythmia in real-time in college athletes complaining of palpitations during exercise.[26] The wider spread implementation of rhythm monitoring in athletes is limited by the variable accuracy of devices based on the nature and intensity of activity.[27,28] Advances in device software including integrating accelerometer data to help filter motion and noise artifact and improved multistep rhythm discrimination algorithms show promise in improving the integrity of diagnosis during exercise.[21] Currently, confirmatory testing of wearable diagnostic data is performed at the discretion of the clinical provider and will remain necessary until more uniformly robust data acquisition is achievable with consumer-grade devices. The utility of wearables in the clinical management of arrhythmias is being acknowledged by professional societies, such as the Heart Rhythm Society, which recently initiated a case-based series highlighting current technologies and shortcomings. This will be serially updated as new digital health technology emerges.[29]

Dyspnea and Chest Pain

The ambulatory assessment of other paroxysmal symptoms such as shortness of breath and chest discomfort is an emerging interest in the application of wearables. Similar to palpitations, these symptoms may be attributable to any number of benign causes, but the detection of symptoms related to a change in cardiovascular hemodynamics has potentially significant clinical implications. Supervised stress testing remains the gold standard for evaluation of these symptoms, although wearables have the potential to provide adjunctive assessment. Aside from the detection of arrhythmias and simple measurement of vitals, several wearable-based indices may provide insight into the cause of these symptoms including cardiopulmonary fitness, intravascular congestion, cardiac output, and ischemia.

Several groups have created multiparameter wearable-based systems to characterize cardiorespiratory fitness and hemodynamic monitoring. One system incorporating measurement of EKG, SpO_2, and heart rate was implemented in the setting of a 6-minute walk test but could have expanded use to characterize maximal aerobic power.[30] A wearable system incorporating ballistocardiogram, seismocardiogram, EKG, and movement detection has been used to monitor for changes in cardiac output and contractility.[31] The incorporation of small form-factor or cuffless blood pressure monitoring into wearables is an ongoing effort. Different methods including traditional oscillometric measurement, radial arterial wall applanation, PPG, pulse-transit time, a piezoelectric-based system, and a flexible pressure sensor incorporating microfluidics have all been proposed as techniques.[32,33] Unfortunately, limitations to their widespread incorporation include form-factor, sensitivity to motion or noise artifact, reliable accuracy compared with reference devices, and validation outside of controlled environment settings. Further hemodynamic characterization with thoracic bioimpedance and remote dielectric sensing technology has been proposed as noninvasive measures of volume status and pulmonary congestion.[34,35] However, changes in thoracic impedance is prone to interference from other noncardiac conditions. These technologies have been largely characterized within the monitoring of heart failure patients, and their utility in monitoring hemodynamic status in other populations is unproven.

Even within athletic populations, wearables could enhance the capability of diagnosing ischemic heart disease. Several feasibility studies have assessed the use of wearables or mobile technology in the detection of myocardial infarction.[36] The ST LEUIS trial compared a smartphone-based device to recreate a multiple lead EKG to standard 12-lead EKG in the diagnosis of ST elevation myocardial infarction or left bundle block. The signal average-derived smartphone EKG demonstrated sensitivity, specificity, and positive and negative predictive value of 89%, 84%, 70%, and 95%, respectively. A two-person case series reported the use of the Apple watch applied to multiple sites to simulate a multilead EKG for the detection of ST elevation.[37] With future refinement of these technologies, it is conceivable that wearables may provide early or subclinical detection of myocardial ischemia and prompt users to seek appropriate care.

Clearance to Play

An additional clinical application of wearables is in the assessment of clearance to play. Participation in physical activity for patients with a known underlying condition or returning to play postinjury is a shared decision-making process. There is widespread interest in developing improved risk stratification tools to inform guidelines to allow meaningful return to participation while mitigating risk for significant morbidity or mortality. Wearables have provided promise as a tool to help monitor athletes activity-associated risk and recovery progress. Obtaining baseline and routine biometric data within athletes can facilitate personalized, longitudinal assessment and identify deviations that may indicate injury or disease. There has been a recent shift in promoting return-to-play among individuals with inherited cardiac disease.[31,38,39] In higher risk patients such as those with long QT syndrome, wearable remote monitoring of QT interval and heart rhythm could be a feasible strategy to assess for arrhythmogenic risk.[40] Similarly, patients with hypertrophic cardiomyopathy could undergo rhythm, heart rate, and hemodynamic monitoring to provide biofeedback to promote safe levels of activity. Wearables have been implemented to monitor global movement, joint-specific movement and strain, assess athletic technique, and measure cardiovascular workload in efforts to prevent injury.[41] Wearables can be used to measure internal and external workloads to predict injury risk and monitor the acute-to-chronic workload ratio to promote safe, gradual return-to-play.[42] In addressing more subtle sequelae of injury in the consideration of return-to-play, wearables can detect changes in heart rate variability, which has been linked to certain diseased states and environmental stress.[43,44] Using this principle, a case report described a decrease in heart rate variability from baseline during low level activity within a concussed athlete, which normalized with injury recovery and return-to-play.[45] These changes have been shown to persist past the symptomatic phase of concussion, although the implications on safe return-to-play remain uncertain.[46] Future research is needed to understand what biosensor data is the most important to monitor during rehabilitation and reengagement with activity to prevent inappropriate clearance to return to competition.

Although the use of diagnostics in these at-risk populations is more clearly established, their use in general preparticipation screening is unclear. Within the United States, professional societal guidelines do not recommend routine diagnostic testing because a part of an athlete's preparticipation evaluation given lack of proven benefit, cost-effectiveness, and implications of false-positive screening. Rather, testing should only be guided by clinical concerns that arise from thorough reviews of personal and family histories and physical examination. In the emerging era of wearables widely adopted by athletes, the utility and logistics of incorporating preexisting patient-generated biometric data into screening evaluations remain unclear. Reviewing a preexisting log of cardiovascular activity, heart rate and rhythm trends, and other logged data could conceivably provide insight into the future risk of athletic participation without the extraneous use of health-care resources. As an example of potential screening utility, one group developed a machine learning algorithm that used PPG biosensor data to detect obstructive hypertrophic cardiomyopathy with 98% accuracy.[47] Although preparticipation EKG screening is not universally performed, mobile EKGs could provide either baseline data or near real-time rhythm assessment at the time of participation. The 1-lead Kardia mobile EKG device has been shown to accurately measure baseline rhythm and intervals compared with standard 12-lead EKG. More recently, the newer 6-lead version of the Kardia mobile EKG device demonstrated even greater correlation with 12-lead EKG. The EKG intervals measured on the mobile EKG were slightly shorter but unlikely to interfere with screening interpretation.[48] Currently, no large-scale data exist that examine the application or benefit of wearables within routine preparticipation screening.

Physical Training and Wellness Support

Aside from facilitating decisions for return-to-play, wearables can provide detailed insight into the global cardiovascular wellness and fitness of athletes and patients looking to mitigate cardiovascular risk. Algorithms to estimate cardiorespiratory fitness based on data collected from wearables has shown promise in correlating with gold standard oxygen consumption testing.[49]

Prescribed independent activity goals are an important aspect of training for athletes as well as the casual patient seeking improved cardiovascular health. Remote monitoring of training activity and the opportunity to provide regular virtual feedback may promote adherence to and efficacy of training programs.[2] Garments with multiple integrated biosensors such as Hexoskin can provide global assessment of cardiorespiratory function during activity.[50] Assessment of these data could feasibly facilitate meaningful feedback and reinforcement in training. Multiple studies have shown that wearables with or without additional feedback approaches can promote increased physical activity and weight loss within the general population. However, sustained results at longer term follow-up have been less clearly demonstrated due to problematic dropout rates.[51] Personalized metrics, such as the personal activity intelligence algorithm, which incorporates activity duration and intensity based on wearable heart rate sensors, have been shown to promote activity and improve cardiovascular outcomes.[52] Metrics such as these can be incorporated into a wearable's data output providing a trackable metric. Emerging wearables afford the opportunity to measure metabolic response to exercise aside from simply monitoring vitals. Several wearable devices using near-infrared light-emitting diode (LED) technology can reliably measure skeletal muscle oxygenation and lactate levels during exertion.[53,54] Wearables that measure other analytes such as the pH or glucose levels in sweat are being developed to measure metabolic health, hydration, and workload capacity.[42] The incorporation of more diverse biometric data can guide further activity recommendations to avoid excessive fatigue, potential injury risk, and monitor for cardiovascular fitness progress.

Stress has long been appreciated as a significant contributor to both psychological and physical disease affecting social interaction and physical performance.[55] However, its quantification and mechanism of impact has been elusive due to its ambiguous definition, its heterogeneous manifestation, and difficulty in real-time assessment. Wearable technology has provided new opportunities in the quantification of stress with hopes of mitigating its long-term contribution to chronic disease. Wearables can provide longitudinal measurement of variables that can indicate increased levels of stress and heightened autonomic activity such as resting heart rate, heart rate variability, body temperature, blood pressure, electrodermal activity, and sleep patterns. Incorporating these data with subjective input, changes in movement or location patterns, and frequency of social media use, calls, or texts have shown correlation with perceived stress.[56–58] Additional biosensors incorporating the detection of cortisol or other inflammatory markers are also under development.[59] These algorithms can improve awareness of high stress states and provide a tool to enable self-guided or health-care-based intervention. Longer term, these wearable applications may help provide insight into the correlation between perceived stress, acute stress response, long-term stress response, and the development of chronic disease.[60]

Many wearables such as the Oura ring have begun to incorporate and emphasize measures of sleep quality, which may have implications on athletic performance or cardiovascular health.[61] PPG devices with movement monitoring have been shown to be able to detect sleep stages with a reasonable degree of accuracy.[62,63] These data could be used to monitor for poor sleep hygiene and potential intervention. The synchronization of wearable sleep data with an app-based cognitive behavioral therapy intervention proved feasible in the treatment of insomnia.[64] The WHOOP band incorporates an algorithm based on activity duration and physiologic markers such as heart rate variability (HRV) to recommend an estimate of the amount of sleep required for adequate recovery.[65] Finally, the prevalence of sleep apnea is increasing and is a known risk factor for progressive cardiovascular disease. The use of remote monitoring technology and wearables poses an attractive method to assess sleep-disordered breathing. The use of PPG as well as heart rate variability has shown to correlate well with polysomnography in the identification of sleep apnea.[66,67] These same remote monitoring technologies can then be applied to assess compliance and improvement with the initiation of noninvasive positive pressure ventilation. These technologies taken together can provide a holistic assessment of factors that contribute to cardiovascular health.

CARDIAC WEARABLES IN THE COVID-19 ERA

The COVID-19 pandemic brought seismic changes to the health-care industry. Although the full scope and duration of these changes is not yet realized, it is safe to assume that a portion of the COVID-era paradigm shifts will affect clinical care into the future.

The Emergence of Telemedicine

One of the most prevalent changes has been the proliferation of virtual medicine. Although the concept of virtual or telemedicine is not new, many health-care systems had been slow to widely adopt its routine use into clinical care. The need for social distancing measures created unprecedented demand for the use of telehealth services.[68] This accelerated the development of virtual clinical infrastructure to conduct remote health care. Health-care systems were tasked with expanding investment in hardware, software, staff training, and clinical workflow algorithms to promote access to remote care. Further, legal constraints, coverage, and reimbursement models for virtual visits were clarified and expanded, paving the way to continue to incorporate this option for clinical care in the future. Within cardiovascular medicine, remote monitoring of cardiovascular implantable electronic devices has been widely adopted and is a pioneering effort in the virtual delivery of longitudinal care.[69] Even before the COVID 19 pandemic, the benefits of telemedicine for cardiovascular disease had been described. These include expanding access to specialty care, high patient satisfaction, and improved communication including patient disease education.[70] Additionally, improved patient outcomes including reduced hospitalization and decreased morbidity have been demonstrated with remote cardiac device monitoring and telehealth management programs for chronic conditions such as congestive heart failure.[69,71] The incorporation of wearable devices and smart technology can serve to expand the utility of telemedicine as a way to provide objective data in the monitoring of cardiovascular disease.[72] For example, with limited inpatient resources during the pandemic, elective admissions such as antiarrhythmic drug loading face potential significant delays. A recent study demonstrated the feasibility of using a consumer EKG device for remote QT-interval monitoring.[73] The continuous, longitudinal measurement of wearable biometric data can provide a personalized model of baseline patient health. These data have also demonstrated correlation with clinical laboratory measurements.[74] Thus, deviations from these baseline values could be used as a marker for disease progression and the need for further assessment.

The Use of Wearables in Detecting Acute Illness

Aside from facilitating monitoring chronic diseases, wearables have also been proposed as a tool for the diagnosis of acute illness. Disturbances in variables such as resting heart rate, temperature, activity level, and sleep that are monitored continuously by wearables correlate with acute illness such as a viral infection.[75] Within the context of COVID 19, several studies validated the correlation between biometric disturbances and symptomatic infectious illness.[76–78] Incorporating wearable device data in addition to presence/absence of fever and reported symptoms had a stronger correlation to COVID 19 testing result than either variable alone. This could prove helpful in resource utilization and identifying patients appropriate for testing. It may also facilitate the identification of presymptomatic infectious individuals, which would be a crucial development in curbing disease transmission. Further, as more data become available, there is the potential to correlate degree or pattern of disturbances in biometrics to disease severity and identify individuals at high risk for severe disease. One feasibility study demonstrated the feasibility of using machine-learning algorithms on data from wearables to not only detect viral infection but also to predict the severity of illness.[79] There are several ongoing efforts to collect large-scale, anonymized wearable device data to track illness trends on a population-based level in near real-time. Should these prove fruitful, it would not only have implications in tracking disease statistics but also facilitate the development and accuracy of predictive models to inform local infection prevention policies. These concepts would likely be expandable to application beyond the current COVID 19 pandemic.

Wearables in COVID-19 Recovery

As the COVID-19 pandemic has progressed, outside of the context of acute critical illness, postinfectious sequelae have emerged as a significant contribution to COVID-19-associated morbidity.[80] Many patients have been found to have evidence of prolonged pulmonary inflammation. COVID long-haulers or post-COVID syndrome has been characterized with protracted symptoms of fatigue, "brain fog," disturbed sleep patterns, and other signs and symptoms suggestive of autonomic dysfunction such as postural orthostatic tachycardia. Neuropsychiatric symptoms have also been described including headache, prolonged alteration in sense of taste and smell, and increased prevalence of psychiatric illness. Cardiovascular manifestations including myocarditis, arrhythmias, and elevated risk for thromboembolic disease have been recognized, including in those who only had mild acute illness. Comparing COVID-positive and COVID-negative patients presenting with viral respiratory illness symptoms, long-term wearable device data showed COVID-19 patients are at risk for prolonged physiologic disturbance in both sleep and resting heart rate. COVID-

19 patients had an initial, transient bradycardia followed by an elevated resting heart rate lasting on average 2 to 3 months.[81] This increases the possibility of remote monitoring, symptom inventory, and follow-up of patients who are at risk for post-COVID complications. Further, data that can feasibly be detected by wearables can inform decision-making for post-COVID return-to-play.[82]

CHALLENGES

Although there are many promising aspects of the rise of consumer wearables in the delivery of cardiovascular care and beyond, their rapid early adoption poses challenges for care providers.

Regulation, Oversight of Consumer Wearables

Currently, the development and marketing of commercial wearables is far outpacing the capacity for independent reliability assessment, validation of devices, and the development of rigorous regulatory oversight. Historically, medical-grade sensors have been regulated by FDA, with most wearables classified as class 1 or 2 noninvasive medical devices. The FDA issued a digital health innovation action plan in 2017 to address the regulation of software as a medical device and most recently launched the Digital Health Center of Excellence as a resource for digital health policy. To date, only a small percentage of wearable devices have obtained FDA clearance. Consumer wearable FDA clearance has largely relied on the accelerated 501(k) pathway that obtains clearance by providing evidence of substantial similarity to a predicate device. AliveCor, Inc, has been a pioneer in obtaining this distinction for their devices. The Kardia 1-lead mobile EKG became the first FDA-cleared Apple Watch medical device accessory when it was approved for the detection of atrial fibrillation. This has led to other companies such as Apple, Fitbit, and Withings to obtain similar distinction. More recently, AliveCor obtained FDA-clearance for their 6-lead mobile EKG and advanced rhythm assessment algorithms for the detection of premature atrial contractions (PACs), premature ventricular contractions (PVCs), and corrected QT (QTc) interval measurement.[83] With the emergence of novel sensors that are not preexisting in clinical care, de novo FDA clearance poses a time-consuming and costly hurdle that may not align with entrepreneurial goals. However, without a designation attesting to the quality of the health data collected, their clinical utility for patient care is uncertain.

Reliability and Actionable Approach of Consumer Wearable Data

For all of the proposed applications of wearables in cardiovascular care, their accuracy and precision are critical to meaningfully inform clinical decision-making. Most devices are calibrated under limited, strictly controlled conditions. However, during real-life activities, multiple studies have demonstrated activity and heart rate monitors can have highly variable performance compared with gold standards.[28,84] Currently, there are no universal standards for an acceptable range of variability compared with reference devices. Further, artificial intelligence (AI)-derived alerts or findings are often considered a "black box" and may be difficult for clinicians to reliably interpret. In the case of using wearables as a screening tool, especially at a large population-base level, one must consider the risk and implications of false-positives and false-negatives. False-positives can lead to anxiety and unnecessary testing or procedures. False-negatives can lead to inappropriate reassurance, delayed diagnosis, and increased risk for morbidity. Even when accurate, the implications of the subclinical detection of abnormalities and whether further investigation is warranted may be unknown. For example, the studies showing increased detection of subclinical atrial fibrillation using wearable devices have yet to demonstrate an improvement in clinical outcomes including decreased stroke or hospitalization. Ultimately, there is limited data regarding the utility and cost-benefit of using wearables to modify health outcomes.

Data Storage, Processing, and Sharing

Similar to the era of big data collection ushered in by the advances in genomics a few decades ago, the proliferation of wearables is generating endless amounts of data that may facilitate remote monitoring and care in near real-time. However, there is a lag in the development of protocols to share, process, review, and create a meaningful actionable plan in response to these data.[85] The onus of processing such large data sets cannot feasibly fall solely on medical providers and will likely rely heavily on consumer-grade software. Health-care systems need to create solutions to be able to interface with these data and incorporate it into patient's medical records. Additionally, these large, population-level data sets provide promising opportunities for clinical research. With such a large array of new wearable technologies, institutional and legal policies will need to be updated to ensure the integrity of patient data storage, use, and privacy.

Medico-legal Responsibility

Beyond the current gaps in incorporating patient-generated wearable data into clinical practice, current legal and clinical guidelines do not specifically address the handling of consumer wearable data. The Health Insurance Portability and Accountability Act of 1996 and the Health Information Technology for Economic and Clinical Health Act of 2009 attempt to outline guidelines for the secure and private handling of patient information and expansion of electronic health records. However, as the consumer health data market has continued to grow, these policies require updating to account for the handling of data generated outside of the context of a health-care system. It is often unclear whether the consumer or the manufacturer owns the data collected by wearables. If an abnormality is detected, is it the medico-legal responsibility of the physician, manufacturer, or patient to acknowledge and follow-up these data? What entities can have access to consumer wearable data and how can these data be used? What are the regulations for secure data handling, storage, and disclosure of breaches that should be required of such a heterogeneous group of companies? These are just a handful of the complex considerations that will need to be addressed before the widespread adoption of consumer wearables as a health information-generating device.

Health-care Equity

Consumer health wearables have a wide price range but remain a luxury item more prevalently adopted among higher income individuals. Should wearables become more integrated into health-care delivery, it poses the risk of becoming a new disparity. Additionally, the clinical infrastructure needed to incorporate telehealth and virtual data into practice may be cost-prohibitive for rural or safety-net health-care systems. The adoption of reimbursement policies by health insurance, Medicare, and Medicaid would likely be necessary to bridge this gap. Beyond potential financial barriers, the available wearable technology needs to be validated in heterogeneous populations. As an example, a recent study showed that pulse oximetry, a commonplace diagnostic tool in clinical medicine, had variable accuracy based on skin tone.[86] Wrist-worn devices have also shown greater error rates in individuals with darker skin tone.[87] Because

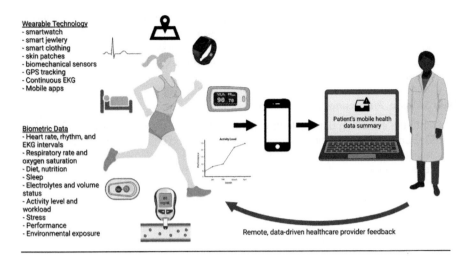

Fig. 2. Depiction of possible future health-care model with patients generating multifaceted biometric data using multiple wearable health devices. These data are stored and organized within the patient's connected smartphone and subsequently forwarded to a healthcare provider who is able to provide targeted feedback and/or implement therapeutic interventions.

wearable device recommendations begin to be included in clinical guidelines, it will be critical to ensure standards of care are accessible to all populations.

FUTURE DIRECTIONS

There are ongoing efforts to address current wearable shortcomings and to expand their capabilities both in obtaining new biometric data as well as interpreting that data to identify healthy and diseased states.

One of the most rapidly developing areas within wearables is a focus on software development to improve the accuracy and feedback of the data collected. By incorporating machine-learning algorithms, wearables have the potential to accommodate for the heterogeneity of input from a diverse population.[17] EKG-based AI algorithms have shown strong concordance in the detection of left ventricular systolic dysfunction, myocardial ischemia, and hypertrophic cardiomyopathy (HCM).[88-90] This could be used as a screening tool to identify patients with cardiovascular diseases associated with significant morbidity and mortality. However, these have been developed with traditional 12-lead EKGs. Their use with wearable EKG monitors would either require adaptation to current single-lead EKGs or to develop wearables that generate additional vectors. Recent research has demonstrated the feasibility of using AI to accurately monitor the QTc interval on a mobile EKG.[91] AI has also been proposed to uncover novel biomarkers including vocal changes in decompensated cardiovascular disease or remote audible detection of agonal breathing and possible integration with emergency notification.[92,93] Incorporating ambulatory wearable health data along with AI and deep-learning algorithms into electronic health records could allow for objective patient surveillance, early identification of disease or decompensation, and the potential avoidance of hospitalization.

New biosensors are focused on expanding the array of measurable biometric data and improving form-factor to allow for use within a dynamic range of activities while minimizing motion and noise artifact. Several emerging technologies were highlighted above. Additionally, an area that is rapidly expanding is the development of wearable sensors to measure the real-time biochemical profile in athletes.[94,95] These sensors have used microfluidics, fluorometric assays, iontophoresis, and electrochemical measurements to analyze saliva and sweat with the goal of optimizing hydration, nutrition, lactate threshold, and thus performance. Electrodermal activity sensors are becoming more prevalent as a measure of autonomic activity as well as a possible indicator of hydration. Flexible patches and tattoos that conform to skin contours are being developed to overcome issues with wearable use during activity and susceptibility to motion and noise artifact.[96] Finally, exposure to harmful environmental factors such as air pollution during training pose increased cardiovascular risk. Future wearable devices may consider environmental sampling to guide safe venue selection for activities.[97] Many more technologies have been developed at the engineering and basic science level but remain untested within clinically relevant systems (**Fig. 2**).

SUMMARY

Health-related wearable technologies are rapidly evolving. Although they pose many exciting possibilities in cardiovascular care, they also pose several uncertainties about their utility and incorporation into clinical practice. Regulatory agencies and guideline experts have recognized the need for ongoing updates to policies to help overcome these obstacles. As clinicians, it is critical to understand the data afforded by these devices, learn to address patient concerns related to these data, and improve preventative care.

CLINICS CARE POINTS

- Wearable-based biofeedback to quantify performance, characterize movement, prevent injuries, and promote short-term weight loss has shown benefit compared with traditional training.
- The AliveCor mobile EKG devices are among the most clinically validated consumer wearables and have the broadest FDA clearance for rhythm discrimination.
- Atrial fibrillation discrimination is a well-studied application of wearables, and an expanding number of devices have obtained FDA clearance to perform this function.
- The utility of wearables in screening large-scale populations for cardiovascular disease remains uncertain.
- The expansion of available wearables has outpaced the development of regulation, rigorous clinical testing, adoption into clinical guidelines, integration into medical records, and mechanisms of reimbursement.

DISCLOSURE

The authors have nothing to disclose.

REFERENCES

1. Bassett DR, Toth LP, LaMunion SR, et al. Step Counting: A Review of Measurement Considerations and Health-Related Applications. Sport Med 2017;47(7): 1303–15.
2. Henriksen A, Mikalsen MH, Woldaregay AZ, et al. Using fitness trackers and smartwatches to measure physical activity in research: Analysis of consumer

wrist-worn wearables. J Med Internet Res 2018;20(3). https://doi.org/10.2196/jmir.9157.

3. Dagher L, Shi H, Zhao Y, et al. Wearables in cardiology: Here to stay. Hear Rhythm 2020;17(5):889–95.

4. Lee R, Mittal S. Utility and limitations of long-term monitoring of atrial fibrillation using an implantable loop recorder. Hear Rhythm 2018;15(2):287–95.

5. Halcox JPJ, Wareham K, Cardew A, et al. Assessment of remote heart rhythm sampling using the AliveCor heart monitor to screen for atrial fibrillation the REHEARSE-AF study. Circulation 2017;136(19):1784–94.

6. Rajakariar K, Koshy A, Sajeev J, et al. Increased Preference of Wearable Devices Compared with Conventional Cardiac Monitoring. Hear Lung Circ 2018;27:S170.

7. Kekade S, Hseieh CH, Islam MM, et al. The usefulness and actual use of wearable devices among the elderly population. Comput Methods Programs Biomed 2018;153:137–59.

8. Muhlestein JB, Anderson JL, Bethea CF, et al. Feasibility of combining serial smartphone single-lead electrocardiograms for the diagnosis of ST-elevation myocardial infarction: Smartphone ECG for STEMI Diagnosis. Am Heart J 2020; 221:125–35.

9. Samol A, Bischof K, Luani B, et al. Single-Lead ECG Recordings Including Einthoven and Wilson Leads by a Smartwatch: A New Era of Patient Directed Early ECG Differential Diagnosis of Cardiac Diseases? Sensors (Basel) 2019;19(20). https://doi.org/10.3390/s19204377.

10. Nielsen JC, Lin YJ, de Oliveira Figueiredo MJ, et al. European Heart Rhythm Association (EHRA)/Heart Rhythm Society (HRS)/Asia Pacific Heart Rhythm Society (APHRS)/Latin American Heart Rhythm Society (LAHRS) expert consensus on risk assessment in cardiac arrhythmias: Use the right tool for the right outcome. Europace 2020;22(8):1147–8.

11. Svennberg E, Engdahl J, Al-Khalili F, et al. Mass screening for untreated atrial fibrillation the STROKESTOP study. Circulation 2015;131(25):2176–84.

12. Perez MV, Mahaffey KW, Hedlin H, et al. Large-Scale Assessment of a Smartwatch to Identify Atrial Fibrillation. N Engl J Med 2019;381(20):1909–17.

13. Guo Y, Wang H, Zhang H, et al. Mobile Photoplethysmographic Technology to Detect Atrial Fibrillation. J Am Coll Cardiol 2019;74(19):2365–75.

14. O'Sullivan JW, Grigg S, Crawford W, et al. Accuracy of Smartphone Camera Applications for Detecting Atrial Fibrillation: A Systematic Review and Meta-analysis. JAMA Netw Open 2020;3(4):e202064. https://doi.org/10.1001/jamanetworkopen.2020.2064.

15. William AD, Kanbour M, Callahan T, et al. Assessing the accuracy of an automated atrial fibrillation detection algorithm using smartphone technology: The iREAD Study. Hear Rhythm 2018;15(10):1561–5.

16. Tarakji KG, Wazni OM, Callahan T, et al. Using a novel wireless system for monitoring patients after the atrial fibrillation ablation procedure: The iTransmit study. Hear Rhythm 2015;12(3):554–9.

17. Lown M, Brown M, Brown C, et al. Machine learning detection of atrial fibrillation using wearable technology. PLoS One 2020;15(1):1–9.

18. Nemati S, Ghassemi MM, Ambai V, et al. Monitoring and detecting atrial fibrillation using wearable technology. Proc Annu Int Conf IEEE Eng Med Biol Soc EMBS 2016;3394–7.

19. Paliakaitė B, Petrėnas A, Sološenko A, et al. Modeling of artifacts in the wrist photoplethysmogram: Application to the detection of life-threatening arrhythmias.

Biomed Signal Process Control 2021;66(February). https://doi.org/10.1016/j.bspc.2021.102421.

20. Corino VDA, Laureanti R, Ferranti L, et al. Detection of atrial fibrillation episodes using a wristband device. Physiol Meas 2017;38(5):787–99.

21. Bashar SK, Han D, Hajeb-Mohammadalipour S, et al. Atrial Fibrillation Detection from Wrist Photoplethysmography Signals Using Smartwatches. Sci Rep 2019;9(1):1–10.

22. McMANUS DD, Chong JW, Soni A, et al. PULSE-SMART: Pulse-Based Arrhythmia Discrimination Using a Novel Smartphone Application. J Cardiovasc Electrophysiol 2016;27(1):51–7.

23. Pevnick JM, Birkeland K, Zimmer R, et al. Wearable technology for cardiology: An update and framework for the future. Trends Cardiovasc Med 2018;28(2):144–50.

24. Sequeira N, D'Souza D, Angaran P, et al. Common wearable devices demonstrate variable accuracy in measuring heart rate during supraventricular tachycardia. Hear Rhythm 2020;17(5):854–9.

25. Reed MJ, Grubb NR, Lang CC, et al. Multi-centre Randomised Controlled Trial of a Smartphone-based Event Recorder Alongside Standard Care Versus Standard Care for Patients Presenting to the Emergency Department with Palpitations and Pre-syncope: The IPED (Investigation of Palpitations in th. EClinicalMedicine 2019;8:37–46.

26. Peritz DC, Howard A, Ciocca M, et al. Smartphone ECG AIDS real time diagnosis of palpitations in the competitive college athlete. J Electrocardiol 2015;48(5):896–9.

27. Gillinov S, Etiwy M, Wang R, et al. Variable accuracy of wearable heart rate monitors during aerobic exercise. Med Sci Sports Exerc 2017;49(8):1697–703.

28. Stahl SE, An H-S, Dinkel DM, et al. How accurate are the wrist-based heart rate monitors during walking and running activities? Are they accurate enough? BMJ Open Sport Exerc Med 2016;2(1):e000106. https://doi.org/10.1136/bmjsem-2015-000106.

29. Wan EY, Ghanbari H, Akoum N, et al. HRS White Paper on Clinical Utilization of Digital Health Technology. Cardiovasc Digit Heal J 2021. https://doi.org/10.1016/j.cvdhj.2021.07.001.

30. Li SH, Lin BS, Wang CA, et al. Design of wearable and wireless multi-parameter monitoring system for evaluating cardiopulmonary function. Med Eng Phys 2017;47:144–50.

31. Etemadi M, Inan OT. Wearable ballistocardiogram and seismocardiogram systems for health and performance. J Appl Physiol 2018;124(2):452–61.

32. Noh S, Yoon C, Hyun E, et al. Ferroelectret film-based patch-type sensor for continuous blood pressure monitoring. Electron Lett 2014;50(3):143–4.

33. Kario K. Management of Hypertension in the Digital Era: Small Wearable Monitoring Devices for Remote Blood Pressure Monitoring. Hypertension 2020;640–50. https://doi.org/10.1161/HYPERTENSIONAHA.120.14742.

34. Malfatto G, Villani A, Rosa F Della, et al. Correlation between trans and intrathoracic impedance and conductance in patients with chronic heart failure. J Cardiovasc Med 2016;17(4):276–82.

35. Amir O, Azzam ZS, Gaspar T, et al. Validation of remote dielectric sensing (ReDS™) technology for quantification of lung fluid status: Comparison to high resolution chest computed tomography in patients with and without acute heart failure. Int J Cardiol 2016;221:841–6. https://doi.org/10.1016/j.ijcard.2016.06.323.

36. Sohn K, Merchant FM, Sayadi O, et al. A novel point-of-care smartphone based system for monitoring the cardiac and respiratory systems. Sci Rep 2017; 7(March):1–10. https://doi.org/10.1038/srep44946.

37. Cobos M. Novel use of Apple Watch 4 to Obtain 3-lead Electrocardiogram and Detect Cardiac Ischemia. Perm J 2020;24(3):99–102.

38. Saberi S, Wheeler M, Bragg-Gresham J, et al. Effect of moderate-intensity exercise training on peak oxygen consumption in patients with hypertrophic cardiomyopathy a randomized clinical trial. J Am Med Assoc 2017;317(13):1349–57.

39. Tobert KE, Bos JM, Garmany R, et al. Return-to-Play for Athletes With Long QT Syndrome or Genetic Heart Diseases Predisposing to Sudden Death. J Am Coll Cardiol 2021;78(6):594–604.

40. Castelletti S, Dagradi F, Goulene K, et al. A wearable remote monitoring system for the identification of subjects with a prolonged QT interval or at risk for drug-induced long QT syndrome. Int J Cardiol 2018;266:89–94.

41. Adesida Y, Papi E, McGregor AH. Exploring the role of wearable technology in sport kinematics and kinetics: A systematic review. Sensors (Switzerland) 2019; 19(7). https://doi.org/10.3390/s19071597.

42. Seshadri DR, Thom ML, Harlow ER, et al. Wearable Technology and Analytics as a Complementary Toolkit to Optimize Workload and to Reduce Injury Burden. Front Sport Act Living 2021;2(January):1–17. https://doi.org/10.3389/fspor.2020. 630576.

43. Electrophysiology TF of the ES of C the NA. Heart Rate Variability. Circulation 1996;93(5):1043–65.

44. Kinnunen H, Rantanen A, Kentt T, et al. Feasible assessment of recovery and cardiovascular health: Accuracy of nocturnal HR and HRV assessed via ring PPG in comparison to medical grade ECG. Physiol Meas 2020;41(4). https://doi.org/10. 1088/1361-6579/ab840a.

45. Lai E, Boyd K, Albert D, et al. Heart rate variability in concussed athletes: A case report using the smartphone electrocardiogram. Hear Case Rep 2017;3(11): 523–6.

46. Abaji JP, Currier D, Moore RD, et al. Persisting effects of concussion on heart rate variability during physical exertion. J Neurotrauma 2016;33(9):811–7. Available at: http://www.embase.com/search/results?subaction=viewrecord&from=expo rt&id=L610404939%0Ahttps://doi.org/10.1089/neu.2015.3989.

47. Green EM, van Mourik R, Wolfus C, et al. Machine learning detection of obstructive hypertrophic cardiomyopathy using a wearable biosensor. Npj Digit Med 2019;2(1):1–4. https://doi.org/10.1038/s41746-019-0130-0.

48. Orchard JJ, Orchard JW, Raju H, et al. Comparison between a 6-lead smartphone ECG and 12-lead ECG in athletes. J Electrocardiol 2021;66:95–7. https://doi.org/10.1016/j.jelectrocard.2021.03.008.

49. Altini M, Casale P, Penders J, et al. Cardiorespiratory fitness estimation using wearable sensors: Laboratory and free-living analysis of context-specific submaximal heart rates. J Appl Physiol 2016;120(9):1082–96. https://doi.org/10. 1152/japplphysiol.00519.2015.

50. Villar R, Beltrame T, Hughson RL. Validation of the Hexoskin wearable vest during lying, sitting, standing, and walking activities. Appl Physiol Nutr Metab 2015; 40(10):1019–24. https://doi.org/10.1139/apnm-2015-0140.

51. Fawcett E, van Velthoven MH, Meinert E. Long-term weight management using wearable technology in overweight and obese adults: Systematic review. JMIR mHealth uHealth 2020;8(3):1–10. https://doi.org/10.2196/13461.

52. Nes BM, Gutvik CR, Lavie CJ, et al. Personalized Activity Intelligence (PAI) for Prevention of Cardiovascular Disease and Promotion of Physical Activity. Am J Med 2017;130(3):328–36. https://doi.org/10.1016/j.amjmed.2016.09.031.

53. Borges NR, Driller MW. Wearable Lactate Threshold Predicting Device is Valid and Reliable in Runners. J Strength Cond Res 2016;30(8):2212–8. https://doi.org/10.1519/JSC.0000000000001307.

54. Ryan TE, Southern WM, Reynolds MA, et al. A cross-validation of near-infrared spectroscopy measurements of skeletal muscle oxidative capacity with phosphorus magnetic resonance spectroscopy. J Appl Physiol 2013;115(12):1757–66. https://doi.org/10.1152/japplphysiol.00835.2013.

55. Cohen S, Janicki-Deverts D, Miller GE. Psychological stress and disease. J Am Med Assoc 2007;298(14):1685–7. https://doi.org/10.1001/jama.298.14.1685.

56. Lee E, Marcucci M, Daniell L, et al. Amphiphysin 2 (Bin1) and T-tubule biogenesis in muscle. Science 2002;297(5584):1193–6. https://doi.org/10.1126/science.1071362.

57. Chopra N, Yang T, Asghari P, et al. Ablation of triadin causes loss of cardiac Ca2+ release units, impaired excitation-contraction coupling, and cardiac arrhythmias. Proc Natl Acad Sci U S A 2009;106(18):7636–41. https://doi.org/10.1073/pnas.0902919106.

58. Yoon S, Sim JK, Cho YH. A Flexible and Wearable Human Stress Monitoring Patch. Sci Rep 2016;6(August 2015):1–11. https://doi.org/10.1038/srep23468.

59. Parlak O, Keene ST, Marais A, et al. Molecularly selective nanoporous membrane-based wearable organic electrochemical device for noninvasive cortisol sensing. Sci Adv 2018;4(7). https://doi.org/10.1126/sciadv.aar2904.

60. Goodday SM, Friend S. Unlocking stress and forecasting its consequences with digital technology. Npj Digit Med 2019;2(1):1–5. https://doi.org/10.1038/s41746-019-0151-8.

61. Baron KG, Duffecy J, Berendsen MA, et al. Feeling validated yet? A scoping review of the use of consumer-targeted wearable and mobile technology to measure and improve sleep. Sleep Med Rev 2018;40:151–9. https://doi.org/10.1016/j.smrv.2017.12.002.

62. Fonseca P, Weysen T, Goelema MS, et al. Validation of photoplethysmography-based sleep staging compared with polysomnography in healthy middle-aged adults. Sleep 2017;40(7). https://doi.org/10.1093/sleep/zsx097.

63. Beattie Z, Oyang Y, Statan A, et al. Estimation of sleep stages in a healthy adult population from optical plethysmography and accelerometer signals. Physiol Meas 2017;38(11):1968–79. https://doi.org/10.1088/1361-6579/aa9047.

64. Kang SG, Kang JM, Cho SJ, et al. Cognitive behavioral therapy using a mobile application synchronizable with wearable devices for insomnia treatment: A pilot study. J Clin Sleep Med 2017;13(4):633–40. https://doi.org/10.5664/jcsm.6564.

65. Sekiguchi Y, Adams WM, Benjamin CL, et al. Relationships between resting heart rate, heart rate variability and sleep characteristics among female collegiate cross-country athletes. J Sleep Res 2019;28(6):1–7. https://doi.org/10.1111/jsr.12836.

66. Arikawa T, Nakajima T, Yazawa H, et al. Clinical Usefulness of New R-R Interval Analysis Using the Wearable Heart Rate Sensor WHS-1 to Identify Obstructive Sleep Apnea: OSA and RRI Analysis Using a Wearable Heartbeat Sensor. J Clin Med 2020;9(10):3359. https://doi.org/10.3390/jcm9103359.

67. Papini GB, Fonseca P, van Gilst MM, et al. Wearable monitoring of sleep-disordered breathing: estimation of the apnea–hypopnea index using wrist-

worn reflective photoplethysmography. Sci Rep 2020;10(1):1–15. https://doi.org/10.1038/s41598-020-69935-7.

68. Varma N, Marrouche NF, Aguinaga L, et al. HRS/EHRA/APHRS/LAHRS/ACC/AHA worldwide practice update for telehealth and arrhythmia monitoring during and after a pandemic. Europace 2021;23(2):313. https://doi.org/10.1093/europace/euaa187.

69. Slotwiner D, Varma N, Akar JG, et al. HRS expert consensus statement on remote interrogation and monitoring for cardiovascular implantable electronic devices. Hear Rhythm 2015;12(7):e69–100. https://doi.org/10.1016/j.hrthm.2015.05.008.

70. Schwamm LH, Chumbler N, Brown E, et al. Recommendations for the Implementation of Telehealth in Cardiovascular and Stroke Care: A Policy Statement from the American Heart Association. Circulation 2017;135(7):e24–44. https://doi.org/10.1161/CIR.0000000000000475.

71. Koehler F, Koehler K, Deckwart O, et al. Efficacy of telemedical interventional management in patients with heart failure (TIM-HF2): a randomised, controlled, parallel-group, unmasked trial. Lancet 2018;392(10152):1047–57. https://doi.org/10.1016/S0140-6736(18)31880-4.

72. Palatini P, Winnicki M, Santonastaso M, et al. Reproducibility of heart rate measured in the clinic and with 24-hour intermittent recorders. Am J Hypertens 2000;13(1 Pt 1):92–8. https://doi.org/10.1016/s0895-7061(99)00170-3.

73. Shah RL, Kapoor R, Bonnett C, et al. Antiarrhythmic drug loading at home using remote monitoring: a virtual feasibility study during COVID-19 social distancing. Eur Hear J - Digit Heal 2021;2(2):259–62. https://doi.org/10.1093/ehjdh/ztab034.

74. Dunn J, Kidzinski L, Runge R, et al. Wearable sensors enable personalized predictions of clinical laboratory measurements. Nat Med 2021;27(6):1105–12. https://doi.org/10.1038/s41591-021-01339-0.

75. Radin JM, Wineinger NE, Topol EJ, et al. Harnessing wearable device data to improve state-level real-time surveillance of influenza-like illness in the USA: a population-based study. Lancet Digit Heal 2020;2(2):e85–93. https://doi.org/10.1016/S2589-7500(19)30222-5.

76. Zhu G, Li J, Meng Z, et al. Learning from Large-Scale Wearable Device Data for Predicting Epidemics Trend of COVID-19. Discret Dyn Nat Soc 2020;2020(Cdc). https://doi.org/10.1155/2020/6152041.

77. Quer G, Radin JM, Gadaleta M, et al. Wearable sensor data and self-reported symptoms for COVID-19 detection. Nat Med 2021;27(1):73–7. https://doi.org/10.1038/s41591-020-1123-x.

78. Smarr BL, Aschbacher K, Fisher SM, et al. Feasibility of continuous fever monitoring using wearable devices. Sci Rep 2020;10(1):1–11. https://doi.org/10.1038/s41598-020-78355-6.

79. Grzesiak E, Bent B, McClain MT, et al. Assessment of the Feasibility of Using Noninvasive Wearable Biometric Monitoring Sensors to Detect Influenza and the Common Cold Before Symptom Onset. JAMA Netw Open 2021;4(9):e2128534. https://doi.org/10.1001/jamanetworkopen.2021.28534.

80. Lopez-Leon S, Wegman-Ostrosky T, Perelman C, et al. More than 50 long-term effects of COVID-19: a systematic review and meta-analysis. Sci Rep 2021;11(1):1–12. https://doi.org/10.1038/s41598-021-95565-8.

81. Radin JM, Quer G, Ramos E, et al. Assessment of Prolonged Physiological and Behavioral Changes Associated With COVID-19 Infection. JAMA Netw Open 2021;4(7):e2115959. https://doi.org/10.1001/jamanetworkopen.2021.15959.

82. Phelan D, Kim JH, Chung EH. A Game Plan for the Resumption of Sport and Exercise After Coronavirus Disease 2019 (COVID-19) Infection. JAMA Cardiol 2020; 5(10):1085–6. https://doi.org/10.1001/jamacardio.2020.2136.

83. FDA Clears First of its Kind Algorithm Suite for Personal ECG. AliveCor. 2020. Available at: https://www.alivecor.com/press/press_release/fda-clears-first-of-its-kind-algorithm-suite-for-personal-ecg/.

84. O'Driscoll R, Turicchi J, Beaulieu K, et al. How well do activity monitors estimate energy expenditure? A systematic review and meta-analysis of the validity of current technologies. Br J Sports Med 2020;54(6):332–40. https://doi.org/10.1136/bjsports-2018-099643.

85. Piwek L, Ellis DA, Andrews S, et al. The Rise of Consumer Health Wearables: Promises and Barriers. Plos Med 2016;13(2):1–9. https://doi.org/10.1371/journal.pmed.1001953.

86. Sjoding MW, Dickson RP, Iwashyna TJ, et al. Racial Bias in Pulse Oximetry Measurement. N Engl J Med 2020;383(25):2477–8. https://doi.org/10.1056/nejmc2029240.

87. Shcherbina A, Mikael Mattsson C, Waggott D, et al. Accuracy in wrist-worn, sensor-based measurements of heart rate and energy expenditure in a diverse cohort. J Pers Med 2017;7(2):1–12. https://doi.org/10.3390/jpm7020003.

88. Attia ZI, Kapa S, Yao X, et al. Prospective validation of a deep learning electrocardiogram algorithm for the detection of left ventricular systolic dysfunction. J Cardiovasc Electrophysiol 2019;30(5):668–74. https://doi.org/10.1111/jce.13889.

89. Ko WY, Siontis KC, Attia ZI, et al. Detection of Hypertrophic Cardiomyopathy Using a Convolutional Neural Network-Enabled Electrocardiogram. J Am Coll Cardiol 2020;75(7):722–33. https://doi.org/10.1016/j.jacc.2019.12.030.

90. Cho Y, Kwon J-M, Kim KH, et al. Artificial intelligence algorithm for detecting myocardial infarction using six-lead electrocardiography. Sci Rep 2020;10(1): 1–10. https://doi.org/10.1038/s41598-020-77599-6.

91. Giudicessi JR, Schram M, Bos JM, et al. Artificial Intelligence-Enabled Assessment of the Heart Rate Corrected QT Interval Using a Mobile Electrocardiogram Device. Circulation 2021;1274–86. https://doi.org/10.1161/CIRCULATIONAHA.120.050231.

92. Chan J, Rea T, Gollakota S, et al. Contactless cardiac arrest detection using smart devices. Npj Digit Med 2019;2(1). https://doi.org/10.1038/s41746-019-0128-7.

93. Maor E, Perry D, Mevorach D, et al. Vocal biomarker is associated with hospitalization and mortality among heart failure patients. J Am Heart Assoc 2020;9(7): 1–11. https://doi.org/10.1161/JAHA.119.013359.

94. Seshadri DR, Li RT, Voos JE, et al. Wearable sensors for monitoring the internal and external workload of the athlete. Npj Digit Med 2019;2(1). https://doi.org/10.1038/s41746-019-0149-2.

95. Alizadeh A, Burns A, Lenigk R, et al. A wearable patch for continuous monitoring of sweat electrolytes during exertion. Lab Chip 2018;18(17):2632–41. https://doi.org/10.1039/c8lc00510a.

96. Seshadri DR, Li RT, Voos JE, et al. Wearable sensors for monitoring the physiological and biochemical profile of the athlete. Npj Digit Med 2019;2(1). https://doi.org/10.1038/s41746-019-0150-9.

97. Münzel T, Hahad O, Daiber A. Running in polluted air is a two-edged sword — physical exercise in low air pollution areas is cardioprotective but detrimental for the heart in high air pollution areas. Eur Heart J 2021;2498–500. https://doi.org/10.1093/eurheartj/ehab227.

Differentiating Physiology from Pathology
The Gray Zones of the Athlete's Heart

Alfred Danielian, MD[a], Ankit B. Shah, MD, MPH[b],*

KEYWORDS

- Exercise physiology • Athlete's heart • Exercise-induced cardiac remodeling
- Hypertrophic cardiomyopathy • Left ventricular noncompaction
- Right ventricular arrhythmogenic cardiomyopathy • Dilated cardiomyopathy

KEY POINTS

- Some athletes with a large cumulative history of vigorous exercise training develop marked cardiac remodeling that can share features with mild forms of cardiomyopathy known as the gray zone.
- Differentiating exercise-induced cardiac remodeling (EICR) from mild forms of cardiomyopathy can be challenging and requires a comprehensive evaluation.
- An integrated clinical approach that factors athlete-specific characteristics (sex, size, sport, ethnicity, and training history) and findings from multimodality imaging are essential to help distinguish between physiologic remodeling from pathologic conditions.
- Hypertrophic cardiomyopathy (HCM), dilated cardiomyopathy (DCM), arrhythmogenic right ventricular (RV) cardiomyopathy, and left ventricular (LV) noncompaction are important differential diagnoses to consider when evaluating athletes who show morphologic and functional changes of the cardiovascular system in response to intense exercise.

INTRODUCTION

Routine vigorous exercise induces structural, functional, and electrical cardiovascular adaptations that are considered physiologic and ultimately, enhance athletic performance. Training-related physiologic changes are more commonly seen in those who exercise vigorously for at least 4 to 8 hours a week.[1] Each sport or athletic pursuit results in a unique set of hemodynamic conditions based on the magnitude of change in cardiac output and peripheral vascular resistance (PVR). These hemodynamic differences can be separated into 2 forms: isotonic or endurance training and isometric

[a] Las Vegas Heart Associates- Affiliated with Mountain View Hospital, 2880 North Tenaya Way Suite 100, Las Vegas, NV 89128, USA; [b] Sports & Performance Cardiology Program, MedStar Health, 3333 North Calvert Street Suite 500 JPB, Baltimore, MD 21218, USA
* Corresponding author.
E-mail address: ankit.b.shah@medstar.net

Clin Sports Med 41 (2022) 425–440
https://doi.org/10.1016/j.csm.2022.02.005
0278-5919/22/© 2022 Elsevier Inc. All rights reserved.

or strength training. Isotonic training requires sustained elevations in cardiac output with normal or reduced PVR that results in a volume challenge for all 4 cardiac chambers. The exercise-induced cardiac remodeling (EICR) in response to this volume challenge is symmetric 4-chamber dilation with minimal increases in cardiac wall thickness or eccentric remodeling (**Fig. 1**).[2] Long-distance running, cycling, or swimming are traditional examples of sports with high isotonic training. This is contrasted by isometric exercise, whereby the predominant hemodynamic effect is large increases in PVR with little change in cardiac output. This type of training can result in marked increases in systolic blood pressure that increase left ventricular (LV) afterload

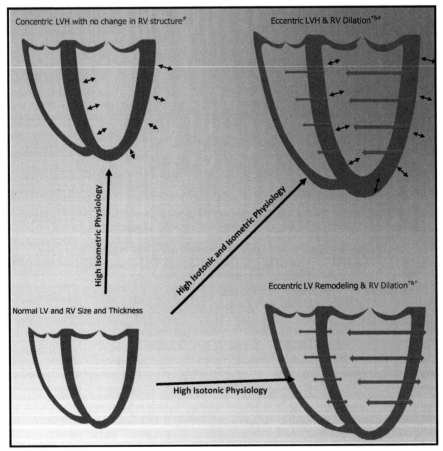

Fig. 1. Spectrum of exercise-induced cardiac remodeling based on the degree of isotonic and isometric physiology. [a]Athletes participating in sports with high isotonic and mixed sports (high isotonic and isometric) are those most likely to display profound remodeling that can create a gray zone with DCM. [b]Athletes participating in sports with high isotonic and mixed sports (high isotonic and isometric) are those most likely to display profound remodeling that can create a gray zone with ARVC. [c]Athletes participating in sports with high isometric and mixed sports (high isometric and isotonic) are those that can display profound remodeling that can create a gray zone with HCM. [d]Athletes participating in sports with high isotonic are those that can display profound remodeling that can create a gray zone with LVNC.

with concentric hypertrophy as the form of EICR.[3] Weightlifting and American-style football are examples of isometric sports.

While volume and pressure are the 2 principle hemodynamic effects, sports are typically not dichotomous and instead most sports use a combination of these 2 hemodynamic influences that result in a spectrum of EICR based on the relative degree of the pressure and volume loads. Thus, classifying sports based on the degree of isotonic and isometric physiology and understanding sport-specific EICR provides a helpful framework when evaluating an athlete with potential cardiovascular pathology.[4–8] While sport type plays an important role in the type of EICR, many other factors influence the magnitude of EICR. Sex is an important variable as female athletes typically have smaller absolute LV dimensions, thickness, mass, and also smaller right ventricular (RV) size compared with male athletes.[9,10,81] However, the LV and RV chamber sizes can be larger in women compared with men when indexed to body surface area (BSA).[9,10] There are no differences in LV or RV systolic or LV diastolic function between sexes. Ethnicity also plays an important role as black athletes have been found to have unique repolarization variants on the electrocardiogram (ECG) and commonly display more pronounced LV hypertrophy compared with white athletes of both sexes.[11] Body size is important as data has shown linear relationships between BSA[7] and height[5] with LV and RV end-diastolic dimensions. Age and exercise exposure which can be quantified as a dose with principal components of duration, intensity, frequency are also important as EICR is not static and progressive remodeling can be seen with continued exercise.[8,12] A genetic predisposition to more robust remodeling likely contributes as well but is not well understood.[13]

In many athletes, EICR is easily distinguished from pathology. However, a small minority of athletes with a high cumulative exercise exposure demonstrates pronounced EICR and sometimes exhibit features of pathologic conditions, making it a challenge to differentiate healthy physiologic remodeling from mild forms of cardiomyopathies. This overlap is considered the diagnostic gray zone. The distinction between physiologic and pathologic changes in the hearts of athletes is of critical importance and has important prognostic and therapeutic implications. A failure to diagnose pathology could lead to catastrophic outcomes, while a misdiagnosis may lead to an unnecessary restriction in training and competition with resultant emotional, psychological, financial, and long-term health consequences. We will review these diagnostic dilemmas and provide a framework to help differentiate extreme forms of physiologic remodeling from mild forms of cardiomyopathies.

DISCUSSION

There are important considerations when evaluating an athlete with pronounced EICR and features of cardiomyopathy regardless of the potential underlying pathology (**Table 1**). Given the expected type and magnitude of EICR is influenced by many factors, it is critical that the consulting cardiologist personally view and interpret imaging studies with the appropriate clinical context. For example, findings of maximal LV wall thickness (LVWT) of 12 mm in an 18-year-old white female endurance runner with a BSA of 1.7 m^2 may warrant further investigation, whereas the same findings in a 24-year-old, black female basketball player with a BSA of 2.2 m^2 may not. We also emphasize that gray zone findings are typically found in those with high cumulative exposure to vigorous exercise and not in the more recreational exercise enthusiast with inconsistent exercise exposure. Discussions on shared decision making and participation in sports with clinically diagnosed cardiomyopathies are out of the scope

Table 1 Common considerations in the evaluation of all gray zone scenarios	
Context	Is the Athlete asymptomatic or did symptoms prompt the evaluation? • Red flag symptoms including chest pain, syncope, cardiac arrest, palpitations, decrease in performance may be more likely to indicate pathology
Sport/Size (BSA)/Sex	Are the imaging findings consistent with the expected remodeling based on the sport, training history (predominantly isometric, mixed physiology, or isotonic), BSA, and sex of the athlete? • Imaging findings that are incongruous with training history, size, and/or sex would favor pathology
Cumulative exercise exposure	Gray zone findings are typically seen in those exercising vigorously over a period of years and should not be considered the norm in a recreational athlete that exercises a few times a week
Family History	A family history of sudden cardiac arrest or death, unexplained syncope or drowning, or genetic cardiomyopathies would favor pathology
Performance-enhancing drugs (PEDs)/substance abuse	Athletes should be specifically asked about the use of PEDs and substances as they can contribute to findings of cardiomyopathy

of this review and the reader is referred to dedicated documents addressing these topics.[14,15]

Gray Zone Scenarios

Scenario #1: dilated left ventricle

Dilated cardiomyopathy (DCM) is characterized by ventricular dilation and depressed myocardial contractility in the absence of abnormal loading conditions such as valvular disease or hypertension.[16] Ventricular dilation as seen by LV end-diastolic diameter (LVEDD) and LV end-diastolic volume (LVEDV) is also commonly seen in athletes, typically in endurance or mixed sports athletes with high levels of isotonic training.[5,8,12,13] One of the hallmarks of an elite endurance athlete is a high peak Vo_2 or pulmonary oxygen uptake. Using the Fick equation, maximal oxygen uptake (VO_{2max}), is determined by the product of maximal cardiac output and maximal arteriovenous oxygen difference. While peak heart rate is not a trainable number, prolonged vigorous aerobic training results in a higher stroke volume with increases in LVEDV. Thus, athletes can maintain cardiac output at rest with heart rates as low as 30 to 40 bpm given this higher stroke volume. While many endurance athletes maintain a normal LV ejection fraction (LVEF), some elite endurance athletes can have a mildly reduced LVEF of 45% to 50%, which can overlap with features of a mild DCM **(Table 2)**.[12,13,17,18]

Athletes with physiologic remodeling generally display normal ECG when using the most recent ECG criteria for athletes, whereas pathologic T-wave inversion (TWI), ST-segment depression, pathologic Q waves, complete left bundle branch block (LBBB), or interventricular conduction delay (IVCD) ≥ 140 ms may be seen in DCM (see **Table 2**).[1,13]

Unfortunately, strict cutoffs for LV dimensions as defined in guidelines are not helpful in differentiating physiology from pathology as in a large cohort (1309) of elite Italian

Table 2
Findings supportive of healthy physiology in each gray zone scenario[a]

	Dilated LV	Dilated RV	LVH	Hypertrabeculation
Gray Zone	Dilated LV, ≥56 mm, and mildly reduced LVEF, <52%	Dilated RV, normal to mildly reduced RV function	LVWT 13–15 mm in men and 12–14 mm in women	Prominent mid-apical LV or RV trabeculations
Sports Type	Endurance/mixed sport	Endurance/mixed sport	Strength/Mixed sport	Particularly endurance sports
Ethnicity	Seen in white and black athletes	White > Black athletes	Black > White athletes	Black > White athletes
ECG	Typically normal based on latest criteria[1]	• Incomplete or complete RBBB <140 ms • Absence of epsilon and/or anterior TWI	Normal based on latest criteria[1]	Normal based on latest criteria[1]
Ambulatory Monitoring	No significant arrhythmias	No significant arrhythmias	No significant arrhythmias	No significant arrhythmias
Echocardiogram	• Symmetric 4 chamber dilation • Normal/Supranormal Diastolic function • GLS > -16%	• Seen with LV dilation • Normal RV morphology • Normal/low normal RVEF • Supranormal LV diastolic function • Normal RVSP and right sided valves	• Concentric LVH • LVEDD > 55 mm • Normal/Supranormal Diastolic function • GLS > -16%	• Normal LVEF • Normal/Supranormal Diastolic function • GLS > -16%
Stress Testing	• Supranormal exercise capacity on CPET • Change LVEF >11% and peak LVEF >63% on stress echocardiogram • No exercise-induced arrhythmias	• Appropriate RV systolic contractile reserve • No exercise-induced arrhythmias	• Supranormal exercise capacity on ETT or CPET • No exercise-induced arrhythmias	• Supranormal exercise capacity on ETT or CPET • No exercise-induced arrhythmias

(continued on next page)

Table 2
(continued)

	Dilated LV	Dilated RV	LVH	Hypertrabeculation
Cardiac MRI	• No pathologic LGE • No wall motion abnormalities	• No pathologic LGE • No regional wall motion abnormalities, aneurysms, or sacculations	• No pathologic LGE • No wall motion abnormalities	• No pathologic LGE • Normal compacted LV wall thickness
Other	NT-proBNP <125pg/mL[21]	N/A	N/A	N/A

[a] Highly trained athletes with pathologic conditions can display some normal findings so a single test/finding should not be used to differentiate physiology from pathology.

athletes, 45% exceeded upper normal limits and 14% of trained athletes showed marked LV enlargement (≥60 mm).[13,19] Maximum LVEDD in elite male athletes has been reported to be as large as 70 to 73 mm.[12,13] The major determinants of cavity dimension were participation in endurance sports and larger BSA. The correlation of BSA and LV dimensions has been reported in professional basketball players as well.[5,7] Age, sex, and training history are also important variables that have been shown to correlate with larger absolute dimensions.[5,8,12,13] While females typically have smaller absolute LV dimensions compared with men, pronounced remodeling can be seen as well with peak an LVEDD range of 61 to 66 mm.[8,10,13,20]

On echocardiographic imaging, athletes with a dilated LV typically have supranormal and robust diastolic function, which is not typical of pathologic LV dilation.[21,22] Additionally, as reviewed above, the increased cardiac output is experienced by all 4 cardiac chambers, so a dilated LV cavity is generally seen with the dilation of the other cardiac chambers in a symmetric fashion with proportionate increases in LV thickness. In combination with other abnormal findings (abnormal diastolic function, LVEF more than mildly reduced), a peak global longitudinal strain (GLS) value of less than −16% supports pathology.[2] With this said, it has been reported that ∼10% of elite athletes had a GLS less than −16% and thus, we would caution making a diagnosis of pathologic LV dilation with an isolated abnormal GLS in absence of other abnormal findings.[21,23] Cardiac magnetic resonance (CMR) imaging can be helpful as pathologic late gadolinium enhancement (LGE) is not routinely seen in gray zone athletes with physiologic remodeling.[21]

Stress testing and ambulatory rhythm monitoring are also important components of the comprehensive work up. Ventricular arrhythmias on ambulatory monitoring or stress testing are more commonly seen in athletes with pathologic LV dilation compared with physiologic LV dilation.[21] On stress echocardiography, augmentation of LVEF greater than 11% and greater than 63% at peak exercise has been shown to favor the diagnosis of EICR over DCM.[21] Cardiopulmonary exercise testing (CPET) has also become an important part of many sports cardiology practices. Athletes with physiologic remodeling should demonstrate supranormal peak V_{O_2} values (reference values used in many laboratories were not derived from an athletic cohort) and normal cardiopulmonary physiology. However, a supranormal peak V_{O_2} does not exclude DCM as highly trained athletes with pathologic dilation may still display excellent functional capacity.[21] However, a reduced or lower than expected exercise capacity may signal pathology. While detraining may help differentiate other gray zone scenarios, it is not recommended in this setting as athletes continue to have dilated chambers even after the cessation of training.[24]

Scenario #2: dilated right ventricle

Remodeling of the RV parallels that of the LV with the most pronounced adaptions seen in endurance or mixed sports athletes with higher cumulative exposure to regular high-intensity isotonic training.[25–27] While the impact of strength training on RV size remains understudied, a prior study reported no change in RV structure among strength-based athletes.[22] Male athletes have larger absolute dimensions compared with female athletes, but when indexed to BSA female athletes may demonstrate larger values.[27] RV enlargement is also part of the criteria for the diagnosis of arrhythmogenic right ventricular cardiomyopathy (ARVC).[28] Thus, physiologic RV enlargement in athletes must be differentiated from pathologic enlargement as vigorous exercise with underlying ARVC can accelerate disease progression, provoke ventricular arrhythmias and increase risk of death.[29] A comprehensive work up may be warranted to help differentiate these 2 etiologies of a dilated right heart.

The ECG favors pathology when anterior TWI (V1–V3) with isoelectric or depressed ST segments are noted or when an epsilon wave is present.[30] When coupled with the other abnormalities, low voltage in the limbs leads and premature ventricular contractions (PVCs) originating from the RV with a superior axis may also suggest pathology. Meanwhile incomplete or complete right bundle branch block (RBBB) with QRS duration less than 140 ms is consistent with athletic remodeling.[1,31] However, a normal ECG does not exclude pathology, as it has been demonstrated that 38% of patients with mild ARVC had a normal ECG.[32]

As seen with the LV, RV dimensions in athletes routinely exceed published cut-offs.[7,19,33,34] In fact, in a cross-sectional study of 1009 Olympic athletes, about one-quarter met criteria for a dilated RV, and 16% and 41% fulfilled the Task Force major and minor criteria, respectively, for the diagnosis of ARVC based on RV outflow tract (RVOT) parasternal long axis (PLAX) measurements.[27,28,35] These numbers decreased to 4% and 32% when indexed to BSA, a finding reported by others,[7] highlighting the importance of taking BSA into consideration when evaluating the RV in athletes. Consistent with prior reports, the authors also found that athletes that participated in endurance sports had the largest RV dimensions.[27] None of the athletes were found to have ARVC after comprehensive evaluation.

Importantly, physiologic RV remodeling is supported by symmetric cardiac enlargement and RV dilation should not be seen in isolation. This is supported by a prior longitudinal study following 29 elite athletes that found that the increase in RV size was seen with a concomitant increase in the LV size and stable RV function.[33] In the prior study on Olympic athletes a positive linear correlation between RV and LV size was described.[27] Thus, absolute RV measurements are generally not helpful in differentiating physiologic from pathologic RV dilation but given the expected balanced ventricular dilation in healthy athletes, a basal end-diastolic RV:LV diameter size ratio of 0.8 ± 0.1 in the long axis on echocardiogram may be used to help differentiate physiologic from pathologic RV dilation.[27,36] In contrast, ARVC is characterized by the disproportional dilation of the RV. Physiologic RV dilation results in proportional increases in RV outflow and inflow such that despite the global enlargement the RV outflow/inflow ratio remains similar to the general population, which is in contrast to a predominant increase in the outflow tract in ARVC.[32,34]

Importantly, dilation of the RV is global and the RV architecture remains normal without aneurysms, sacculations, or regional wall motion abnormalities. RV function is commonly normal but a mild reduction in RV function has been reported.[37,38] Marked RV systolic dysfunction and regional wall motion abnormalities suggest pathology. Myocardial deformation by speckle tracking echocardiography and tissue Doppler in elite endurance athletes has been normal, albeit slightly lower compared with nonathletes.[39] Thus, use of global RV strain has been recommended to be used as part of the diagnostic algorithm given it is typically reduced in ARVC but normal in athletes.[35,40] Importantly, many of the RV imaging parameters are influenced by recent high-intensity training so imaging should be conducted when the athlete is well hydrated and has refrained from exercise for at least 6 hours, and even longer if participating in ultra-endurance events, before the examination.[41]

If diagnostic uncertainty remains, CMR can better assess for focal akinesia, dyskinesia, aneurysms, and for the presence of LGE as ARVC criteria are not solely based on RV size but require morphologic abnormalities as well.[28] While most of the endurance athletes have no evidence of LGE, focal LGE at the RV insertion points has been reported in endurance athletes that have a higher cumulative exercise exposure and lower RVEF.[42–44] The significance of this finding remains an active area of research but at present isolated LGE at the RV insertion points should not be considered pathologic.[30]

Athletes with physiologic RV dilation and mild reduction in RV systolic function should show appropriate contractile reserve during stress echocardiography.[45] Absence of contractile reserve or increase in ventricular ectopy with exercise should raise concern for pathology. There is insufficient data on the impact of detraining on the RV in highly trained athletes and detraining should not be used to differentiate physiologic from pathology RV remodeling at this time.

Scenario #3: left ventricular hypertrophy

Physiologic left ventricular hypertrophy (LVH) with little change in LV cavity size is traditionally seen with strength/power or isometric-based training with sports such as weightlifting, American-style football (especially linemen), track and field throwing, or shot put. However, elite mixed-sports athletes (rowers, cyclists) display the greatest degree of LVH.[46] The expected degree and pattern of LVWT for a particular athlete is influenced by age, sex, ethnicity, body size, sports type, and intensity. Studies have shown that the LVWT in athletes rarely exceeds 12 mm in men and 11 mm in women.[11,47] Among 947 elite Italian athletes who were exclusively Caucasian, only 1.7% had LVWT ≥ 13 mm, a finding that was corroborated in a study of 3500 British athletes whereby only 1.5% had LVWT ≥ 13 mm.[47,48] In both studies, none of the athletes had an LVWT greater than 16 mm and LVH was seen with LV cavity dilatation supporting physiologic remodeling. Importantly, black athletes can display more pronounced LVH with 18% of black male athletes reported to have an LVWT greater than 12 mm compared with 4% of white male athletes.[49] Additionally, 3% of black male athletes had a wall thickness ≥ 15 mm. Similar findings are seen in females whereby 3% of black athletes showed LVWT ≥ 11 mm compared with zero white female athletes.[11] Thus, only a small minority of athletes develop pronounced LVH (13–15 mm in men and 12–14 mm in women) that can overlap with mild forms of hypertrophic cardiomyopathy (HCM).[7,49,50]

HCM is characterized by abnormal thickening of the LV defined as an LVWT ≥ 15 mm in any segment of the LV on echocardiography or CMR imaging in the absence of another cardiac, systemic, or metabolic cause for the hypertrophy in adults.[51] A lesser degree of LVH (13–14 mm) can be diagnostic when genotype positive or when present in family members of a relative with HCM.[51] Differentiating physiologic from pathologic LVH is critical as HCM remains a leading cause of sudden cardiac arrest/death in young athletes.[52–54]

Athletes with gray zone LVH and red flag symptoms, concerning family history (see **Table 1**), or dynamic/provocable murmurs raise concern for pathologic LVH. The ECG can be helpful as over 90% of individuals with HCM have abnormal findings.[55,56] Deep TWI, especially in the inferolateral leads, ST-segment depressions, pathologic Q waves, profound intraventricular conduction delays (≥140 ms), and complete LBBB are commonly seen in HCM but not considered normal physiologic findings in athletes.[1] Pathologic TWI (excludes leads aVR, III, and V1 and in V1–V4 when preceded by domed ST segment in asymptomatic black athletes) are common, ~50% of the time, associated with cardiac pathology with HCM being the most common.[57] Meanwhile, isolated voltage criteria for LVH is common in athletes and does not correlate with pathology when there are no other associated ECG abnormalities.[1] Furthermore, given the age-related variable penetrance of HCM, it is recommended that all athletes with abnormal ECG but normal initial investigations be routinely monitored with serial comprehensive evaluations.[1]

Echocardiography can be instrumental in differentiating LVH due to EICR from pathology. Accurate measurement of LVWT is of paramount importance and primary imaging should be reviewed to ensure that there has not been erroneous inclusion of RV trabeculation, papillary muscles, or moderator band in the measurements. The LVH in athletes is commonly symmetric so findings of focal or segmental LVH or abnormalities of the mitral valve should raise concern for pathologic LVH.[51] Athletes with gray zone LVH typically have proportionate increases in LV cavity size while the LVEDD in HCM is frequently small (usually < 45 mm) and studies have suggested that LVEDD may be a useful discriminator with greater than 55 mm suggesting EICR.[55,58,59]

LV diastolic function in healthy athletes is almost always normal or supranormal and usually abnormal in individuals with HCM. However, strength-trained athletes, those who are most likely to develop concentric LVH and represent the group most difficult to distinguish from individuals with HCM, were not well represented in studies that evaluated diastolic function in athletes. A recent study of American-style football players showed impairment of diastolic function in those with concentric LVH, which was felt to possibly be explained by resting systemic hypertension in this population.[22,60] Furthermore, athletes with HCM can also have normal LV diastolic parameters, limiting the role of LV diastolic function in isolation as a reliable parameter to differentiate EICR from pathology.[55]

GLS is reduced in individuals with HCM compared with healthy athletes.[55] However, minor reductions in GLS have been shown in healthy athletes and a decrease in GLS has also been seen in athletes that develop concentric remodeling.[61,62] One study, compared patients with sedentary HCM with athletes with HCM and athletes without HCM. There was no difference in resting GLS between the athletes with HCM and the athletes without HCM, but a significant decrease in GLS in the sedentary HCM individuals.[63] The authors did show that mechanical dispersion of longitudinal strain did differentiate the athletes with HCM from the athletes without HCM, potentially serving as a promising tool to differentiate gray zone LVH.

CMR allows for superior visualization of the entire heart, including identifying focal areas of hypertrophy that can be missed by echocardiography, especially when limited to the anterior free wall, posterior septum, and apex.[57,64,65] In addition to providing more accurate quantification of ventricular wall thickness, mass, volume, and function, it has the additional advantage of evaluating for myocardial fibrosis. LGE, suggestive of fibrosis or scar, can be seen in up to 75% of individuals with HCM most often in the area of maximal LVWT and at the anteroseptal and inferoseptal segments of insertion of the right ventricle.[66] LGE in young, healthy athletes should be considered abnormal with the possible exception of LGE at RV insertion sites whereby less is known about its significance.[67]

Metabolic stress testing using CPET may be helpful in differentiating physiologic LVH from HCM. While a reduced or lower than expected peak Vo_2 may signal pathology, a normal or supranormal peak Vo_2 does not exclude HCM as fit athletes with mild HCM can display robust peak Vo_2 values.[68] Additionally, stress echocardiography can help assess the hemodynamic response to exercise, functional capacity, provocable LV outflow tract gradient, and systolic anterior motion of the mitral valve, and while not diagnostic of HCM these findings can be valuable when integrated all of the data.

The diagnostic dilemma of the gray zone may persist despite a comprehensive diagnostic evaluation. In these cases, detraining and follow-up cardiac imaging to assess for regression of LVH can be considered. Limited evidence suggests approximately 2 to 3 months of detraining may result in the reduction of LVWT.[69] This approach has mostly been shown in a small number of athletes documenting regression of eccentric LVH.[24,69] While a very small study of strength-trained athletes with concentric LVH showed significant regression of LVWT and LV mass during detraining, the degree to which there may be the regression of LVWT in athletes with HCM has not been reliably validated.[70] Importantly, athletes with regression of gray zone LVH on detraining should be followed longitudinally as some will develop clear phenotypic HCM in serial follow-up.

Scenario #4: hypertrabeculation

Hypertrabeculation of the LV apex with normal LVWT is a common and benign finding in athletes.[71,72] It is suggested that a chronic increase in cardiac preload in the setting of isotonic physiology may be a stimulus for trabecular enlargement.[2] In contrast, left ventricular noncompaction (LVNC) is a rare, inherited cardiomyopathy characterized by the presence of increased trabeculation and deep intertrabecular recesses in the LV with a thin layer of compact myocardium (CM) and a thicker layer of noncompacted myocardium (NCM) that can result in heart failure, systemic thromboembolism, LV dilation, ventricular arrhythmias, and sudden death.[73,74]

In a study of 1146 healthy, highly trained athletes, LV trabeculations were more commonly seen in athletes compared with controls, 18.3% versus 7%, respectively.[75] Additionally, 8.1% of the athletes fulfilled published criteria for LVNC.[76] LV hypertrabeculation was more common in endurance athletes and in African/Afro-Caribbean athletes compared with Caucasian athletes (28.8% vs 16.3%). A recent study evaluating physical activity in the general population showed that LVNC phenotype based on MRI criteria was higher in those exercising at the highest vigorous physical activity quintile (30.5%) compared with participants engaging in no vigorous physical activity, 14.2%.[77,78] The finding that 14.2% of subjects performing no vigorous exercise met MRI criteria for LVNC also highlights a concern of overdiagnosing LVNC based on solely on findings of hypertrabeculation that meet published cut-points for LVNC.[76,78,79]

While there are no specific criteria to differentiate hypertrabeculation as a component of EICR from LVNC, a comprehensive evaluation using history, ECG, echocardiography, exercise stress testing, ambulatory monitoring, and CMR can help identify high-risk features. Athletes with physiologic hypertrabeculation typically have normal ECGs while inferolateral TWI, ST-segment depression, pathologic Q waves, profound IVCD, LBBB favor a diagnosis of LVNC.[1,80]

Echocardiography remains the first-line imaging modality as physiologic hypertrabeculation is typically seen with robust diastolic function and normal LV systolic function. Marked abnormalities in strain imaging should raise concern for pathologic hypertrabeculations.[80] CMR is superior to echocardiography in identifying regions of NCM, allowing for more accurate measurements of both, the CM and NCM, and also for identifying LGE. Findings of hypertrabeculation when associated with a thin CM (<5 mm), marked impairment of LV systolic function, and LGE on CMR may suggest LVNC.[2,75] Failure of appropriate LV augmentation on stress echocardiography, exercise-induced ventricular tachyarrhythmias, and a Vo_{2max} less than 100% predicted on CPET also favor a diagnosis of LVNC over EICR.[80]

SUMMARY

In many athletes, healthy, physiologic EICR is easily distinguished from pathology. However, a small minority of athletes with high cumulative exercise exposures demonstrate pronounced EICR that can overlap with features of cardiomyopathies. The distinction between physiologic and pathologic changes in the hearts of athletes can be challenging and typically requires a comprehensive evaluation. For athletes with gray zone findings, a single test or finding does not typically exclude the diagnosis of cardiomyopathy but instead, the final diagnosis requires an integration of all of the available data. Athletes with gray zone findings that are ultimately deemed to be physiologic should be followed serially to assess for pathologic phenotypic changes.

AUTHOR CONTRIBUTIONS

All authors read and approved the final version of the article.

CLINICS CARE POINTS

- Dilated left ventricle-Pronounced left ventricular dilation is typically found in those with high cumulative exposure to vigorous endurance exercise and not expected in the more casual athlete.
- Dilated right ventricle-38% of patients with mild ARVC have a normal ECG, highlighting the importance of a comprehensive evaluation to help differentiate EICR from ARVC.
- Left ventricular hypertrophy-Pronounced LVH in athletes (> 13-15 mm in men and > 12-14 mm in women) is seen only in a minority of athletes and may overlap with mild forms of HCM.
- Hypertrabeculation-Athletes with physiologic hypertrabeculation typically have a normal ECG, normal left ventricular systolic and diastolic function, and normal thickness compacted myocardium.

CONFLICTS OF INTEREST

The authors certify that there is no commercial or financial conflict of interest regarding the material discussed in the article.
    Funding: none.

DISCLOSURE

The authors have nothing to disclose.

REFERENCES

1. Sharma S, Drezner JA, Baggish A, et al. International Recommendations for Electrocardiographic Interpretation in Athletes. J Am Coll Cardiol 2017;69:1057–75.
2. Baggish AL, Battle RW, Beaver TA, et al. Recommendations on the Use of Multimodality Cardiovascular Imaging in Young Adult Competitive Athletes: A Report from the American Society of Echocardiography in Collaboration with the Society of Cardiovascular Computed Tomography and the Society for Cardiovascular Magnetic Resonance. J Am Soc Echocardiogr 2020;33:523–49.
3. Weiner RB, Baggish AL. Exercise-induced cardiac remodeling. Prog Cardiovasc Dis 2012;54:380–6.
4. Wasfy MM, Weiner RB, Wang F, et al. Endurance Exercise-Induced Cardiac Remodeling: Not All Sports Are Created Equal. J Am Soc Echocardiogr 2015;28: 1434–40.
5. Engel DJ, Schwartz A, Homma S. Athletic Cardiac Remodeling in US Professional Basketball Players. JAMA Cardiol 2016;1:80–7.
6. Wasfy MM, Weiner RB, Wang F, et al. Myocardial Adaptations to Competitive Swim Training. Med Sci Sports Exerc 2019;51:1987–94.
7. Shames S, Bello NA, Schwartz A, et al. Echocardiographic Characterization of Female Professional Basketball Players in the US. JAMA Cardiol 2020;5:991–8.

8. Churchill TW, Petek BJ, Wasfy MM, et al. Cardiac Structure and Function in Elite Female and Male Soccer Players. JAMA Cardiol 2021;6:316–25.

9. D'Ascenzi F, Biella F, Lemme E, et al. Female Athlete's Heart: Sex Effects on Electrical and Structural Remodeling. Circ Cardiovasc Imaging 2020;13:e011587.

10. Finocchiaro G, Dhutia H, D'Silva A, et al. Effect of Sex and Sporting Discipline on LV Adaptation to Exercise. JACC Cardiovasc Imaging 2017;10:965–72.

11. Rawlins J, Carre F, Kervio G, et al. Ethnic differences in physiological cardiac adaptation to intense physical exercise in highly trained female athletes. Circulation 2010;121:1078–85.

12. Abergel E, Chatellier G, Hagege AA, et al. Serial left ventricular adaptations in world-class professional cyclists: implications for disease screening and follow-up. J Am Coll Cardiol 2004;44:144–9.

13. Pelliccia A, Culasso F, Di Paolo FM, et al. Physiologic left ventricular cavity dilatation in elite athletes. Ann Intern Med 1999;130:23–31.

14. Maron BJ, Zipes DP, Kovacs RJ. Eligibility and Disqualification Recommendations for Competitive Athletes With Cardiovascular Abnormalities: Preamble, Principles, and General Considerations: A Scientific Statement From the American Heart Association and American College of Cardiology. J Am Coll Cardiol 2015;66:2343–9.

15. Baggish AL, Ackerman MJ, Putukian M, et al. Shared Decision Making for Athletes with Cardiovascular Disease: Practical Considerations. Curr Sports Med Rep 2019;18:76–81.

16. Yancy CW, Jessup M, Bozkurt B, et al. ACCF/AHA guideline for the management of heart failure: a report of the American College of Cardiology Foundation/American Heart Association Task Force on Practice Guidelines. J Am Coll Cardiol 2013;62:e147–239.

17. Bar-Shlomo BZ, Druck MN, Morch JE, et al. Left ventricular function in trained and untrained healthy subjects. Circulation 1982;65:484–8.

18. Bekaert I, Pannier JL, Van de Weghe C, et al. Non-invasive evaluation of cardiac function in professional cyclists. Br Heart J 1981;45:213–8.

19. Lang RM, Badano LP, Mor-Avi V, et al. Recommendations for cardiac chamber quantification by echocardiography in adults: an update from the American Society of Echocardiography and the European Association of Cardiovascular Imaging. J Am Soc Echocardiogr 2015;28:1–39 e14.

20. Pelliccia A, Maron BJ, Culasso F, et al. Athlete's heart in women. Echocardiographic characterization of highly trained elite female athletes. JAMA 1996;276:211–5.

21. Millar LM, Fanton Z, Finocchiaro G, et al. Differentiation between athlete's heart and dilated cardiomyopathy in athletic individuals. Heart 2020;106:1059–65.

22. Baggish AL, Wang F, Weiner RB, et al. Training-specific changes in cardiac structure and function: a prospective and longitudinal assessment of competitive athletes. J Appl Physiol (1985) 2008;104:1121–8.

23. Caselli S, Montesanti D, Autore C, et al. Patterns of left ventricular longitudinal strain and strain rate in Olympic athletes. J Am Soc Echocardiogr 2015;28:245–53.

24. Pelliccia A, Maron BJ, De Luca R, et al. Remodeling of left ventricular hypertrophy in elite athletes after long-term deconditioning. Circulation 2002;105:944–9.

25. Scharhag J, Schneider G, Urhausen A, et al. Athlete's heart: right and left ventricular mass and function in male endurance athletes and untrained individuals determined by magnetic resonance imaging. J Am Coll Cardiol 2002;40:1856–63.

26. Scharf M, Brem MH, Wilhelm M, et al. Cardiac magnetic resonance assessment of left and right ventricular morphologic and functional adaptations in professional soccer players. Am Heart J 2010;159:911–8.

27. D'Ascenzi F, Pisicchio C, Caselli S, et al. RV Remodeling in Olympic Athletes. JACC Cardiovasc Imaging 2017;10:385–93.

28. Marcus FI, McKenna WJ, Sherrill D, et al. Diagnosis of arrhythmogenic right ventricular cardiomyopathy/dysplasia: proposed modification of the task force criteria. Circulation 2010;121:1533–41.

29. Prior D, La Gerche A. Exercise and Arrhythmogenic Right Ventricular Cardiomyopathy. Heart Lung Circ 2020;29:547–55.

30. Sanz-de la Garza M, Carro A, Caselli S. How to interpret right ventricular remodeling in athletes. Clin Cardiol 2020;43:843–51.

31. Kim JH, Noseworthy PA, McCarty D, et al. Significance of electrocardiographic right bundle branch block in trained athletes. Am J Cardiol 2011;107:1083–9.

32. Bauce B, Frigo G, Benini G, et al. Differences and similarities between arrhythmogenic right ventricular cardiomyopathy and athlete's heart adaptations. Br J Sports Med 2010;44:148–54.

33. D'Ascenzi F, Pelliccia A, Corrado D, et al. Right ventricular remodelling induced by exercise training in competitive athletes. Eur Heart J Cardiovasc Imaging 2016;17:301–7.

34. Oxborough D, Sharma S, Shave R, et al. The right ventricle of the endurance athlete: the relationship between morphology and deformation. J Am Soc Echocardiogr 2012;25:263–71.

35. Lang RM, Badano LP, Mor-Avi V, et al. Recommendations for cardiac chamber quantification by echocardiography in adults: an update from the American Society of Echocardiography and the European Association of Cardiovascular Imaging. Eur Heart J Cardiovasc Imaging 2015;16:233–70.

36. Phelan D, Kim JH, Elliott MD, et al. Screening of Potential Cardiac Involvement in Competitive Athletes Recovering From COVID-19: An Expert Consensus Statement. JACC Cardiovasc Imaging 2020;13:2635–52.

37. D'Andrea A, Riegler L, Morra S, et al. Right ventricular morphology and function in top-level athletes: a three-dimensional echocardiographic study. J Am Soc Echocardiogr 2012;25:1268–76.

38. Prakken NH, Velthuis BK, Teske AJ, et al. Cardiac MRI reference values for athletes and nonathletes corrected for body surface area, training hours/week and sex. Eur J Cardiovasc Prev Rehabil 2010;17:198–203.

39. Teske AJ, Prakken NH, De Boeck BW, et al. Echocardiographic tissue deformation imaging of right ventricular systolic function in endurance athletes. Eur Heart J 2009;30:969–77.

40. Saberniak J, Leren IS, Haland TF, et al. Comparison of patients with early-phase arrhythmogenic right ventricular cardiomyopathy and right ventricular outflow tract ventricular tachycardia. Eur Heart J Cardiovasc Imaging 2017;18:62–9.

41. Qasem M, George K, Somauroo J, et al. Right ventricular function in elite male athletes meeting the structural echocardiographic task force criteria for arrhythmogenic right ventricular cardiomyopathy. J Sports Sci 2019;37:306–12.

42. La Gerche A, Burns AT, Mooney DJ, et al. Exercise-induced right ventricular dysfunction and structural remodelling in endurance athletes. Eur Heart J 2012;33:998–1006.

43. Aengevaeren VL, Caselli S, Pisicchio C, et al. Right Heart Remodeling in Olympic Athletes During 8 Years of Intensive Exercise Training. J Am Coll Cardiol 2018;72:815–7.

44. Bohm P, Schneider G, Linneweber L, et al. Right and Left Ventricular Function and Mass in Male Elite Master Athletes: A Controlled Contrast-Enhanced Cardiovascular Magnetic Resonance Study. Circulation 2016;133:1927–35.

45. La Gerche A, Burns AT, D'Hooge J, et al. Exercise strain rate imaging demonstrates normal right ventricular contractile reserve and clarifies ambiguous resting measures in endurance athletes. J Am Soc Echocardiogr 2012;25: 253–262 e1.

46. Sharma S. Athlete's heart–effect of age, sex, ethnicity and sporting discipline. Exp Physiol 2003;88:665–9.

47. Pelliccia A, Maron BJ, Spataro A, et al. The upper limit of physiologic cardiac hypertrophy in highly trained elite athletes. N Engl J Med 1991;324:295–301.

48. Basavarajaiah S, Wilson M, Whyte G, et al. Prevalence of hypertrophic cardiomyopathy in highly trained athletes: relevance to pre-participation screening. J Am Coll Cardiol 2008;51:1033–9.

49. Basavarajaiah S, Boraita A, Whyte G, et al. Ethnic differences in left ventricular remodeling in highly-trained athletes relevance to differentiating physiologic left ventricular hypertrophy from hypertrophic cardiomyopathy. J Am Coll Cardiol 2008;51:2256–62.

50. Kim JH, Baggish AL. Differentiating Exercise-Induced Cardiac Adaptations From Cardiac Pathology: The "Grey Zone" of Clinical Uncertainty. Can J Cardiol 2016; 32:429–37.

51. Ommen SR, Mital S, Burke MA, et al. AHA/ACC Guideline for the Diagnosis and Treatment of Patients With Hypertrophic Cardiomyopathy: Executive Summary: A Report of the American College of Cardiology/American Heart Association Joint Committee on Clinical Practice Guidelines. Circulation 2020;142:e533–57.

52. Maron BJ, Shirani J, Poliac LC, et al. Sudden death in young competitive athletes. Clinical, demographic, and pathological profiles. JAMA 1996;276:199–204.

53. Maron BJ. Sudden death in young athletes. N Engl J Med 2003;349:1064–75.

54. Peterson DF, Kucera K, Thomas LC, et al. Aetiology and incidence of sudden cardiac arrest and death in young competitive athletes in the USA: a 4-year prospective study. Br J Sports Med 2021;55:1196–203.

55. Sheikh N, Papadakis M, Schnell F, et al. Clinical Profile of Athletes With Hypertrophic Cardiomyopathy. Circ Cardiovasc Imaging 2015;8:e003454.

56. Rowin EJ, Maron BJ, Appelbaum E, et al. Significance of false negative electrocardiograms in preparticipation screening of athletes for hypertrophic cardiomyopathy. Am J Cardiol 2012;110:1027–32.

57. Schnell F, Riding N, O'Hanlon R, et al. Recognition and significance of pathological T-wave inversions in athletes. Circulation 2015;131:165–73.

58. Caselli S, Maron MS, Urbano-Moral JA, et al. Differentiating left ventricular hypertrophy in athletes from that in patients with hypertrophic cardiomyopathy. Am J Cardiol 2014;114:1383–9.

59. Maron BJ. Distinguishing hypertrophic cardiomyopathy from athlete's heart: a clinical problem of increasing magnitude and significance. Heart 2005;91: 1380–2.

60. Weiner RB, Wang F, Isaacs SK, et al. Blood pressure and left ventricular hypertrophy during American-style football participation. Circulation 2013;128:524–31.

61. Lin J, Wang F, Weiner RB, et al. Blood Pressure and LV Remodeling Among American-Style Football Players. JACC Cardiovasc Imaging 2016;9:1367–76.

62. Swoboda PP, Erhayiem B, McDiarmid AK, et al. Relationship between cardiac deformation parameters measured by cardiovascular magnetic resonance and aerobic fitness in endurance athletes. J Cardiovasc Magn Reson 2016;18:48.

63. Schnell F, Matelot D, Daudin M, et al. Mechanical Dispersion by Strain Echocardiography: A Novel Tool to Diagnose Hypertrophic Cardiomyopathy in Athletes. J Am Soc Echocardiogr 2017;30:251–61.

64. Maron MS, Maron BJ, Harrigan C, et al. Hypertrophic cardiomyopathy phenotype revisited after 50 years with cardiovascular magnetic resonance. J Am Coll Cardiol 2009;54:220–8.

65. Sheikh N, Papadakis M, Panoulas VF, et al. Comparison of hypertrophic cardiomyopathy in Afro-Caribbean versus white patients in the UK. Heart 2016;102: 1797–804.

66. Rudolph A, Abdel-Aty H, Bohl S, et al. Noninvasive detection of fibrosis applying contrast-enhanced cardiac magnetic resonance in different forms of left ventricular hypertrophy relation to remodeling. J Am Coll Cardiol 2009;53:284–91.

67. Wilson M, O'Hanlon R, Prasad S, et al. Diverse patterns of myocardial fibrosis in lifelong, veteran endurance athletes. J Appl Physiol (1985) 2011;110:1622–6.

68. Sharma S, Elliott PM, Whyte G, et al. Utility of metabolic exercise testing in distinguishing hypertrophic cardiomyopathy from physiologic left ventricular hypertrophy in athletes. J Am Coll Cardiol 2000;36:864–70.

69. Maron BJ, Pelliccia A, Spataro A, et al. Reduction in left ventricular wall thickness after deconditioning in highly trained Olympic athletes. Br Heart J 1993;69:125–8.

70. Weiner RB, Wang F, Berkstresser B, et al. Regression of "gray zone" exercise-induced concentric left ventricular hypertrophy during prescribed detraining. J Am Coll Cardiol 2012;59:1992–4.

71. Caselli S, Attenhofer Jost CH, Jenni R, et al. Left Ventricular Noncompaction Diagnosis and Management Relevant to Pre-participation Screening of Athletes. Am J Cardiol 2015;116:801–8.

72. Poscolieri B, Bianco M, Vessella T, et al. Identification of benign form of ventricular non-compaction in competitive athletes by multiparametric evaluation. Int J Cardiol 2014;176:1134–6.

73. Arbustini E, Favalli V, Narula N, et al. Left Ventricular Noncompaction: A Distinct Genetic Cardiomyopathy? J Am Coll Cardiol 2016;68:949–66.

74. Brosnan MJ, Rakhit D. Differentiating Athlete's Heart From Cardiomyopathies - The Left Side. Heart Lung Circ 2018;27:1052–62.

75. Gati S, Chandra N, Bennett RL, et al. Increased left ventricular trabeculation in highly trained athletes: do we need more stringent criteria for the diagnosis of left ventricular non-compaction in athletes? Heart 2013;99:401–8.

76. Jenni R, Oechslin E, Schneider J, et al. Echocardiographic and pathoanatomical characteristics of isolated left ventricular non-compaction: a step towards classification as a distinct cardiomyopathy. Heart 2001;86:666–71.

77. de la Chica JA, Gomez-Talavera S, Garcia-Ruiz JM, et al. Association Between Left Ventricular Noncompaction and Vigorous Physical Activity. J Am Coll Cardiol 2020;76:1723–33.

78. Petersen SE, Selvanayagam JB, Wiesmann F, et al. Left ventricular non-compaction: insights from cardiovascular magnetic resonance imaging. J Am Coll Cardiol 2005;46:101–5.

79. Chin TK, Perloff JK, Williams RG, et al. Isolated noncompaction of left ventricular myocardium. A study of eight cases. Circulation 1990;82:507–13.

80. Gati S, Sharma S. CardioPulse: the dilemmas in diagnosing left ventricular non-compaction in athletes. Eur Heart J 2015;36:891–3.

81. Rao Shiavax, Shah Ankit. Exercise and the Female Heart. Clinical Therapeutics 2021;44(1):41–9. https://doi.org/10.1016/j.clinthera.2021.11.018. In press.

Exercise Stress Testing in Athletes

Gary Parizher, MD, Michael S. Emery, MD, MS*

KEYWORDS

- Exercise stress test • Athlete's heart • Sports cardiology
- Hypertrophic cardiomyopathy • Congenital coronary anomaly
- Cardiopulmonary exercise testing

KEY POINTS

- There are unique indications for exercise stress testing in athletes that typically emphasize evaluating the risk of intense training/competition.
- Treadmill protocols used for the general population are often poorly suited for athletes.
- A cycle ergometer, which integrates smoothly with cardiopulmonary exercise testing, can provide additional information.
- Extensive customization of an exercise protocol may be necessary for a complete evaluation.

INTRODUCTION

Exercise stress testing (EST) is an established noninvasive method for assessment of cardiac function in the general population. Diagnosis of coronary disease, assessment of exercise capacity, risk-stratification for cardiac events, and prognostication in the context of cardiac pathologic condition are all possible with modern EST modalities.[1] Athletes, by virtue of their training, exhibit different performance characteristics on EST compared with their untrained counterparts.[2] EST protocols in athletes are therefore necessarily different compared with protocols used in the general population. Although athletes share indications for stress testing with the general population, there are indications that are unique to the competitive athlete, such as providing the athlete with information about overall fitness and informing training regimens. In the sports cardiology community, indications for EST in athletes also revolve around assessment of risk of sudden cardiac death (SCD) during athletic activities, estimated at 1 in 50,000 athletes per year at the NCAA level.[3] Although rare, these events are tragic, and efforts in the sports cardiology community to refine risk-stratification strategies are ongoing.

Sports Cardiology Center, Heart, Vascular, and Thoracic Institute, Cleveland Clinic, Cleveland, OH, USA
* Corresponding author. Sports Cardiology Center, Heart, Vascular, and Thoracic Institute, Cleveland Clinic, 9500 Euclid Avenue, Desk J2-4, Cleveland, OH 44195, USA
E-mail address: emerym2@ccf.org

Stress tests can play a crucial role in this assessment, so understanding their performance in an athlete is essential for the practitioner caring for this population.

GENERAL INDICATIONS FOR EXERCISE STRESS TESTING IN ATHLETES

EST offers a useful demonstration of exercise capacity and can evaluate fitness and inform exercise regimens.[4] In athletes presenting with abnormal signs and symptoms, such as dyspnea, chest pain, or evidence of conduction disease, clinicians can use stress testing to diagnose a cardiac/pulmonary condition just as in the general population.[5] The deliberate provocation of symptoms using prescribed exercise under monitored conditions offers both a diagnostic and a prognostic yield. Stress testing can be used to quantify exercise capacity, monitor the hemodynamic response to exercise, or determine the mechanism underlying impaired performance in trained athletes. In addition, athletes with known cardiovascular abnormalities are at increased risk for exertion-related SCD compared with their healthy counterparts. Therefore, an EST that identifies a cardiovascular abnormality can also provide information to impact risk-stratification and eligibility for athletic competition.[6,7] In fact, deliberate provocation of arrhythmias, hemodynamic changes, and symptoms in athletes with known cardiovascular conditions to determine safety of competition is a unique indication for EST in this population.[4] Many conditions, including arrhythmias and coronary abnormalities, can be evaluated with EST; a detailed discussion of specific indications can be found in a later section of this review.

HOW TO APPROACH EXERCISE TESTING IN ATHLETES: PROTOCOLS, MODALITIES, AND EQUIPMENT

When performing EST in athletes, it is important to reproduce the physiologic conditions under which they experience symptoms and/or conditions they experience in competition and training.[4] Multiple graded-workload and fixed-workload exercise treadmill tests have been compared in their ability to elicit a subject's maximal exercise capacity.[8–10] The Bruce protocol, which evolved during the 1950s, is the most commonly performed treadmill exercise test in the United States and can predict cardiovascular risk in the general population.[11–13] The Bruce treadmill protocol uses sequential 90-second intervals with increments in both speed and grade. Trained athletes, often capable of withstanding a longer stress test than members of the general population, can progress to higher grades at which point local leg muscle fatigue can be limiting.[14] This can result in premature test termination before achievement of maximum cardiovascular stress, thereby rendering a nondiagnostic test. The Astrand and Costill/Fox protocols, which start at higher speeds and change grades more gently, more reliably elicit maximal cardiovascular stress in individuals with athletic training and can still be completed within 10 to 12 minutes.[14–17]

Although treadmill stress tests yield a maximal oxygen consumption 8% to 12% higher than that from a bicycle ergometer test, the latter still has its place in the testing of athletes.[18–20] Despite limitations, cycle ergometers offer several advantages in comparison to treadmills: decreased noise on electrocardiographic (ECG) tracings owing to reduced upper-body movement, direct measurement of subjects' power output, lower equipment cost, easier measurement of blood pressure, ease of simultaneous echocardiography, and a smaller footprint in the testing room.[21] In fact, athletes who are accustomed to cycling as a form of training and/or competition may be able to use their own bicycles connected to a validated commercially available ergometer unit.[22] Manual braking cycle ergometers maintain an adjustable steady resistance, resulting in a constant workload as long as the subject can maintain pedaling speed, whereas more modern electronic braking models automatically adjust resistance to maintain a specified workload independent of pedaling speed.[23] This unique functionality enabled the pioneering of ramp protocols in the 1980s, in which the work rate increases in steady linear fashion over the course of the exercise test.[24] Grades can be customized to elicit test durations of approximately 10 minutes, and ramp tests can more precisely quantify exercise capacity than tests using arbitrarily chosen difficulty intervals.[25] The flexibility inherent to a ramp protocol is important in customizing a stress test for athletes. Moreover, ramp tests lend themselves well to cardiopulmonary exercise testing (CPX). Examples of testing protocols are shown in **Table 1**.

Ultimately, neither a treadmill nor a cycle ergometer may be the best equipment to mimic the workload an athlete encounters in competition or training. Alternative methods may be necessary for a more faithful reproduction of an athlete's peak exertion, and customized exercise protocols have demonstrated improvement in diagnostic yield.[26] For example, exercise tolerance in cross-country skiers has been assessed with a rollerski treadmill.[27] A stationary rowing ergometer has been used to assess competitive rowers.[28] A variety of agility and jumping tests have been described to test basketball players.[29] Burst interval stress tests have demonstrated improved diagnostic utility in a small cohort of patients with catecholaminergic polymorphic ventricular tachycardia.[30] ECG data could be gathered easily (albeit possibly with increased noise), and echo images can be obtained at rest and immediately after cessation of exercise during the recovery period. In some cases, arrhythmias may be

Table 1
Selected exercise stress tests and their characteristics

Exercise Stress Test	Characteristics
Treadmill	
Bruce protocol	• Most common exercise treadmill test performed in the United States • Leg fatigue from prolonged test and high treadmill grade can render test suboptimal in athletes
Cornell protocol	• Common exercise treadmill test in the general population • More gentle increments in metabolic demand compared with the Bruce protocol
Astrand protocol	• Constant speed (5 mph) with sequential increase in grade • Duration limited more by cardiovascular reserve than leg fatigue in trained individuals
Costill/Fox protocol	• Constant speed (9 mph) with sequential increase in grade • Highly demanding test; used to quantify metabolic demands in elite marathon runners
Cycle ergometer	• Smaller footprint in testing room • Less motion artifact on electrocardiography and echocardiography • May underrepresent exercise capacity in athletes not accustomed to cycling • Typically yields maximum oxygen consumption approximately 10% lower than treadmill exercise tests • Ideal for ramp protocols and cardiopulmonary exercise testing
Custom/unconventional stress test	• Useful to accurately reproduce conditions of training and competition • Typically used to provoke symptoms and/or arrhythmias • Requires flexibility in equipment use and data acquisition • Examples include burst/sprint tests, agility tests, and others

detected with a wearable heart monitor applied during exercise with data captured remotely. Examples of athletes undergoing stress testing are shown in **Fig. 1.**

Standard equipment for conducting stress testing, in addition to the exercise machine, includes a blood pressure cuff, ECG monitors, and potentially imaging equipment, such as an echocardiography machine depending on the question the test is meant to address. Gas exchange equipment is necessary for conduction of cardiopulmonary testing. A lactate monitor can be useful during nongraded or ramp exercise testing to help identify the lactate threshold, which in turn can help interpret the athlete's fitness level, discussed in more detail later.[31–33] Exercise nuclear tests, typically used to evaluate coronary artery disease in adults, can be useful in the evaluation of young athletes with congenital anomalies of the coronary arteries.[34] In addition, resuscitative equipment, including an external defibrillator, should be present at all times during stress testing in case of life-threatening emergencies, such as arrhythmias.[35]

STRESS TESTING IN SPECIFIC CONDITIONS
Hypertrophic Cardiomyopathy

Hypertrophic cardiomyopathy (HCM) is the most common cause of SCD in athletes in the United States, and engaging in competitive sports is an independent risk factor for SCD in patients with HCM.[7,36,37] EST is demonstrably safe and useful in HCM despite previous guidelines suggesting it is relatively contraindicated in this condition.[38] Normal physiologic ventricular remodeling that takes place in response to loading conditions imposed by athletic training can be difficult to distinguish from pathologic hypertrophy.[39] In established cases of HCM, stress testing is recommended to provoke a dynamic left ventricular outflow tract (LVOT) gradient and determine its contribution to symptoms, evaluate exercise capacity, and assess response to therapy.[40] Although EST is appropriate to perform in athletes with HCM to manage their pathologic condition, the ability to predict overt risk of SCA during sporting activity is limited. Traditionally, athletes who manifest a definite HCM phenotype, as determined by echocardiography and/or cardiac MRI, are recommended not to participate in most competitive sports regardless of stress testing results, with the exception of low-intensity sports.[41,42] However, more contemporary data have been discordant with regards to risk of SCA during sporting activities attributable to HCM, and the recently updated HCM guidelines focused more on a shared decision-making approach to sporting participation after a comprehensive evaluation with an expert provider, which should include an EST.[40]

Coronary Pathologic Condition

The second most common cause of SCD in young athletes in the United States is congenital coronary anomalies.[7] This pathologic condition is a challenge for clinicians because, although it can manifest with typical exertional angina and abnormal EST, it can also be asymptomatic, and indeed the index presentation may be SCD.[43] EST can be falsely negative among people with these anomalies, and echocardiography will only detect some, so contrast-enhanced computed tomography and/or coronary angiography remain the gold standard in diagnosis.[44–47] However, EST still plays an important role in the management of coronary anomalies once they are identified. Athletes with an anomalous origin of a right coronary artery from the left sinus of Valsalva are recommended to undergo EST for risk-stratification, as those without symptoms or abnormal findings can be permitted to compete bearing in mind the risk of a false-negative test.[48] Those with an abnormal stress test and those with an anomalous origin of a left coronary artery from the right sinus of Valsalva should be restricted from competition in all except low-intensity sports until surgical repair. Anomalous origin of

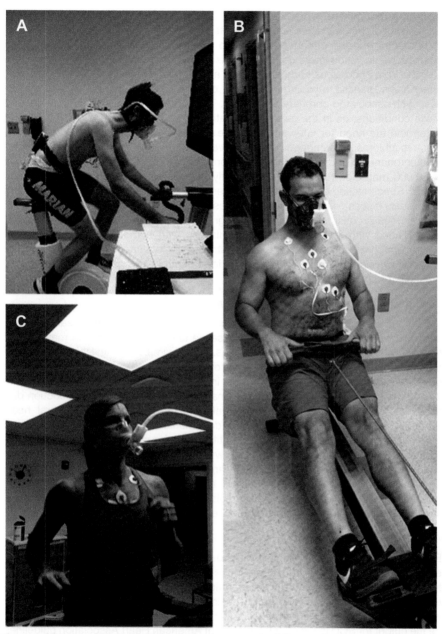

Fig. 1. Athletes undergoing SCD using a cycle ergometer (*A*), a rowing ergometer (*B*), and a treadmill (*C*). Displayed with permission from the athletes.

a coronary artery from the pulmonary artery is rare and usually results in myocardial infarction in early childhood.[49] Because of cardiac compromise, these patients are unlikely to engage in rigorous athletic training and competition; nonetheless, guidelines recommend restricting participation in low-intensity sports until surgical revascularization. Three months after surgical correction of congenital coronary anomalies, guidelines recommend repeat stress testing; asymptomatic individuals with reassuring results can be counseled and participate with lifted restrictions. Notably, exercise or dobutamine is the preferred stressor to assess anomalous coronary arteries, as pharmacologic vasodilators do not mimic ischemic physiology in this condition.[50,51]

Aside from anomalous coronary origins, athletes can manifest atherosclerotic coronary artery disease, myocardial bridging, coronary artery spasm, or Kawasaki disease with associated coronary aneurysms. The role of stress testing in athletes with these conditions, as in the general population, is to quantify exercise capacity and determine the need for intervention before participation in strenuous exercise.[52] In masters athletes, who engage in competitive sport in midlife and beyond, atherosclerotic coronary artery disease is the most common relevant form of heart disease. One in 50,000 marathon runners, predominantly men, is estimated to suffer SCD each year.[53] Stress testing can be used in masters athletes to render a de novo diagnosis of coronary disease, evaluate the status of established coronary disease to assess risk of strenuous exercise, and monitor for progression of known stable disease via serial tests. Those with established coronary disease with hemodynamically significant obstruction are recommended to be restricted to low-intensity sports, as acute vigorous physical exertion may trigger sudden death or myocardial infarction in the presence of coronary obstruction.[54]

Conduction, Valvular, and Congenital Disease

Indications for EST in athletes with manifest structural congenital heart disease, valvular heart disease, and conduction disease are similar to those in members of the general population with these conditions.[55,56] Maximal EST with Doppler echocardiography can be used to confirm absence of symptoms or elevated pulmonary artery pressures, which may otherwise constitute indications for correction of the abnormality and restriction on competition.[57] In management of athletes with conduction disease, such as bradyarrhythmia, rare ventricular ectopy without structural heart disease, or manifest accessory pathways, documented resolution of the ECG abnormality with exercise suggests that competition may be safe.[58,59] Provocation of arrhythmias or other ECG abnormalities with stress testing, on the other hand, suggests the need for further evaluation and treatment before lifting restrictions on training and competition.[60] For example, athletes with catecholaminergic polymorphic ventricular tachycardia should be restricted from all but low-intensity sports if stress testing provokes ventricular ectopy, even in asymptomatic individuals.[61]

Asymptomatic Athletes

EST in the asymptomatic individual with no known cardiovascular or pulmonary disease is the subject of ongoing debate in the Sports Cardiology community.[62] The International Olympic Committee and Federation International Football Association both mandate ECG stress testing as part of their preparticipation screening protocols for athletes ≥35 years old.[63] As atherosclerotic coronary artery disease is more likely to be the culprit for SCD in older athletes, current American Heart Association guidelines recommend routine EST as part of preparticipation evaluation in asymptomatic men age ≥40 to 45 years of age and women age ≥50 to 55 years of age with at least 1 coronary risk factor.[53,54] European guidelines also recommend routine stress testing before participation in sports for selected high-risk individuals, with age being an important risk factor.[64] On the other hand, in the robust Italian government-mandated national preparticipation program, prospective studies have demonstrated a benign prognosis in younger asymptomatic athletes in the absence of structural heart disease regardless of EST results.[65,66] Although sensitivity of preparticipation evaluation for cardiac pathologic condition improves with the inclusion of routine EST, the positive predictive value of EST drops. At present, there is no guideline recommendation to perform EST in young asymptomatic athletes without established structural heart disease or risk factors for coronary artery disease.

CARDIOPULMONARY EXERCISE TESTING IN ATHLETES

CPX involves the use of specialized equipment to directly measure minute ventilation (VE) as well as partial pressures of expired gasses on a breath-by-breath basis, thereby yielding rates of oxygen consumption (V_{O_2}) and carbon dioxide production (V_{CO_2}) during exercise. Commercially available equipment and software packages gather and display extensive data in multiple graphical formats, which can be intimidating to the unfamiliar provider, resulting in underutilization of this useful testing modality. However, when applied to the competitive athlete, CPX can provide important diagnostic information to elucidate causes of symptoms as well as assist in assessing fitness and creating a specific prescription for exercise. An exhaustive discussion of the performance and interpretation of CPX is beyond the scope of this review but can be found in published guidelines.[67–69] Nonetheless, several key variables assessed by CPX merit attention in the application of exercise testing to athletes.

The maximal rate of oxygen consumption during exercise (peak V_{O_2} or $V_{O_{2max}}$) is considered the metric that defines the limits of the cardiopulmonary system and is commonly interpreted to represent overall aerobic conditioning in athletes.[70] Peak V_{O_2} is typically limited in large part by the rate at which oxygen can be supplied to skeletal muscles and is closely correlated to maximum cardiac output, which is augmented by increased stroke volume in trained athletes.[71] This variable reflects the combined function of cardiac, pulmonary, and skeletal muscle systems, so it can be abnormal in a variety of conditions and therefore does not assist the clinician in distinguishing the specific cause of dyspnea or exercise intolerance. Moreover, although $V_{O_{2max}}$ is closely associated with aerobic performance, alone it does not account for competitive success, as exercise economy (oxygen consumption at a given exercise intensity) and lactate threshold, along with many other factors, also influence athletic performance.[72–74]

As exercise intensity increases, the energy demands of skeletal muscle exceed the oxygen delivery capacity of the cardiac and pulmonary systems, resulting in increasing contributions of anaerobic glycolysis to meet metabolic demands. This results in lactate accumulation with subsequent increased carbon dioxide production in excess of rising oxygen consumption. The point in the exercise test at which lactate begins to accumulate is referred to interchangeably in the literature as the anaerobic threshold, ventilatory threshold (VT), and lactate threshold; although these events are related, they are not physiologically identical.[75] VT can be identified with CPX by detecting the point at which the relationship between VE and V_{O_2} changes, as the excess carbon dioxide production drives an increase in VE disproportionate to the increase in V_{O_2}. Three manifestations of this time point are a change in the relationship between VCO_2 and V_{O_2} from linear to exponential, a progressive increase in the VE/V_{O_2} ratio without a corresponding increase in VE/VCO_2, and an increase in the end-tidal oxygen concentration without a corresponding decrease in the end-tidal carbon dioxide concentration.[76] The exercise intensity at which VT takes place, typically 50% to 65% of peak V_{O_2} (but sometimes higher in well trained athletes), is thought to represent the maximum workload that an athlete can sustain for an extended period.[77] VT is commonly used to guide exercise prescription in a highly individualized manner, and serial measurements of VT can be useful to assess change in exercise tolerance with training.[77,78]

Although achieving a specific diagnosis may not be possible, CPX can aid in the distinction between cardiovascular and pulmonary patterns of exercise limitation.[79] Basic spirometry measurements are built into CPX packages. Measurements of forced expiratory volume in 1 second before and after exercise can elucidate exercise-induced bronchoconstriction.[80] The maximum VE during exercise can be compared with maximum voluntary ventilation (MVV), which is calculated from a maneuver of deep and rapid breathing at rest. Although maximal VE approaching MVV, that is, a VE/MVV ratio $\geq$0.80 to 0.90, can be indicative of an athlete approaching his/her limits of pulmonary reserve during exercise, it is not necessarily abnormal in highly trained endurance athletes.[81,82] A cardiac cause of exercise intolerance can be suspected with an abnormal relationship between change in Vo_2 and change in exercise intensity. This relationship can be derived from a plot of Vo_2 and exercise wattage (W); however, it requires a lower-extremity exercise ergometer for direct measurement of power output.[83] In healthy adults, Vo_2 increases linearly and steadily with increasing work, yielding a $\Delta Vo_2/\Delta W$ slope, which is independent of an athlete's training level. A depressed $\Delta Vo_2/\Delta W$ slope is suggestive of cardiac dysfunction, and an inflection point in the $\Delta Vo_2/\Delta W$ relationship can indicate the onset of myocardial ischemia during exercise testing.[84] Normal values fall at approximately 10 ± 1 mL/min/W, and a lower limit of normal of 8.4 mL/min/W has been proposed for detection of cardiac pathologic condition.[85]

Some athletes experience symptoms when returning to competition after detraining; in these individuals, a decreased Vo_2 and VT in the absence of other abnormalities may suggest deconditioning. Suboptimal effort during EST can also be identified with CPX. The peak respiratory exchange ratio, defined as the highest recorded VCO_2/Vo_2 ratio, indicates an excellent exercise effort if the value falls at or above 1.10.[86] A plateau in Vo_2 despite increasing exercise intensity can also suggest maximal effort. These are more reliable indicators of exercise effort than the arbitrary 85% of maximal age-predicted heart rate.[87]

SUMMARY

The design of an EST for an athlete must take into account the unique demands of the athlete's training and competition, the presence and timing of symptoms, the question being asked of the clinician, and the available equipment. In the symptomatic athlete, every effort should be made to reproduce the conditions that provoke symptoms. Creative effort and unconventional methods are sometimes necessary to accomplish this objective. Apart from indications to evaluate symptoms, stress testing can provide valuable information about an athlete's fitness and inform training regimens, especially with the addition of comprehensive cardiopulmonary testing equipment. Interpretation of EST must also take into account how the results impact the athlete's eligibility to train and compete in high-intensity sports. Restricting an athlete's eligibility to compete can cause major deleterious effects on the athlete's mental health and career.[88] However, testing can also detect modifiable abnormalities, allowing the athlete to return to play unrestricted once successful treatment is completed. In this high-stakes decision, a well-done stress test can provide invaluable information to the treating clinician and remains a mainstay of the evaluation of the athletic heart.

CLINICS CARE POINTS

- Stress testing in an athlete needs to be tailored to the individual athlete's sport/training as well as to the scenario that provokes any symptoms being evaluated.

- An exercise stress test in an athlete should be taken to a true maximal level of exertion and not terminated at arbitrary stopping points (eg, 85% of age predicted maximal heart rate).
- Cardiopulmonary exercise testing is a valuable tool to investigate the integrative physiology of athletic performance (cardiac, pulmonary, musculoskeletal) as well as provide training zones in athletes with and without cardiac disorders.

DISCLOSURE

The authors have no financial competing interests to disclose.

REFERENCES

1. Gibbons RJ, Balady GJ, Beasley JW, et al. ACC/AHA guidelines for exercise testing: executive summary. a report of the American College of Cardiology/ American Heart Association Task Force on Practice Guidelines (Committee on Exercise Testing). Circulation 1997;96(1):345–54.
2. Lollgen H, Leyk D. Exercise testing in sports medicine. Dtsch Arztebl Int 2018; 115(24):409–16.
3. Harmon KG, Drezner JA, Wilson MG, et al. Incidence of sudden cardiac death in athletes: a state-of-the-art review. Br J Sports Med 2014;48(15):1185–92.
4. Sarma S, Levine BD. Beyond the Bruce protocol: advanced exercise testing for the sports cardiologist. Cardiol Clin 2016;34(4):603–8.
5. Garner KK, Pomeroy W, Arnold JJ. Exercise stress testing: indications and common questions. Am Fam Physician 2017;96(5):293–9.
6. Maron BJ, Zipes DP, Kovacs RJ, et al. Eligibility and disqualification recommendations for competitive athletes with cardiovascular abnormalities: preamble, principles, and general considerations: a scientific statement from the American Heart Association and American College of Cardiology. Circulation 2015;132(22): e256–61.
7. Maron BJ, Doerer JJ, Haas TS, et al. Sudden deaths in young competitive athletes: analysis of 1866 deaths in the United States, 1980-2006. Circulation 2009;119(8):1085–92.
8. Froelicher VF Jr, Brammell H, Davis G, et al. A comparison of three maximal treadmill exercise protocols. J Appl Physiol 1974;36(6):720–5.
9. Froelicher VF Jr, Brammell H, Davis G, et al. A comparison of the reproducibility and physiologic response to three maximal treadmill exercise protocols. Chest 1974;65(5):512–7.
10. Lukaski HC, Bolonchuk WW, Klevay LM. Comparison of metabolic responses and oxygen cost during maximal exercise using three treadmill protocols. J Sports Med Phys Fitness 1989;29(3):223–9.
11. Bruce RA, Blackmon JR, Jones JW, et al. Exercising testing in adult normal subjects and cardiac patients. Pediatrics 1963;32:742–56.
12. Stuart RJ Jr, Ellestad MH. National survey of exercise stress testing facilities. Chest 1980;77(1):94–7.
13. Shaw LJ, Peterson ED, Shaw LK, et al. Use of a prognostic treadmill score in identifying diagnostic coronary disease subgroups. Circulation 1998;98(16):1622–30.
14. Kang J, Chaloupka EC, Mastrangelo MA, et al. Physiological comparisons among three maximal treadmill exercise protocols in trained and untrained individuals. Eur J Appl Physiol 2001;84(4):291–5.

15. Costill DL, Fox EL. Energetics of marathon running. Med Sci Sports Exerc 1969; 1(2):81–6.
16. Davies B, Daggett A, Jakeman P, et al. Maximum oxygen uptake utilising different treadmill protocols. Br J Sports Med 1984;18(2):74–9.
17. Astrand PO, Saltin B. Oxygen uptake during the first minutes of heavy muscular exercise. J Appl Physiol 1961;16:971–6.
18. McKay GA, Banister EW. A comparison of maximum oxygen uptake determination by bicycle ergometry at various pedaling frequencies and by treadmill running at various speeds. Eur J Appl Physiol Occup Physiol 1976;35(3): 191–200.
19. Wicks JR, Sutton JR, Oldridge NB, et al. Comparison of the electrocardiographic changes induced by maximam exercise testing with treadmill and cycle ergometer. Circulation 1978;57(6):1066–70.
20. Niederberger M, Bruce RA, Kusumi F, et al. Disparities in ventilatory and circulatory responses to bicycle and treadmill exercise. Br Heart J 1974;36(4):377–82.
21. Lear SA, Brozic A, Myers JN, et al. Exercise stress testing. an overview of current guidelines. Sports Med 1999;27(5):285–312.
22. Lillo-Bevia JR, Pallares JG. Validity and reliability of the Cycleops hammer cycle ergometer. Int J Sports Physiol Perform 2018;13(7):853–9.
23. Pina IL, Balady GJ, Hanson P, et al. Guidelines for clinical exercise testing laboratories. a statement for healthcare professionals from the committee on exercise and cardiac rehabilitation, American Heart Association. Circulation 1995;91(3): 912–21.
24. Whipp BJ, Davis JA, Torres F, et al. A test to determine parameters of aerobic function during exercise. J Appl Physiol Respir Environ Exerc Physiol 1981; 50(1):217–21.
25. Myers J, Bellin D. Ramp exercise protocols for clinical and cardiopulmonary exercise testing. Sports Med 2000;30(1):23–9.
26. Churchill TW, Disanto M, Singh TK, et al. Diagnostic yield of customized exercise provocation following routine testing. Am J Cardiol 2019;123(12):2044–50.
27. Losnegard T, Mikkelsen K, Ronnestad BR, et al. The effect of heavy strength training on muscle mass and physical performance in elite cross country skiers. Scand J Med Sci Sports 2011;21(3):389–401.
28. Otter RT, Brink MS, Lamberts RP, et al. A new submaximal rowing test to predict 2,000-m rowing ergometer performance. J Strength Cond Res 2015;29(9): 2426–33.
29. Puente C, Abian-Vicen J, Salinero JJ, et al. Caffeine improves basketball performance in experienced basketball players. Nutrients 2017;9(9).
30. Roston TM, Kallas D, Davies B, et al. Burst exercise testing can unmask arrhythmias in patients with incompletely penetrant catecholaminergic polymorphic ventricular tachycardia. JACC Clin Electrophysiol 2021;7(4):437–41.
31. Coyle EF, Coggan AR, Hopper MK, et al. Determinants of endurance in well-trained cyclists. J Appl Physiol 1985;64(6):2622–30.
32. Abe D, Sakaguchi Y, Tsuchimochi H, et al. Assessment of long-distance running performance in elite male runners using onset of blood lactate accumulation. Appl Human Sci 1999;18(2):25–9.
33. Sjodin B, Jacobs I. Onset of blood lactate accumulation and marathon running performance. Int J Sports Med 1981;2(1):23–6.
34. Cremer PC, Mentias A, Koneru S, et al. Risk stratification with exercise N(13)-ammonia PET in adults with anomalous right coronary arteries. Open Heart 2016;3(2):e000490.

35. Link MS, Myerburg RJ, Estes NA 3rd, et al. Eligibility and disqualification recommendations for competitive athletes with cardiovascular abnormalities: task force 12: emergency action plans, resuscitation, cardiopulmonary resuscitation, and automated external defibrillators: a scientific statement from the American Heart Association and American College of Cardiology. Circulation 2015;132(22): e334–8.

36. Maron BJ, Ommen SR, Semsarian C, et al. Hypertrophic cardiomyopathy: present and future, with translation into contemporary cardiovascular medicine. J Am Coll Cardiol 2014;64(1):83–99.

37. Maron BJ. Clinical course and management of hypertrophic cardiomyopathy. N Engl J Med 2018;379(20):1977.

38. Drinko JK, Nash PJ, Lever HM, et al. Safety of stress testing in patients with hypertrophic cardiomyopathy. Am J Cardiol 2004;93(11):1443–4. A1412.

39. Maron BJ, Pelliccia A, Spirito P. Cardiac disease in young trained athletes. Insights into methods for distinguishing athlete's heart from structural heart disease, with particular emphasis on hypertrophic cardiomyopathy. Circulation 1995;91(5):1596–601.

40. Ommen SR, Mital S, Burke MA, et al. AHA/ACC guideline for the diagnosis and treatment of patients with hypertrophic cardiomyopathy: a report of the American College of Cardiology/American Heart Association Joint Committee on clinical practice guidelines. Circulation 2020;142(25):e558–631.

41. Levine BD, Baggish AL, Kovacs RJ, et al. Eligibility and disqualification recommendations for competitive athletes with cardiovascular abnormalities: task force 1: classification of sports: dynamic, static, and impact: a scientific statement from the American Heart Association and American College of Cardiology. J Am Coll Cardiol 2015;66(21):2350–5.

42. Maron BJ, Udelson JE, Bonow RO, et al. Eligibility and disqualification recommendations for competitive athletes with cardiovascular abnormalities: task force 3: hypertrophic cardiomyopathy, arrhythmogenic right ventricular cardiomyopathy and other cardiomyopathies, and myocarditis: a scientific statement from the American Heart Association and American College of Cardiology. Circulation 2015;132(22):e273–80.

43. Frommelt PC. Congenital coronary artery abnormalities predisposing to sudden cardiac death. Pacing Clin Electrophysiol 2009;32(2):S63–6.

44. Edwards CP, Yavari A, Sheppard MN, et al. Anomalous coronary origin: the challenge in preventing exercise-related sudden cardiac death. Br J Sports Med 2010;44(12):895–7.

45. Brothers JA, Frommelt MA, Jaquiss RDB, et al. Expert consensus guidelines: anomalous aortic origin of a coronary artery. J Thorac Cardiovasc Surg 2017; 153(6):1440–57.

46. Frommelt P, Lopez L, Dimas VV, et al. Recommendations for multimodality assessment of congenital coronary anomalies: a guide from the American Society of Echocardiography: developed in collaboration with the Society for Cardiovascular Angiography and Interventions, Japanese Society of Echocardiography, and Society for Cardiovascular Magnetic Resonance. J Am Soc Echocardiogr 2020;33(3):259–94.

47. Osaki M, McCrindle BW, Van Arsdell G, et al. Anomalous origin of a coronary artery from the opposite sinus of Valsalva with an interarterial course: clinical profile and approach to management in the pediatric population. Pediatr Cardiol 2008; 29(1):24–30.

48. Van Hare GF, Ackerman MJ, Evangelista JA, et al. Eligibility and disqualification recommendations for competitive athletes with cardiovascular abnormalities: task force 4: congenital heart disease: a scientific statement from the American Heart Association and American College of Cardiology. Circulation 2015; 132(22):e281–91.

49. Lardhi AA. Anomalous origin of left coronary artery from pulmonary artery: a rare cause of myocardial infarction in children. J Fam Community Med 2010;17(3): 113–6.

50. Chu E, Cheitlin MD. Diagnostic considerations in patients with suspected coronary artery anomalies. Am Heart J 1993;126(6):1427–38.

51. Lameijer H, Ter Maaten JM, Steggerda RC. Additive value of dobutamine stress echocardiography in patients with an anomalous origin of a coronary artery. Neth Heart J 2015;23(2):139–40.

52. Thompson PD, Myerburg RJ, Levine BD, et al. Eligibility and disqualification recommendations for competitive athletes with cardiovascular abnormalities: task force 8: coronary artery disease: a scientific statement from the American Heart Association and American College of Cardiology. J Am Coll Cardiol 2015;66(21): 2406–11.

53. Kim JH, Malhotra R, Chiampas G, et al. Cardiac arrest during long-distance running races. N Engl J Med 2012;366(2):130–40.

54. Maron BJ, Araujo CG, Thompson PD, et al. Recommendations for preparticipation screening and the assessment of cardiovascular disease in masters athletes: an advisory for healthcare professionals from the working groups of the World Heart Federation, the International Federation of Sports Medicine, and the American Heart Association Committee on Exercise, Cardiac Rehabilitation, and Prevention. Circulation 2001;103(2):327–34.

55. Stout KK, Daniels CJ, Aboulhosn JA, et al. AHA/ACC Guideline for the management of adults with congenital heart disease: a report of the American College of Cardiology/American Heart Association Task Force on clinical practice guidelines. Circulation 2018;139(14):e698–800.

56. Otto CM, Nishimura RA, Bonow RO, et al. ACC/AHA guideline for the management of patients with valvular heart disease: a report of the American College of Cardiology/American Heart Association Joint Committee on Clinical Practice Guidelines. Circulation 2020;143(5):e72–227.

57. Bonow RO, Nishimura RA, Thompson PD, et al. Eligibility and disqualification recommendations for competitive athletes with cardiovascular abnormalities: task force 5: valvular heart disease: a scientific statement from the American Heart Association and American College of Cardiology. J Am Coll Cardiol 2015;66(21): 2385–92.

58. Zipes DP, Link MS, Ackerman MJ, et al. Eligibility and disqualification recommendations for competitive athletes with cardiovascular abnormalities: task force 9: arrhythmias and conduction defects: a scientific statement from the American Heart Association and American College of Cardiology. Circulation 2015; 132(22):e315–25.

59. Lampert R. Evaluation and management of arrhythmia in the athletic patient. Prog Cardiovasc Dis 2012;54(5):423–31.

60. Makimoto H, Nakagawa E, Takaki H, et al. Augmented ST-segment elevation during recovery from exercise predicts cardiac events in patients with Brugada syndrome. J Am Coll Cardiol 2010;56(19):1576–84.

61. Ackerman MJ, Zipes DP, Kovacs RJ, et al. Eligibility and disqualification recommendations for competitive athletes with cardiovascular abnormalities: task force

10: the cardiac channelopathies: a scientific statement from the American Heart Association and American College of Cardiology. J Am Coll Cardiol 2015;66(21): 2424–8.

62. La Gerche A, Baggish AL, Knuuti J, et al. Cardiac imaging and stress testing asymptomatic athletes to identify those at risk of sudden cardiac death. JACC Cardiovasc Imaging 2013;6(9):993–1007.

63. Ljungqvist A, Jenoure P, Engebretsen L, et al. The International Olympic Committee (IOC) consensus statement on periodic health evaluation of elite athletes March 2009. Br J Sports Med 2009;43(9):631–43.

64. Heidbuchel H, Adami PE, Antz M, et al. Recommendations for participation in leisure-time physical activity and competitive sports in patients with arrhythmias and potentially arrhythmogenic conditions: part 1: supraventricular arrhythmias. a position statement of the section of sports cardiology and exercise from the European Association of Preventive Cardiology (EAPC) and the European Heart Rhythm Association (EHRA), both associations of the European Society of Cardiology. Eur J Prev Cardiol 2020;28(14):1539–51.

65. Verdile L, Maron BJ, Pelliccia A, et al. Clinical significance of exercise-induced ventricular tachyarrhythmias in trained athletes without cardiovascular abnormalities. Heart Rhythm 2015;12(1):78–85.

66. Zorzi A, Vessella T, De Lazzari M, et al. Screening young athletes for diseases at risk of sudden cardiac death: role of stress testing for ventricular arrhythmias. Eur J Prev Cardiol 2020;27(3):311–20.

67. Balady GJ, Arena R, Sietsema K, et al. Clinician's guide to cardiopulmonary exercise testing in adults: a scientific statement from the American Heart Association. Circulation 2010;122(2):191–225.

68. Guazzi M, Adams V, Conraads V, et al. EACPR/AHA scientific statement. Clinical recommendations for cardiopulmonary exercise testing data assessment in specific patient populations. Circulation 2012;126(18):2261–74.

69. Guazzi M, Arena R, Halle M, et al. Focused update: clinical recommendations for cardiopulmonary exercise testing data assessment in specific patient populations. Circulation 2016;133(24):e694–711.

70. Saltin B, Astrand PO. Maximal oxygen uptake in athletes. J Appl Physiol 1967; 23(3):353–8.

71. Levine BD. VO2max: what do we know, and what do we still need to know? J Physiol 2008;586(1):25–34.

72. Martin DE, Vroon DH, May DF, et al. Physiological changes in elite male distance runners training for Olympic competition. Phys Sportsmed 1986;14(1):152–206.

73. Conley DL, Krahenbuhl GS. Running economy and distance running performance of highly trained athletes. Med Sci Sports Exerc 1980;12(5):357–60.

74. Coyle EF, Feltner ME, Kautz SA, et al. Physiological and biomechanical factors associated with elite endurance cycling performance. Med Sci Sports Exerc 1991;23(1):93–107.

75. Wasserman K, Beaver WL, Whipp BJ. Gas exchange theory and the lactic acidosis (anaerobic) threshold. Circulation 1990;81(1 Suppl):II14–30.

76. Santos EL, Giannella-Neto A. Comparison of computerized methods for detecting the ventilatory thresholds. Eur J Appl Physiol 2004;93(3):315–24.

77. Arena R, Sietsema KE. Cardiopulmonary exercise testing in the clinical evaluation of patients with heart and lung disease. Circulation 2011;123(6):668–80.

78. Amann M, Subudhi AW, Walker J, et al. An evaluation of the predictive validity and reliability of ventilatory threshold. Med Sci Sports Exerc 2004;36(10):1716–22.

79. Weisman IM, Zeballos RJ. An integrated approach to the interpretation of cardiopulmonary exercise testing. Clin Chest Med 1994;15(2):421–45.
80. Crapo RO, Casaburi R, Coates AL, et al. Guidelines for methacholine and exercise challenge testing-1999. This official statement of the American Thoracic Society was adopted by the ATS board of directors, July 1999. Am J Respir Crit Care Med 2000;161(1):309–29.
81. Miyachi M, Shibayama H. Ventilatory capacity and exercise-induced arterial desaturation of highly trained endurance athletes. Ann Physiol Anthropol 1992; 11(3):263–7.
82. Hopkins SR, McKenzie DC, Schoene RB, et al. Pulmonary gas exchange during exercise in athletes. I. Ventilation-perfusion mismatch and diffusion limitation. J Appl Physiol 1985;77(2):912–7.
83. Palange P, Carlone S, Forte S, et al. Cardiopulmonary exercise testing in the evaluation of patients with ventilatory vs circulatory causes of reduced exercise tolerance. Chest 1994;105(4):1122–6.
84. Belardinelli R, Lacalaprice F, Carle F, et al. Exercise-induced myocardial ischaemia detected by cardiopulmonary exercise testing. Eur Heart J 2003; 24(14):1304–13.
85. Sietsema KE, Sue DY, Stringer WW, et al. Wasserman & Whipp's principles of exercise testing and interpretation 2021.
86. Ramos-Jimenez A, Hernandez-Torres RP, Torres-Duran PV, et al. The respiratory exchange ratio is associated with fitness indicators both in trained and untrained men: a possible application for people with reduced exercise tolerance. Clin Med Circ Respirat Pulm Med 2008;2:1–9.
87. Jain M, Nkonde C, Lin BA, et al. 85% of maximal age-predicted heart rate is not a valid endpoint for exercise treadmill testing. J Nucl Cardiol 2011;18(6):1026–35.
88. Putukian M. The psychological response to injury in student athletes: a narrative review with a focus on mental health. Br J Sports Med 2016;50(3):145–8.

Myocarditis in the Athlete
A Focus on COVID-19 Sequelae

John D. Symanski, MD[a],*, Jason V. Tso, MD[b],
Dermot M. Phelan, MD, PhD[a], Jonathan H. Kim, MD, MSc[b]

KEYWORDS

- Myocarditis • Athletes • Cardiac magnetic resonance imaging • SARS-CoV-2
- COVID-19

KEY POINTS

- Myocarditis is an inflammatory disease of the myocardium, frequently caused by viral infections, with a broad spectrum of clinical presentations from mild self-resolving symptoms to fulminant heart failure, arrhythmias, and death. It is an important cause of sudden cardiac death in athletes.
- Higher than expected prevalence of myocardial injury associated with severe adverse events in hospitalized patients with COVID-19 raised concern regarding the risk of return-to-play in athletes recovered from infection. Screening strategies were established to identify evidence of cardiac injury in such athletes.
- Small, single-center reports of minimally symptomatic SARS-CoV-2–infected athletes using cardiac MRI as a screening tool reported a wide range of incidence of cardiac injury. These studies have highlighted the importance of the judicious use of advanced imaging in such evaluations.
- Large multicenter registries of athletes have demonstrated a low incidence of significant cardiac injury, which is consistent with the observed prevalence of adverse events in this population. These reassuring data have lead to revision of screening recommendations in athletes post-COVID-19, with increasing focus on only evaluating those with clinical suspicion for myocarditis.
- On-going research is required to define the long-term risk of "subclinical myocarditis," the impact of COVID-19 variants, and the optimal evaluation and treatment of post-acute sequalae of COVID-19.

INTRODUCTION

Myocarditis is an inflammatory disease of the myocardium with wide-ranging clinical presentations from mild self-limited cardiac symptoms to the presence of cardiac

[a] Sanger Heart & Vascular Institute, Atrium Health, 1237 Harding Place, Suite 5100, Charlotte, NC 28204, USA; [b] Emory University School of Medicine, Emory Clinical Cardiovascular Research Institute, 1462 Clifton Road, NE, Suite 502, Atlanta, GA 30311, USA
* Corresponding author.
E-mail address: John.Symanski@atriumhealth.org

Clin Sports Med 41 (2022) 455–472
https://doi.org/10.1016/j.csm.2022.02.007
0278-5919/22/© 2022 Elsevier Inc. All rights reserved.
sportsmed.theclinics.com

dysfunction and possible fulminant heart failure.[1] Myocarditis is frequently due to acute viral infection and has become a focus of concern during the coronavirus disease 2019 (COVID-19) pandemic.[1–3] Among competitive athletes and highly active individuals, exercise during active viral myocarditis may exacerbate myocardial inflammation with precipitation of malignant ventricular arrhythmias. Indeed, myocarditis is a leading cause of sudden cardiac death (SCD) in athletes.[4–7] In consideration of return-to-play (RTP) for competitive athletes diagnosed with myocarditis, consensus guidelines exist that emphasize temporal abstinence from exercise training coupled with complete resolution of myocardial inflammation, normalization of cardiac function, and absence of ventricular arrhythmias with exertion.[8,9]

In the general population, infection with SARS-CoV-2 may lead to severe cardiac sequalae, especially in older individuals with significant underlying comorbidities.[10–13] Recognition of the high prevalence of clinically relevant cardiac injury among hospitalized patients with COVID-19 that was documented to be associated with poor outcomes led to significant apprehension in the care of competitive athletes. Whether athletes with asymptomatic or mild-COVID-19 infection might harbor myocarditis and remain at high risk for adverse cardiac events after recovery was of particular concern.[13–15] Since the early stages of the pandemic, considerable data have been acquired to provide sports medicine practitioners with updated prevalence estimates of cardiac injury in competitive athletes convalesced from COVID-19.[16–26] In this review, the authors detail the pathophysiology and clinical evaluation of athletes diagnosed with clinical myocarditis. They also discuss key developments focused on athletes infected by COVID-19. They aim to provide an evidence-based rationale in the care of athletes and highly active individuals for sports medicine and cardiology practitioners in the context of myocarditis- and COVID-19–related cardiac injury.

PATHOPHYSIOLOGY

Viruses are the most common pathogens known to cause myocarditis. Endomyocardial biopsy samples have revealed adenovirus, enteroviruses (Coxsackie type B and cytomegalovirus), parvovirus B-19 (B19V), and human herpesvirus 6 to be most frequent, with variations in prevalence by geographic regions.[1–3] Bacterial, fungal, and protozoal infections; drug-induced hypersensitivity eosinophilic reactions; and other autoimmune conditions represent less frequent causes of myocarditis.[1–3,27] With infection, usually from the upper respiratory system or gastrointestinal tract, viral myocarditis is thought to progress over 3 phases: (1) an *acute phase* typically lasting 3 to 7 days during which the virus gains entry to myocardial and vascular endothelial cells via viral-specific mechanisms or receptors followed by viral replication and subsequent myocyte necrosis; (2) a *subacute phase* of approximately 1 to 3 months with host immune cells and cytokine activation causing further cardiac damage and potential impairments in cardiac function. Although most myocarditis cases will resolve spontaneously, a minority will progress to (3) a *chronic phase* (chronic myocarditis or chronic inflammatory cardiomyopathy) characterized by myocyte abnormalities (variations in cell diameter), focal or diffuse fibrosis, and inflammatory cell infiltrates, which seem to be mediated through autoimmune processes rather than persistent viral-mediated injury.[2,27]

Myocarditis has been implicated in 3% to 10% of cases of SCD in young athletes.[4–7] Athletes may be particularly vulnerable to myocarditis, given the repetitive physical exhaustion associated with exercise training as well as the ancillary stresses that accompany competitive sports participation.[6,28] Prolonged intense physical exertion such as marathon running and training may lead to impaired immune responses and increased susceptibility to infection for 3 to 72 hours.[29] In addition, in murine models, forced exercise following coxsackievirus infection increases viral titers and the cytotoxic T-cell response, leading to increased myocardial necrosis and mortality.[30,31]

MYOCARDITIS CLINICAL PRESENTATION

The clinical presentation of myocarditis can be variable. Fulminant myocarditis often presents with acute, severe heart failure symptoms (dyspnea, chest pain) and potentially catastrophic malignant arrhythmias, heart block,[7] or cardiogenic shock.[32] In more typical cases of myocarditis, clinical symptoms are generally less severe but may still manifest angina, dyspnea, palpitations, or syncope. In some cases, specific complaints may be absent or attributed to the initial systemic symptoms of seasonal viral infections. Athletes may be more attuned to minor physiologic disturbances and complain of nonspecific symptoms such as fatigue, myalgias, or exercise intolerance.[28] Highlighting the variability in symptomatic myocarditis presentation, a recent analysis of 97 myocarditis-related sudden death cases in young individuals (mean age 19.3 ± 6.2 years) determined that only 47% reported symptoms before death.[7] These data should be interpreted cautiously, however, as retrospective evaluation of symptoms in autopsy-based studies may be unreliable.

MYOCARDIAL INJURY AND COVID-19

With the emergence of the COVID-19 pandemic, initial reports detailed an alarmingly high prevalence of myocardial injury in hospitalized patients.[11–15] These observational reports indicated biomarker evidence of cardiac injury was common among hospitalized patients with COVID-19 and that those with cardiac injury were at particularly high risk of mortality.[11,12] Importantly, patients included in these studies had severe illness (reason for hospitalization), were older, and displayed a high incidence of comorbid conditions.[11–15] Nevertheless, this high rate of cardiac involvement suggested a possible SARS-CoV-2 tropism for cardiac cells and raised concerns for individuals experiencing asymptomatic or mild COVID-19 infection.[33,34] Entry of the virus via the ACE-2 receptor in respiratory and cardiac tissue was purported as a potential underlying mechanism leading to the high prevalence of observed cardiac injury.[35] However, subsequent autopsy-based studies have noted absence of lymphocytic predominant myonecrosis[36,37] and classic histologic evidence of myocarditis associated with COVID-19 infection.[36] Given these data, mechanisms underlying COVID-19–related cardiac injury seem multifactorial, and caution is required in the clinical interpretation of patients diagnosed with COVID-19 myocarditis.

COVID-19 CARDIAC INJURY IN ATHLETES

Clinical diagnosis of myocarditis in athletes can be extremely challenging (**Figs. 1** and **2**).[7,28,38] As the compilation of COVID-19 data in athletes has evolved over time, differentiating clinically relevant cardiac injury and presumed myocarditis from subclinical injury of unclear clinical significance remains a critically important issue. Given early concerns taken from observational data in hospitalized patients with COVID-19,[10–15] prior expert consensus recommendations advised a postinfection screening evaluation in athletes, beginning with a focused medical history and examination, no earlier than 10 days after COVID-19 test positivity.[39] Inclusion of so-called "triad" testing (electrocardiogram [ECG], troponin, and echocardiography) was also recommended as the cornerstone of the RTP evaluation. However, as clinical outcomes of athletes

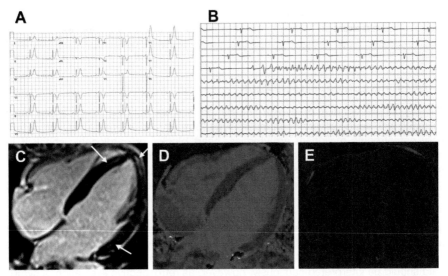

Fig. 1. Case 1. A 34-year-old former professional rugby player and recreational cyclist, presenting with cardiac arrest. Two week earlier, he suffered a witnessed spell during sleep with erratic breathing, loss of bladder continence, and transient unresponsiveness. He woke shortly before arrival of emergency responders and felt otherwise normal. Initial evaluation including 12-lead ECG (A), head CT and EEG, high sensitivity troponin, transthoracic echocardiography, and coronary CT angiography (not shown) were unremarkable. The patient was discharged with an event monitor and maintained his exercise routine without symptom limitation. Two days after cycling 80 miles, he suffered a ventricular fibrillation arrest captured on the event monitor (B); again, recognized by erratic breathing during sleep. Following successful resuscitation, he experienced transient LV dysfunction requiring circulatory support with V-A ECMO. Ventricular function normalized by hospital day 2 and the patient was weaned from cardiopulmonary support. Serial COVID-19 testing was negative. Cardiac MRI 1 week after admission revealed normal cardiac chamber dimensions, LV wall thickness, and biventricular function (EF 65%). Delayed gadolinium enhancement images (C) revealed a midmyocardial stripe of LGE (arrows) involving the mid- and distal septum and basal and apical lateral walls (quantitative scar burden 8%). Parametric mapping demonstrated diffusely elevated native T1 (D, E) and T2 values. Clinical history and MRI features were most consistent with myocarditis.

convalesced from COVID-19 and prevalence of cardiac injury in this population were reported, it became clearer that (1) most competitive athletes experienced either asymptomatic or mild COVID-19 symptoms, (2) prevalence of cardiac injury was low in this population, and (3) those diagnosed with clinical myocarditis usually report cardiopulmonary symptoms consistent with myocarditis.[40] As such, it must be emphasized that COVID-myocarditis in the athlete remains a *clinical diagnosis* associated with high pretest probability of disease.

As with other causes of myocarditis, presenting symptoms in individuals with cardiac involvement due to COVID-19 may include chest pain, dyspnea, palpitations, and syncope. For athletes who have RTP, a decline in the athlete's peak performance, prolonged dyspnea, or persistence of an elevated heart rate during recovery from exercise might herald the existence of myocardial inflammation and may require ongoing clinical investigation to exclude the presence of cardiac injury if there is sufficient clinical suspicion. The highly fit and competitive athlete may be less inclined to

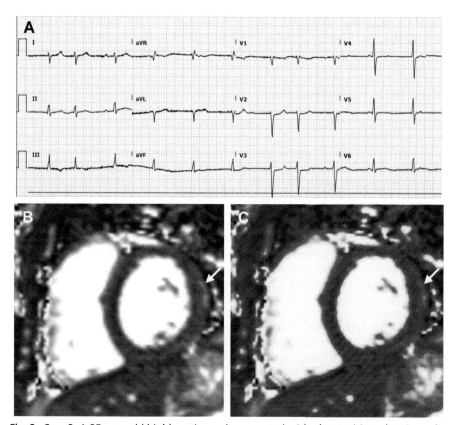

Fig. 2. Case 2. A 25-year-old highly active male presented with pharyngitis and an irregular pulse. ECG (*A*) showed a junctional rhythm with occasional atrial activity and a variable PR interval. He reported no chest discomfort or shortness of breath. High-sensitivity troponin was elevated at 5452 ng/L, and COVID-19 testing was positive. Echocardiography revealed normal left ventricular chamber and wall thickness with low to normal LV systolic function (EF 53%). No regional wall motion abnormalities were evident, and global longitudinal strain was normal at −17.3%. RV size and function were normal, and a trivial posterior pericardial effusion was noted. Troponin levels normalized within 2 weeks. Cardiac MRI performed 3 weeks after presentation revealed a mildly dilated LV chamber with normal wall thickness and an LVEF of 67%. Subepicardial LGE was present in the basal to apical inferior and apical lateral segments (*B*) with a scar size of 14%. Native T1 values were mildly elevated along the lateral segments (*C*) and normal in all other regions. T2 values were normal.

acknowledge symptoms due to concern of being withheld from training and competition or loss of team standing/position. Therefore, it is imperative for coaches, trainers, and team physicians to encourage athletes to remain attentive and be forthright with suggestive symptoms.

CLINICAL EVALUATION OF MYOCARDITIS
Electrocardiogram

The 12-lead ECG may provide invaluable clues in patients with myocarditis, although this test is limited by poor sensitivity (47%) and specificity.[41–43] Suggestive features may include subtle increases in resting heart rate, PR and QRS interval durations, premature ventricular contraction burden, or reduction of QRS amplitude (**Table 1**). More striking abnormalities include new bundle branch blocks or fractionated QRS (>120 msec), sinus arrest, high-grade AV block, complex ventricular ectopy, and ST-segment changes mimicking acute myocardial infarction. The incidence of abnormal ECG findings varies by study population, severity of symptoms, and extent and distribution of myocardial inflammation. In a contemporary series of 443 mostly young (median age 34 years) and highly symptomatic patients with acute myocarditis from the Lombardy region of Italy, ST-segment elevation was the most common ECG finding (57.5%), with other ST-segment abnormalities noted in an additional 23.5%.[44] Harris and colleagues[7] suggested that among lethal cases of myocarditis, inflammatory involvement of the conduction system is relatively common (38%) and may result in sudden death from heart block.

By contrast, ECG abnormalities appear infrequently among athletes with myocarditis following COVID-19 infection. In the 2 largest series of athletes evaluated after COVID-19 infection, ECG changes were uncommon, even among those with CMRI findings of myocarditis.[23,26] The Big 10 COVID-19 Registry (N = 1597 athletes) identified 37 individuals with clinical or subclinical myocarditis using CMRI.[23] Overall, 4 of 9 athletes (44%) with clinical symptoms of myocarditis (chest pain, dyspnea, and palpitations) and just 1 of 28 (14%) without cardiac symptoms exhibited abnormal ECG findings. The Outcomes Registry for Cardiac Conditions in Athletes identified 21 cases with myocardial or pericardial involvement by CMRI from screening of 3018 post-COVID athletes with mostly mild or moderate symptoms. ECG abnormalities were rare (4/21 or 19%) with T-wave inversion in V_{5-6} observed in just one case.[26] Because many athletes exhibit ST-segment or T-wave alterations, which can simulate pathologic findings, adherence to standardized interpretation guidelines for athletes and direct comparison with previously obtained ECG tracings is crucial.[45]

CLINICS CARE POINT

- Abnormal ECG findings occur infrequently among athletes following COVID-19 infection, even when MRI features that suggest acute myocarditis are present.

Cardiac Biomarkers

In the clinical assessment of myocarditis, high-sensitivity troponin is the preferred biomarker (alternatively early generation troponin or creatine kinase-myocardial band assays) to assess myocyte necrosis along with C-reactive protein.[41,44] The differential complete blood count may show eosinophilia in the presence of eosinophilic myocarditis.[46] Peripheral blood serologic and virologic tests are frequently unrevealing, except with suspected Lyme disease or human immunodeficiency virus.[41] Antinuclear antibody testing may be appropriate in patients with known or suspected history of autoimmune disorders.[47] When considering biomarker interpretation in athletes diagnosed with COVID-19, it is important to consider the training history, as recent physical activity may precipitate troponin release (see **Table 1**).[48] It has been recommended that high-sensitivity troponin assessment not be performed within ~24 to 48 hours of exercise.[40]

Recently, a novel circulating micro-RNA produced by cardiac myosin–specific type 17 helper lymphocytes has been identified in mice and humans with myocarditis. The human homologue, designated hsa-miR-Chr8:96, may have the potential to differentiate patients with myocarditis from those with acute coronary syndromes. Although

Table 1
Comparison of typical training effects on the heart versus "red flag" findings raising suspicion for acute viral-related cardiac injury/myocarditis

	Athletic Remodeling/Training Effects	"Red Flags" Suggesting Disease
Symptoms	• None	• Chest pain, abnormal shortness of breath beyond normal exercise-induced symptoms, palpitations, presyncope or syncope, decrement in performance
ECG	• Changes related to high vagal tone (such as bradycardia, early repolarization, first degree heart block, or Mobitz type I AV block) or athletic remodeling (LVH, atrial enlargement)	• Any pathologic changes compared with prior study • Frequent or multiform premature ventricular beats or arrhythmias • ST and T-wave changes • Left bundle branch block • Advanced AV block
Biomarkers	• Troponin and BNP/NT-Pro BNP may be mildly elevated immediately after strenuous exercise but return to normal quickly (<48 h)	• Persistent (>48 h) or more than mild elevation in cardiac biomarkers • Elevation in C-reactive protein, erythrocyte sedimentation rate, and leukocytosis
Echocardiography	• Symmetric dilation of all 4 cardiac chambers without regional wall motion abnormalities • Symmetric eccentric LV hypertrophy • Normal or low-normal EF with normal diastolic function • Normal augmentation of biventricular function with exercise (≥10% with exercise) • Normal/low-normal global longitudinal strain, better than −16%. • Prominent LV apical trabeculations with normal LVEF and wall thickness	• Disproportionate LV or RV enlargement • Asymmetric wall thickening (>2 mm between contiguous segments) • Any segmental wall motion abnormalities • Abnormal EF (<50% LVEF, <44% RVEF) particularly if associated with low tissue Doppler/abnormal diastolic function • Failure to augment biventricular function with exercise • Abnormal global longitudinal strain, worse than −16% • >Trivial pericardial effusion
Cardiac MRI	• Morpho-functional changes outlined in the earlier echocardiographic section • LGE is absent with possible exception of right ventricular insertion point LGE • Parametric maps are normal	• Morpho-functional changes outlined in the earlier echocardiographic section. • LGE in a mid- or subepicardial distribution • >Trivial pericardial effusion with prominent pericardial enhancement • Abnormal T1 or T2 mapping

Abbreviations: BNP, B-type natriuretic peptide; EF, ejection fraction; LGE, late gadolinium enhancement; LV, left ventricle; LVH, left ventricle hypertrophy; RVEF, right ventricular ejection fraction.

promising, further studies are necessary (including patients with dilated cardiomyopathy) in order to validate the suitability of this novel biomarker in clinical practice.[49]

CLINICS CARE POINT

- Intense physical activity may precipitate cardiac biomarker release, high-sensitivity troponin testing in athletes recovered from COVID-19 should generally not be performed within ~24 to 48 hours of exercise.

Echocardiography

Echocardiography remains an integral part of the evaluation of athletes with suspected myocarditis.[2,28,38] Early on, although left ventricular ejection fraction (LVEF) typically remains normal, findings such as increased LV wall thickness and enhanced myocardial echogenicity, mild regional hypokinesis (particularly in the inferior and inferolateral segments), and abnormalities of tissue-Doppler and regional strain imaging may be recognized.[2,50,51] Right ventricular (RV) dysfunction may also be evident, especially in those with severe pulmonary injury.[28] Pericardial effusions have been observed with varying frequencies. In the early phases of myocarditis, LV dimensions are generally normal, even when the EF is reduced. LV dilation often implies chronicity, with the caveat that the athlete's type of exercise training (particularly endurance modalities) and corollary cardiovascular adaptations may affect chamber dimensions (see **Table 1**). Recognition of LV dysfunction should also continue to prompt the clinician to consider potential effects of performance enhancing (anabolic steroid, amphetamines) and recreational drugs (cocaine). Finally, prominent LV apical trabeculations are increasingly recognized as nonpathologic findings in athletes and are likely to be encountered with broader application of post-COVID-19 cardiovascular imaging.[52]

Endomyocardial Biopsy

Endomyocardial biopsy (EMB) remains the "gold standard" for a confirmatory diagnosis of myocarditis.[1,2,41,53] However, given the invasive nature and risk of complications, EMB is generally reserved for defining treatment in severely affected individuals. In experienced hands, the risk of complications (perforation, tamponade, severe dysrhythmias) is acceptably low (~1%–2%).[54] An additional shortcoming of EMB is potential sampling error, as myocardial inflammation may be patchy or confined to regions inaccessible by RV sampling (ie, lateral LV wall). The timing of sampling relative to phase of illness may also affect the diagnostic yield of EMB.[53]

Cardiac MRI

CMRI has evolved into the most sensitive and comprehensive noninvasive diagnostic tool for assessment of myocardial tissue characterization, including recognition and quantitation of inflammation and replacement fibrosis resulting from acute myocarditis.[55] CMRI also serves as the reference standard for quantitation of cardiac mass, cardiac chamber dimensions, and EF assessment. CMRI is recommended (class I) for patients with *clinically* suspected acute myocarditis or in patients with chest pain, normal coronary arteries, and elevated troponin (myocardial infarction with non-obstructive coronary arteries).[56] CMRI is not only a powerful diagnostic tool but also provides important information regarding risk stratification during recovery from acute myocarditis. The absence of late gadolinium enhancement (LGE) post-myocarditis portends an excellent prognosis, whereas multiple trials have shown that the presence of LGE is associated with an increased risk of major adverse cardiac events.[57–59] Whether the presence of LGE in athletes post-COVID-19 proves to be a substrate of ventricular arrhythmias is unknown.

CMRI should ideally be performed within 2 to 3 weeks from onset of symptoms and/ or detection of biomarker abnormalities, as diagnostic accuracy may be reduced during the first days of illness or beyond this temporal window. In the context of recent controversies surrounding the utility of CMRI screening for athletes post-COVID-19 infection and because of the exquisite high sensitivity for detection of subtle abnormalities of myocardial tissue characterization, there remains uncertainty regarding the clinical relevance of subtle abnormal CMRI findings in asymptomatic patients or those without ECG, biomarker, or echocardiographic abnormalities.

The original Lake Louise Criteria, published in 2009, designated 3 key elements of myocardial inflammation detected by CMRI: (1) *hyperemia*—identified by intense signal on early gadolinium enhancement images; (2) *edema*—indicated by increased myocardial T2 relaxation time or increased signal intensity on T2-weighted images; and (3) *necrosis/fibrosis*—as exhibited on LGE images.[60] In this first iteration, abnormal findings in 2 of the 3 elements diagnosed acute myocarditis with a 74% sensitivity and 86% specificity.[61] The addition of novel parametric (T1 and T2) mapping techniques has been shown to improve the diagnostic accuracy of CMRI for acute myocarditis. The 2018 Updated Lake Louise Criteria include T2-mapping for edema and native T1 mapping and extracellular volume (ECV) for inflammatory injury.[55] One study examining the updated criteria reported enhanced sensitivity (87.5%) while preserving high specificity (96.2%) for diagnosis of acute myocarditis.[62]

At present, there have been 11 separate reports, primarily small observational case series, detailing CMRI findings in athletes following COVID-19 infection (**Table 2**). These studies vary in terms of subject age, sex, race, ethnicity, geographic distribution, sporting discipline, and symptomatology, and detailed correlations of ECG, biomarker, and echocardiographic findings have been inconsistent. Indications for CMRI, either clinically directed or universally mandated, and timing relative to symptom onset or COVID-19 positivity have also been nonuniform. Further, scanner type (1.5 vs 3 T), imaging protocols/sequences, and the experience of the interpreter have not been standardized. Finally, although prior studies incorporated the updated Lake Louise criteria, absence of case-control comparative groups of noninfected athletes and nonathletes represent a critical omission in most of these studies. Additional limitations are present in careful review of these studies. First, there is stark discrepancy in the observed frequency of CMRI-defined myocarditis with rates ranging between 0% and 17%.[16–26] In the Big Ten COVID-19 Registry (N = 1597 athletes), among the 13 participating institutions, incidence rates for myocarditis varied by site from 0% to 7.6%.[23] A second limitation of CMRI studies in athletes has been the lack of standardized CMRI interpretation by a core laboratory to validate abnormal findings. As such, given the expertise required for CMRI interpretation, interpreter bias is a clear, critical limitation. For example, although Brito and colleagues[21] observed a high prevalence of pericardial enhancement and associated effusions in 39.5% (N = 19) of a cohort of convalesced COVID-19 athletes (N = 48), in no other CMR-based athletic study has this degree of presumed pericarditis been replicated.

Fibrosis confirmed by LGE is often observed in myocarditis (see **Table 2**). Yet, whether LGE reported in prior COVID-19 convalesced athlete case series data represents recent COVID-19 injury is unknown in the absence of comparative baseline CMRI data. Prior investigators appropriately excluded focal septal RV insertion site fibrosis as an indicator of COVID-19 injury, given the increasing recognition of this

Table 2
MRI studies in athletes diagnosed with COVID-19

Reference	Site	Cohort	Timing of MRI after Diagnosis and Symptom Frequency	MRI Parameters	Frequency of Abnormal MRI Findings	Additional Observations
Rajpal et al. *JAMA Card* (Published Online Sept 11, 2020)	Ohio State University	26 collegiate athletes Mean age: 19.5 y Female: 42.3%	(11–53 d) Mild: 12 (46%) None: 14 (54%)	Cine, T1/T2, ECV, & LGE (1.5 T)	Myocarditis: 4/26 (15%); pericardial effusion: 2	No ↑ troponin, LGE in 12 (46%): 4 with & 8 without ↑ T2
Brito et al. *JACC CV Imag* (Published Online Nov 4, 2020)	W. Virginia University	54 collegiate athletes Mean age: 19 y; female: 15%	Symptoms: None: 16 (30%) Mild: 36 (66%) Moderate: 2 (4%)	Serial MRI in 48 (89%)	Abnormal: 27 (56.3%) Pericardial effusion or LGE: 19 (39.5%)	6 (12.5%) ↓ GLS and/or ↑ native T1; LGE in 1, ↓EF w/s ↑ T1; normal T2 in all, ↑ Troponin 1 (3%)
Vago et al. *JACC CV Imag* (Published Online Dec 16, 2020)	Hungary	12 pro athletes Median age: 23 y Female: 83.3% [15 athletic & 15 healthy controls]	(Median: 67 d [female], 90 d [male]) Symptoms: None: 2 (17%) Mild to mod: 10 (83%)	Cine, T1 &T2, (1.5 T)	No myocarditis/LGE, normal T1 and T2	—
Clark et al. *Circulation* (Published Online Dec 17, 2020)	Vanderbilt University	59 collegiate athletes; 60 athletic controls; 27 healthy controls	(10–162 d; median 21.5 d)	Cine, T1/T2 mapping, & ECV (1.5 T)	Myocarditis: 2 (3%) but no symptoms, 1 late ↓ EF (45%)	Focal infero-septal LGE in 22% COVID (+) vs 24% athletic controls
Starekova et al. *JAMA Card* (Published Online Jan 14, 2021)	Univ. of Wisconsin	145 collegiate & high school athletes Female: 25.5%	(11–194; median 15 d) Symptoms: None: 24 (16.6%) Mild: 71 (49%); Moderate: 40 (27.6%)	(1.5 or 3 T)	Myocarditis: 2 (1.4%) 1 with extensive LGE, ↑T2, & (+) troponin; 1 with mild LGE & (−) troponin	—

Study	Location	Population	Time	MRI sequence	Findings	Notes
Malek et al. *J Mag Res Imag* (Jan 20, 2021)	Warsaw, Poland	26 Olympic & pro athletes Mean age: 24 y Female: 81%	(1–2 mo)	Cine, T1/T2, dark blood T2, LGE (1.5 T)	Abnormal: 19% (5/26), No myocarditis by MRI	4 with borderline myocardial edema, 1 with LGE and pleural-pericardial effusion
Martinez et al. *JAMA Card* (Online Mar 4, 2021)	US	789 pro athletes [MLS, MLB, NHL, NFL, WNBA] Male: 98.5% MRI in 27	(3–156 d)	NS*	Abnormal MRI in 5 (0.6%): myocarditis 3 (0.4%) pericarditis 2 (0.3%)	
Hendrickson et al. *Circulation* (May 11, 2021)	Univ. of Tennessee	137 D-I, II, III (age 18–27) Male: 68% MRI in 5	(Median: 16 d) 87% mild or moderate symptoms	Cine, T2, LGE	No (0/5) abnormal MRI	Trace of small effusions in 4 athletes T1/T2 mapping & ECV not on all
Daniels et al. *JAMA Card* (Online May 27, 2021)	13 Big Ten Universities	1597 collegiate athletes male: 60.3%	(10–77 days)	Cine, T1 & T2	37 (2.3%) Clinical myocarditis: 9 Subclinical:28 31 Fulfilled LL Criteria	MRI yield 7.4x > f/u MRI in 27: Resolution ↑T2 in all & LGE in 11
Hwang et al. *Clin J Sport Med* (Published Online June 24, 2021)	Stanford University	55 collegiate athletes MRI in 8 for abnormal screening	NS	NS*	Myocarditis: (1) Pericarditis: (1) + CP	
Moulson et al. *Circulation* (July 27, 2021)	US (ORCCA Registry)	3,018 COVID (+) collegiate athletes - 42 US schools CI-MRI: (119) 1°-MRI: (198)	(18–63 days; Median 33 days)	NS*	Definite, possible, or probable cardiac involvement in 21/ 3018 (0.7%)	CI: -15/2820 (0.5%) Dx yield 4.2x higher when MRI CI: -15/119 (12.6%) CI -6/198 (3%) in 1° screening MRI

finding as a likely benign marker in athletes, particularly masters-level endurance athletes.[63,64] A recent report demonstrated focal nonischemic fibrosis in 17% of asymptomatic triathletes, which seemed to correlate with exercise-induced hypertension and competition history.[63] Another study identified focal LGE in 37.6% of healthy endurance athletes versus 2.8% in healthy control subjects ($P < 0.001$), with a typical pattern in the RV insertion points.[64] In each of these studies, athletes with LGE also tended to exhibit higher ECV in remote, nonfibrotic myocardium assessed with T1 mapping.

The significance of "subclinical" myocarditis detailed with CMR-based screening remains uncertain. Present short-term cardiac outcomes are reassuring after RTP in competitive athletes, and to-date, no sports-related cardiac events clearly linked to COVID-19 have been confirmed in any athlete included in published registry data.[23,26] Another reassuring observation from the Big-10 Registry was derived from a subset of 27 athletes who underwent follow-up CMRI and demonstrated normalization of T2 elevation in all subjects with resolution of LGE in 11 (40.7%).[23] In addition to evidence suggesting CMRI-based screening does not improve athlete health outcomes, we must also acknowledge the legitimate concerns of costs in implementing widespread CMRI screening, limited scanner availability, and inappropriate health care resource allocation as separate reasons why CMRI screening for all athletes convalesced from COVID-19 is not practical. Future unfortunate and tragic athlete SCD cases will undoubtedly still occur, just as before the COVID-19 pandemic; this emphasizes the importance of careful adjudication of follow-up data from US and multinational registries, avoidance of overreaching correlation with potential prior COVID-19 infection, and continued vigilance with emergency preparedness to prevent such tragic events.

CLINICS CARE POINT

- Cardiac MRI is recommended for athletes with *clinically* suspected acute myocarditis, including those with chest pain, elevated high-sensitivity troponin levels, and abnormal ECG changes in the absence of obstructive or anomalous coronary arteries. Imaging should typically be performed within 2 to 3 weeks of symptom onset and/or abnormal biomarker or ECG findings with interpretation by experienced imaging specialists.

ACTIVITY RESTRICTION AND RETURN-TO-PLAY

As exercise may augment pathogen virulence in other acute viral infections, it is prudent to assume this may also be the case with SARS-CoV2.[29–31] Although RTP algorithms for athletes diagnosed with COVID-19 are continually evolving, most expert opinions have recommended athletes refrain from vigorous exercise, especially while symptomatic.[39,40,65,66] Early recommendations prescribed a period of rest for all athletes diagnosed with COVID-19 as well as further cardiac workup in those with any symptoms.[39,65] Subsequent recommendations have refined RTP strategies to be tailored to symptom severity, with more severe symptoms warranting a longer period of rest and more extensive cardiac risk stratification.[40,66]

An important unaddressed clinical issue is whether athletes with a remote history of COVID-19 and have fully recovered should undergo cardiovascular risk assessment; this also applies to those found to have a positive COVID-19 antibody test without any history of prior clinical symptoms. Currently, definitive outcomes data to address this issue are lacking. However, there are currently no data to suggest that athletes with prior COVID-19 infection are suffering from increased rates of SCD or incident heart failure.[16–26] Future recommendations based on athlete registry data[23,26] will be forthcoming and may offer further guidance on which athletes warrant activity restriction and advanced evaluation.

Athletes diagnosed with clinical myocarditis, whether due to COVID-19 or other causes, should generally follow current American College of Cardiology/American Heart Association sports eligibility guidelines for myocarditis.[8] These athletes should be restricted from physical training for at least 3 to 6 months following resolution of initial symptoms. After this period of convalescence, cardiac enzyme and ventricular systolic function should be reevaluated and ambulatory rhythm monitoring and exercise testing should be performed. If these tests reveal no biomarker evidence of ongoing cardiac injury/inflammation, normalization of LV function, and no significant rhythm disturbances, athletes can gradually return to training.[8] The use of CMRI for follow-up imaging of athletes diagnosed with myocarditis, based on previous abnormal CMRI findings, may be preferred. Although persistent LGE following clinical recovery still has unclear clinical implications, improvement of inflammatory findings on CMRI after 3 to 6 months of exercise abstinence is a reassuring finding and therefore reasonable to proceed with RTP after careful shared risk and decision-making between practitioner, athlete, and other key stakeholders.

MYOCARDITIS TREATMENT

A severe clinical presentation of myocarditis, or fulminant myocarditis, includes the presence of cardiogenic shock or unstable arrythmias and warrants emergent transfer for intensive cardiac care at an experienced medical center. Clinical management may include initiation of mechanical circulatory support, extracorporeal membrane oxygenation, parenteral inotropic therapy, and EMB.[2,32] The empirical use of corticosteroids may be considered, although clear outcomes data are lacking on the effectiveness of steroid or immunotherapy in nonspecific cases of myocarditis. For specific autoimmune conditions such as giant-cell or sarcoid myocarditis, corticosteroids and advanced immunosuppressive regimens are indicated and recommended by most experts.[65,66] If clinical myocarditis as a consequence of an active viral infection is suspected, specific antiviral therapy may be considered, although evidence-based treatment courses are not well established.[3] For all patients presenting with acute myocarditis and reduced EF, regardless of cause, medical management for heart failure is the cornerstone of treatment. Consultation with a cardiology or heart failure specialist is recommended, and medications should be initiated in accordance with contemporary heart failure guidelines, including β-blocker, angiotensin receptor and neprilysin inhibitor, mineralocorticoid antagonist, sodium-glucose cotransporter-2 inhibitor, and diuretics as indicated.[67]

FUTURE RESEARCH DIRECTIONS

Numerous clinical uncertainties relevant to athletes convalesced from COVID-19 infection persist. First, although LGE is an established risk factor in patients with cardiomyopathy, the natural history and predictive value of nonspecific LGE observed in athletes is unclear. Second, in the context of subclinical myocarditis detected by CMRI, ongoing follow-up of long-term clinical outcomes of athletes convalesced from COVID-19 remains imperative. Although cardiac outcomes to date are reassuring, unknown long-term outcomes concomitant with emerging COVID-19 variants necessitate ongoing scientific vigilance and maintenance of current registry data. Finally, the emergence of postacute sequalae of COVID-19 (PASC), or "long-haul"

COVID-19, represents a critical challenge in sports medicine and cardiology. Ruling out myocarditis as a cause of persistent symptoms is a key first step; however, delineating underlying mechanisms and best practices for clinical management of athletes suffering from PASC is a pressing challenge in the care of recovered athletes post-COVID-19.

CONCLUSIONS

Concern for acute myocarditis warrants thorough investigations and thoughtful clinical judgment for athletes in consideration of RTP. Advanced cardiac imaging, although increasing test sensitivity for myocarditis, has also introduced a new element of clinical uncertainty in the evaluation of athletes convalesced from COVID-19. Athletes diagnosed with COVID-19 should undergo cardiac testing based on clinical presentation, with specific attention paid to the presence of cardiopulmonary symptoms. Athletes with higher pretest probability for myocarditis should undergo appropriate cardiac testing, including selective consideration for CMRI before RTP versus a universal screening approach. Emerging conundrums in the care of athletes throughout the COVID-19 pandemic include the challenges presented by PASC, which requires continued follow-up in large athletic registry cohorts, and the concern for new COVID-19 variants, which requires ongoing vigilance in assessing potential untoward cardiac outcomes in recovered athletes after COVID-19 infection.

DISCLOSURES

The authors have reported that they have no relationships relevant to the contents of this paper to disclose.

REFERENCES

1. Fung G, Luo H, Qiu Y, et al. Myocarditis. Circ Res 2016;118:496–514.
2. Ammirati E, Frigerio M, Adler E, et al. Management of acute myocarditis and chronic inflammatory cardiomyopathy. Circ Heart Fail 2020;13e:007405.
3. Law Y, Lai A, Chen S, et al. Diagnosis and management of myocarditis in children. a scientific statement from the American Heart Association. Circulation 2021;144:e123–35.
4. Harmon KG, Asif IM, Maleszewski JJ, et al. Incidence, cause, and comparative frequency of sudden cardiac death in national collegiate athletic association athletes. Circulation 2015;132:10–9.
5. Peterson DF, Kucera K, Thomas LC, et al. Aetiology and incidence of sudden cardiac arrest and death in young competitive athletes in the USA: a 4-year prospective study. Br J Sports Med 2021;55:1196–203.
6. Maron BJ, Doerer JJ, Haas TS, et al. Sudden deaths in young competitive athletes. Circulation 2009;119:1085–92.
7. Harris K, Mackey-Bojack S, Bennett, et al. Sudden unexpected death due to myocarditis in young people, including athletes. Am J Cardiol 2021;143:131–4.
8. Maron BJ, Udelson JE, Bonow RO, et al. Eligibility and disqualification recommendations for competitive athletes with cardiovascular abnormalities: task force 3: hypertrophic cardiomyopathy, arrhythmogenic right ventricular cardiomyopathy and other cardiomyopathies, and myocarditis. Circulation 2015;132:e273–80.
9. Pelliccia A, Solberg EE, Papadakis M, et al. Recommendations for participation in competitive and leisure time sport in athletes with cardiomyopathies, myocarditis,

and pericarditis: position statement of the sport cardiology section of the European Association of Preventive Cardiology (EAPC). Eur Heart J 2019;40:19–33.

10. Clerkin KJ, Fried JA, Raikhelkar J, et al. COVID-19 and cardiovascular disease. Circulation 2020;141:1648–55.

11. Shi S, Qin M, Shen B, et al. Association of cardiac injury with mortality in hospitalized patients with COVID-19 in Wuhan, China. JAMA Cardiol 2020;5:802–10.

12. Guo T, Fan Y, Chen M, et al. Cardiovascular implications of fatal outcomes of patients with coronavirus disease 2019 (COVID-19). JAMA Cardiol 2020;5:811–8.

13. Pinney S, Giustino G, Halperin J, et al. Coronavirus historical perspective, disease mechanisms, and clinical outcomes. J Am Coll Cardiol 2020;76:1999–2010.

14. Puntman V, Carerj M, Wieters I, et al. Outcomes of cardiovascular magnetic resonance imaging in patients recently recovered from coronavirus disease 2019 (COVID-19). JAMA Cardiol 2020;5:1265–73.

15. Huang L, Zhao P, Tang D, et al. Cardiac involvement in patients recovered from COVID-2019 identified using magnetic resonance imaging. JACC Cardiovasc Imaging 2020;13:2330–9.

16. Rajpal S, Tong MS, Borchers J, et al. Cardiovascular magnetic resonance findings in competitive athletes recovering from COVID-19 infection. JAMA Cardiol 2021;6:116–8.

17. Starekova J, Bluemke DA, Bradham WS, et al. Evaluation for myocarditis in competitive student athletes recovering from coronavirus disease 2019 with cardiac magnetic resonance imaging. JAMA Cardiol 2021;6:945–50.

18. Małek ŁA, Marczak M, Miłosz-Wieczorek B, et al. Cardiac involvement in consecutive elite athletes recovered from Covid-19: a magnetic resonance study. J Magn Reson Imaging 2021;53:1723–9.

19. Clark DE, Parikh A, Dendy JM, et al. COVID-10 myocardial pathology evaluation in athletes with cardiac magnetic resonance (COMPETE CMR). Circulation 2021; 143:609–12.

20. Martinez MW, Tucker AM, Bloom OJ, et al. Prevalence of inflammatory heart disease among professional athletes with prior COVID-19 infection who received systematic return-to-play cardiac screening. JAMA Cardiol 2021;4:E1–8. Published online March.

21. Brito D, Meester S, Yanamala N, et al. High prevalence of pericardial involvement in college student athletes recovering from COVID-19. JACC Cardiovasc Imaging 2021;14:541–55.

22. Hendrickson BS, Stephens RE, Chang JV, et al. Cardiovascular evaluation after COVID-19 in 137 collegiate athletes. Results of an algorithm-guided screening. Circulation 2021;143:1926–8.

23. Daniels CJ, Rajpal S, Greenshields JT, et al. Prevalence of clinical and subclinical myocarditis in competitive athletes with recent SARS-CoV-2 infection: results from the big ten COVID-19 cardiac registry. JAMA Cardiol 2021;27:E1–10. Published online May.

24. Vago H, Szabo L, Dohy Z, et al. Cardiac magnetic resonance findings in patients recovered from COVID-19. Initial experience in elite athletes. JACC Cardiovasc Imaging 2021;14:1279–81.

25. Hwang CE, Kussman A, Christle JW, et al. Findings form cardiovascular evaluation of national collegiate athletic association division I collegiate student-athletes after asymptomatic or mildly symptomatic SARS-CoV-2 infection. Clin J Sport Med 2022;(32):103–7.

26. Moulson N, Petek BJ, Drezner JA, et al. Outcomes registry for cardiac conditions in athletes investigators. SARS-CoV-2 cardiac involvement in young competitive athletes. Circulation 2021;144:256–66.

27. Kindermann I, Barth C, Mahfoud F, et al. Update on myocarditis. J Am Coll Cardiol 2012;59:779–92.

28. Halle M, Binzenhöfer L, Mahrholdt H, et al. Myocarditis in athletes: a clinical perspective. Eur J Prev Cardiol 2020;3. Published online March.

29. Nieman DC. Marathon training and immune function. Sports Med 2007;37:412–5.

30. Kiel R, Smith F, Chason J, et al. Coxsackie-virus B3 myocarditis in C3H/HeJ mice: description of an inbred model and the effect of exercise on virulence. Eur J Epidemiol 1989;5:348–50.

31. Gatmaitan B, Chason J, Lerner A. Augmentation of the virulence of murine coxsackie-virus B-3 myocardiomyopathy by exercise. J Exp Med 1970;131: 1121–36.

32. Kociol RD, Cooper LT, Fang JC, et al. Recognition and initial management of fulminant myocarditis. Circulation 2020;141:e69–92.

33. Madjid M, Safavi-Naeini P, Solomon SD, et al. Potential effects of coronaviruses on the cardiovascular system: a review. JAMA Cardiol 2020;5:831–40.

34. Yancy CW, Fonarow GC. Coronavirus Disease 2019 (COVID-19) and the heart-is heart failure the next chapter? JAMA Cardiol 2020;5:1216–7.

35. Vaduganathan M, Vardeny O, Michel T, et al. Renin-angiotensin-aldosterone system inhibitors in patients with Covid-19. N Engl J Med 2020;382:1653–9.

36. Kawakami R, Sakamoto A, Kawai K, et al. Pathological evidence for SARS-CoV-2 as a cause of myocarditis: JACC review topic of the week. J Am Coll Cardiol 2021;77:314–25.

37. Basso C, Leone O, Rizzo S, et al. Pathological features of COVID-19-associated myocardial injury: a multicentre cardiovascular pathology study. Eur Heart J 2020;41:3827–35.

38. Eichhorn C, Bière L, Schnell F, et al. Myocarditis in athletes is a challenge. JACC Cardiovasc Imaging 2020;13:494–507.

39. Phelan D, Kim JH, Chung EH. A game plan for the resumption of sport and exercise after coronavirus disease 2019 (COVID-19) Infection. JAMA Cardiol 2020;5: 1085–6.

40. Phelan D, Kim J, Elliott M, et al. Screening of potential cardiac involvement in competitive athletes recovering from COVID-19. An expert consensus statement. JACC Cardiovasc Imaging 2020;13:2635–52.

41. Carforio A, Pankuweit S, Arbustini E, et al. Current state of knowledge on etiology, diagnosis, management, and therapy of myocarditis: A position statement of the european society of cardiology working group on myocardial and pericardial disease. Eur Heart J 2013;34:2636–2648a.

42. Ukena C, Mahfoud F, Kindermann I, et al. Prognositic electrocardiographic parameters in patients with suspected myocarditis. Eur J Heart Fail 2011;13: 398–405.

43. Mogera T, Di Lenarda A, Dreas L, et al. Electrocardiography of myocarditis revisited: Clinical and prognostic ssignificance of electrocardiographic changes. Am Heart J 1992;124:455–67.

44. Ammirati E, Cipriani M, Moro C, et al. Clinical presentation and outcome in a contemporary cohort of patients with acute myocarditis: multicenter lombardy fegistry. Circulation 2018;138:1088–99.

45. Sharma S, Drezner J, Baggish A, et al. International recommendations for electrocardiographic interpretation in athletes. J Am Coll Cardiol 2017;69:1057–75.

46. Brambatti M, Matassini MV, Adler ED, et al. Eosinophic myocarditis: characteristics, treatment, and outcomes. J Am Coll Cardiol 2017;70:2363–75.
47. Carforio A, Marcolongo R, Jahns R, et al. Immune-mediated and autoimmune myocarditis: clinical presentation, diagnosis, and management. Heart Fail Rev 2013;18:715–32.
48. Shave R, Baggish A, George K, et al. Exercise-induced cardiac troponin elevation. Evidence, mechanisms, and implications. J Am Coll Cardiol 2010;56:169–76.
49. Blanco-Dominguez R, Sanchez-Diaz R, de la Fuente H, et al. A novel circulating microRNA for the detection of acute myocarditis. N Engl J Med 2021;384:2014–27.
50. Ammirati E, Veronese G, Brambatti M, et al. Fulminant versus acute nonfulminant myocarditis in patients with left ventricular systolic dysfunction. J Am Coll Cardiol 2019;74:299–311.
51. Hsiao J, Koshino Y, Bonnichsen C, et al. Speckle tracking echocardiography in acute myocarditis. Int J Cardiovasc Imaging 2013;29:275–84.
52. Caselli S, Ferreira D, Kanawati E, et al. Prominent left ventricular trabeculations in competitive athletes: A proposal for risk stratification and management. Int J Cardiol 2016;223:590–5.
53. Cooper L, Baughman K, Feldman A, et al. The role of endomyocardial biopsy in the management of cardiovascular disease: a scientific statement from the American Heart Association, the American College of Cardiology, and the European Society of Cardiology: endorsed by the Heart Failure Society of America and the Heart Failure Association of the European Society of Cardiology. J Am Coll Cardiol 2007;50:1914–31.
54. Yilmaz A, Kindermann I, Kindermann M, et al. Comparative evaluation of left and right ventricular endomyocardial biopsy: differences in complication rate and diagnostic performance. Circulation 2010;122:900–9.
55. Ferreira V, Schulz-Menger J, Holmvang G, et al. Cardiovascular magnetic resonance in nonischemic myocardial inflammation: expert recommendations. J Am Coll Cardiol 2018;72:3158–76.
56. Pasupathy S, Air T, Dreyer R, et al. Systematic review of patients presenting with suspected myocardial infarction and non-obstructive coronary arteries. Circulation 2015;131:861–70.
57. Grani C, Eichhorn C, Biere L, et al. Prognostic value of cardiac magnetic resonance tissue characterization in risk stratifying patients with suspected myocarditis. J Am Coll Cardiol 2017;70:1964–76.
58. Aquaro G, Perfetti M, Camastra G, et al. Cardiac magnetic resonance working group of the Italian Society of Cardiology. Cardiac MR with late gadolinium enhancement in acute myocarditis with preserved systolic function: ITAMY study. J Am Coll Cardiol 2017;70:1977–87.
59. Di Marco A, Anguera I, Schmitt M, et al. Late gadolinium enhancement and the risk for ventricular arrhythmias or sudden death in dilated cardiomyopathy: systematic review and meta-analysis. JACC Heart Fail 2017;5:28–38.
60. Frierich M, Sechtem U, Schulz-Menger, et al. Cardiovascular magnetic resonance in myocarditis: a JACC white paper. J Am Coll Cardiol 2009;53:1475–87.
61. Pan JA, Lee YJ, Salerno M. Diagnostic performance of extracellular volume, native T1, and T2 mapping versus Lake Louise criteria by cardiac magnetic resonance for detection of acute myocarditis: a meta-analysis. Circ Cardiovasc Imaging 2018;11:e007598. Published online July 16.

62. Luetkens JA, Faron A, Isaak A, et al. Comparison of the original and the 2018 Lake Louise criteria for diagnosis of acute myocarditis: results of a validation cohort. Radiol Cardiothorac Imaging 2019;1:e190010. Published online July 25.

63. Tahir E, Starekova J, Muellerleile K, et al. Myocardial fibrosis in competitive triathletes detected by contrast-enhanced CMR correlates with exercise-induced hypertension and competition history. JACC Cardiovasc Imaging 2018;11:1260–70.

64. Domenech-Ximenos B, Sanz-de la Garza M, Prat-Gonzalez S, et al. Prevalence and pattern of cardiovascular magnetic resonance late gadolinium enhancement in highly trained endurance athletes. J Cardiovasc Magn Reson 2020;22:62.

65. Kandolin R, Lehtonen J, Salmenkivi K, et al. Diagnosis, treatment, and outcome of giant-cell myocarditis in the era of combined immunosuppression. Circ Heart Fail 2013;6:15–22.

66. Fussner L, Karlstedt E, Hodge D, et al. Management and outcomes of cardiac sarcoidosis: a 20-year experience in two tertiary care centres. Eur J Heart Fail 2018;20:1713–20.

67. Writing Committee, Maddox TM, Januzzi JL Jr, Allen LA, et al. 2021 Update to the 2017 ACC expert consensus decision pathway for optimization of heart failure treatment: answers to 10 pivotal issues about heart failure with reduced ejection fraction: a report of the American College of Cardiology solution set oversight committee. J Am Coll Cardiol 2021;77:772–810.

Hypertrophic Cardiomyopathy and Exercise: Mutually Exclusive or Beneficial?

Matthew W. Martinez, MD[a,b,*]

KEYWORDS

- Hypertrophic cardiomyopathy • Exercise • Athlete • Sports cardiology

KEY POINTS

- Sudden cardiac arrest is rare during exercise.
- HCM is an important cause of this rare event.
- Exercise prescription is an important part of HCM care.
- HCM risk stratification has improved significantly allowing improved risk determination.
- Shared decision making is an important part of all HCM care including recommendations for exercise and potential risk.

INTRODUCTION

Hypertrophic cardiomyopathy (HCM) is a common heterogeneous cardiac disorder.[1] Only a small subset of patients with HCM will experience sudden cardiac arrest (SCA) with most HCM patients having normal longevity.[2] Cardiorespiratory fitness reduces all-cause and cardiovascular mortality with exercise being the standard of care for most patients with cardiovascular disease to improve functional capacity and reduce morbidity and mortality. These facts are in opposition to the historic restrictive approach to sports activity for HCM patients,[3,4] which has led individuals with HCM to largely abstain from exercise for fear of worsening hypertrophy and increasing risk of SCA.[1,4] Recent studies illustrate that sudden cardiac death, in both the general population and athletes,[5,6] is more likely to occur with structurally normal hearts than with HCM. Despite that, management guidelines, primarily based on case studies and expert opinion, exclude patients with HCM from intensive physical activity and

[a] Department of Cardiovascular Medicine, Atlantic Health, Morristown Medical Center, Morristown, NJ 07960, USA; [b] Sports Cardiology and Hypertrophic Cardiomyopathy
* 111 Madison Avenue, Suite 301, Morristown, NJ 07960.
E-mail address: Matthew.Martinez@atlantichealth.org
Twitter: @mmartinezheart (M.W.M.)

Clin Sports Med 41 (2022) 473–484
https://doi.org/10.1016/j.csm.2022.02.011
0278-5919/22/© 2022 Elsevier Inc. All rights reserved.

exercise.[7] This review aims to review existing data and discuss an approach to further efforts to determine how best to advocate exercise and HCM.

ATHLETE AND SUDDEN CARDIAC ARREST

The incidence of SCA among athletes is low and not different than age-matched nonathlete populations. Several studies have shown the absolute number of sudden deaths associated with exertion in the general population exceeds that observed among young competitive athletes.[8,9] As mentioned earlier, several studies have shown that sudden cardiac death[5,6] is more likely to occur with structurally normal hearts than with HCM. The proposed mechanism for the reported events in athletes thought to be malignant arrhythmias related to the physiologic demands of intense athletics. Dias and colleagues[10] discussed in detail that instantaneous risk of cardiac arrhythmias may be increased during exercise secondary to the combined actions of elevated sympathetic drive, myocardial stretch, and myocardial ischemia. Male athletes are consistently found to be at greater risk, with a nearly 10:1 higher representation of Black male athletes in those with SCA.[11–14] Studies offer conflicting data regarding the proportion of SCA due to HCM; however, HCM is considered to be the most common structural heart disease responsible for SCA in the young.[4–6,15] Maron and colleagues[16] showed that 36% of SCA in young competitive athletes with an autopsy-confirmed cardiovascular diagnosis were due to HCM. Highly visible events in young athletes garner significant attention; however, most of the exercise-associated events occur during recreational activities.[8] The mechanism of SCA is thought to be from ventricular arrhythmias due to myocardial disarray, interstitial collagen deposition, and scarring after myocyte death from microvascular dysfunction and ischemia, thus creating an unpredictable, arrhythmogenic substrate.[17] Although regular physical activity is effective for primary and secondary prevention of numerous chronic diseases,[18] the concern is that exercise and high-intensity sports may cause maladaptive remodeling, ventricular arrhythmias, and SCA among individuals with HCM.[10] In contrast, studies have shown two-thirds of SCA in younger individuals with HCM died during routine activities, rest, or sleep.[19,20] In the United Kingdom, a study examined the circumstances and demographics of SCA in 184 patients with HCM who underwent a postmortem examination by an expert cardiac pathologist between 1994 and 2014. The study found that nearly 80% of deaths occurred at rest and only 11% of patients were involved in recreational or competitive athletics[21], only 20% of patients had an antemortem diagnosis of HCM. An important note when counseling patients is that although a smaller proportion died during activity, the amount of time spent during the day in activity is less than the time at rest.

EXERCISE RISK IN HYPERTROPHIC CARDIOMYOPATHY

In general population studies, most of the exercise-related SCA attributable to HCM occurs in individuals who are undiagnosed.[21,22] In fact, exercise-related SCA incidence among HCM patients in the general population is rare. In the general population study of those aged 10 to 45 years in Ontario, in 70 million person-years of follow-up, there were 53 sudden deaths attributable to HCM with only 17% of HCM-related SCAs related to moderate or vigorous exercise.[22] This calculates into an incidence rate of HCM-related SCA associated with exercise is 0.064 per 1000 HCM person-years. Although low, it is 10-fold higher than the overall risk of cardiac arrest during competitive sport in the general population aged 12 to 45 years, of 0.76 per 100,000 person-years.[23] Ontario does not have programmatic cardiac screening, so this may be the best representative data of a true natural history of exercise-related death related to

HCM. In addition, the proportion of SCAs related to exercise was similar regardless of whether they had an antemortem diagnosis of HCM. Therefore, exercise restriction of identified persons is unlikely to explain the observed low frequency of exercise-related SCA. Similarly, a prospective study on sudden death in young adults (aged ≤35 years) conducted in Australia found that most SCAs in HCM occurred during rest or light exercise.[20] As these studies included the general population, it is reasonable to assume that most individuals were not athletes and likely engaged in exercise for less than 5% of their time. Not to leave the reader thinking exercise is unrelated to a risk of SCA, the fact that 15% to 20% of SCAs were exercise related suggests there is some association of exercise with increased instantaneous risk of SCA.

EXERCISE IS MEDICINE IN HYPERTROPHIC CARDIOMYOPATHY

A high level of cardiorespiratory fitness reduces the risk of all-cause and cardiovascular mortality in the general population regardless of gender.[24,25] As a result, exercise has become a standard of care for most patients with cardiovascular disease to improve functional capacity and reduce morbidity/mortality. If HCM patients are managed using the contemporary guideline-driven management strategies, HCM-related mortality is reported as low as 0.5% per year,[26,27] and most deaths among HCM patients are unrelated to HCM. Individuals with HCM have long been advised to participate in mild regular physical activity as an effective method for the prevention of additional chronic diseases[18] that can worsen symptoms and outcomes in HCM. These comorbid chronic conditions include a reduction in known cardiovascular risk factors such as hypertension, diabetes mellitus, hyperlipidemia, and obesity. A study of 426 patients with HCM undergoing exercise echocardiography from the Cleveland Clinic found that despite reporting being asymptomatic or only minimally symptomatic by history, 82% of patients achieved less than 100% of age-sex–predicted metabolic equivalent tasks (METs).[28] This reflects that HCM patients often adopt a sedentary lifestyle with survey data of individuals with HCM indicating they are less active, more obese, and negatively affected emotionally compared with normal controls.[29–33] Compared to inactivity, whether moderate-intensity exercise confers any greater risk for sudden cardiac death is not clear. However, there is a strong signal that reduced levels of cardiorespiratory fitness is a marker for adverse future events in patients with HCM. The largest HCM study of cardiopulmonary exercise testing found that both $\dot{V}o_{2max}$ and $\dot{V}co_2$ (minute volume of expired CO_2) are independent predictors of heart failure and cardiac transplantation but NOT of SCA, sustained ventricular arrhythmias, or appropriate implantable cardioverter-defibrillator (ICD) therapies. Notably, this applies equally to patients with and without resting left ventricular (LV) outflow tract obstruction and underscores the importance of exercise in those with HCM.[34]

In most of the patients with HCM, exercise capacity is limited[35] demonstrated by a lower peak oxygen consumption ($\dot{V}o_{2peak}$) than age-matched competitive and recreational athletes. This persists even if the individual with HCM engages in regular and endurance sport.[36] Small impediments to diastolic filling may compromise with resultant reduction in exercise stroke volume[37] and reduced exercise capacity. A minority of athletes with HCM can achieve superior peak oxygen consumption levels that allow for competitive performance at the national or international level in sports requiring a high degree of fitness.[38]

Although reduced activity may be due to exercise inherent limitations related to HCM, there is some onus related to the lack of routine exercise prescriptions given to those with HCM as well as inconsistent clinician messages regarding the benefits of exercise in HCM. The AHA, the American College of Cardiology (ACC; 36th

Bethesda Conference), and the European Society of Cardiology (ESC) have produced consensus documents (predominantly expert opinion recommendations) that advocate competitive sport restriction in trained athletes affected by a variety of genetic and acquired cardiovascular diseases.[3,4] As a result, patients and clinicians appear to focus on activities that individuals with HCM should avoid rather than identifying individual risk and risk tolerance to develop an optimal dose/amount of physical activity with continued sport participation.[10,31]

The chronic effects of exercise training have been shown to be cardioprotective in animal models of HCM and in humans for a variety of cardiac diseases. Increased parasympathetic tone, reduced sympathetic tone, and improved myocardial energetics (compared with sedentary state) conferred by regular aerobic training result in a substantially lower risk of life-threatening arrhythmias than observed in sedentary persons or animals with similar underlying substrate.[17,24,25,39] Most exercise data in HCM patients come from largely sedentary individuals, there are several studies that evaluated HCM in athletes. Several studies have demonstrated the benefits of regular, moderate exercise while maintaining safety in those with HCM. A small prospective nonrandomized study of 20 symptomatic patients (35% NYHA class 2 and 65% with NYHA class 3, mean age of 50 years) showed that a structured exercise training program (exercise intensity was gradually increased from 50% to 85% of the HR reserve) led to improvement in functional capacity with increase in METs from 4.77 ± 2.2 to 7.2 ± 2.8 ($P = .01$) and in NYHA class by ≥ 1 grade in 10 patients (50%). No adverse events or sustained ventricular arrhythmias occurred during the training program and none of the patients experienced deterioration during follow-up.[40] Although not powered for safety, no serious events such as sudden death or sustained VA occurred. Dejgaard and colleagues[41] demonstrated that vigorous activity was associated with larger LV volumes, favorable diastolic function, and no increase in ventricular arrhythmias in 132 HCM patients, 11 were competitive athletes. In an observational study, Sheikh and colleagues[38] demonstrated that competitive athletes with HCM had lower mean LV wall thickness, larger LV end-diastolic diameter and volume, more normal indices of diastolic function, lower LV outflow tract gradients, less mitral regurgitation, a lower incidence of systolic anterior motion, and similar proportion with late gadolinium enhancement (LGE) when compared to nonathletes with HCM. Like the Dejgaard study mentioned earlier, it is unclear whether these are a result of training or indicators of less severe disease, which allows for high-level athletic training.

RESET-HCM, a recent randomized 16-week study of 136 patients with HCM (mean age of 64 years), showed a modest but statistically significant increase in oxygen capacity (peak Vo_2 compared with placebo) and quality-of-life physical function among patients who engaged in moderate-intensity exercise.[42] It is noteworthy that the study included high-risk patients; more than 30% had ICDs, and 4% had a history of sustained VT or cardiac arrest. No patient with HCM experienced a major adverse cardiovascular event during the study period. Although there were no deaths, aborted SCD, ICD discharges, or sustained ventricular arrhythmias, 3 participants did experience symptomatic nonsustained VT (one of whom had an ICD).[42]

Pelliccia and colleagues[43] showed that among 35 mostly low-risk athletes with HCM, there was no difference in the incidence of symptoms or major events between athletes who stopped exercise and those who continued competitive sports. This group published a follow-up study of predominantly low-risk, white athletes demonstrating no difference in symptoms or freedom from SCA between HCM-trained and detrained patients. They noted that similar results may not be seen in populations that are younger, racially diverse, or have more severe phenotypes, more data are needed in this regard.[44]

The majority of those included in these studies are older subjects, as a result, widespread applicability to young individuals with HCM is not certain or whether these studies can be extended to high-intensity exercise. However, the ICD Sports Registry of 440 athletes with ICDs, shed some insight when they reported no deaths or external resuscitations during or after sports and the likelihood of receiving a shock was similar between competition and other physical activity among individuals with HCM.[45]

Whether or not long-term exercise, especially if begun at a young age, modifies, attenuates, or worsens the structural abnormalities associated with HCM remains unknown. Even if exercise does not alter the structural abnormalities associated with HCM, it may improve prognosis via the various mechanisms attributed to the known benefits of exercise on cardiovascular, autonomic, and metabolic function.[46] More data are needed to appropriately comment on the efficacy and safety of high-intensity exercise in this population.

RISK STRATIFICATION

Risk stratification in HCM can be challenging.[1] Sudden death risk markers in HCM patients have been identified and have resulted in improved outcomes in those with HCM at risk for SCA through ICD implantation (**Fig. 1**). Maron and colleagues[26,47] have demonstrated that SCA risk stratification has improved over time and the risk of SCA in those deemed "low risk" is extremely low. In this cohort, they found their contemporary risk factor strategy had a sensitivity of 95% to reliably identify those at at-risk for SCA and would benefit from an ICD implantation. They used contemporary risk factors that are independent of exercise/sports participation to determine risk. This strategy was at the heart of the ACC/AHA 2020 guideline algorithm and explanation of how to best utilize these risk factors to determine those at risk and provide an ICD recommendation (see **Fig. 1**).[1,47] The risk factors include recent unexplained syncope with or without outflow obstruction; family history of HCM-related sudden death in a close relative; thin-walled akinetic/dyskinetic LV apical aneurysm with regional scarring; repetitive and/or prolonged episodes of nonsustained ventricular tachycardia on ambulatory monitoring; extensive LGE including end-stage progression; and massive left ventricular hypertrophy (wall thickness $\geq$30 mm). There were no single risk markers that applied to all patients at risk for SCA.[47] The ESC had previously published a model to estimate the individual 5-year risk of SCA to provide guidance on the need for prophylactic ICDs. Notably, this was not created for athletes specifically and may not represent the true risk of SCA for athletes with HCM. In addition, further study found the ESC HCM model to have a low sensitivity for SCA and argued that the calculator, based on mathematical population models, leaves many individuals vulnerable.[48,49] It also does not account for LGE presence, reduced systolic function or an LV apical aneurysm which limits its contemporary application including exercise risk assessment. Using the criteria noted earlier has resulted in a robust ability to identify those HCM patients at risk for SCA. Maron and colleagues[47] followed 2094 patients with HCM over 17 years and showed that the ESC risk score was less sensitive compared with an enhanced ACC/AHA risk factor strategy. Risk stratification scenarios can involve a measure of ambiguity when data are insufficient to allow definitive recommendations. Predictive power of individual sudden death risk factors is also influenced by age, with risk markers most relevant in young and middle-aged patients. In stable HCM adults older than 60 years, the identified sudden death rate is 0.2% per year.[50]

Risk assessment is an ongoing process to help identify HCM patients with high-risk features that place them at increased risk some of whom may benefit from an ICD

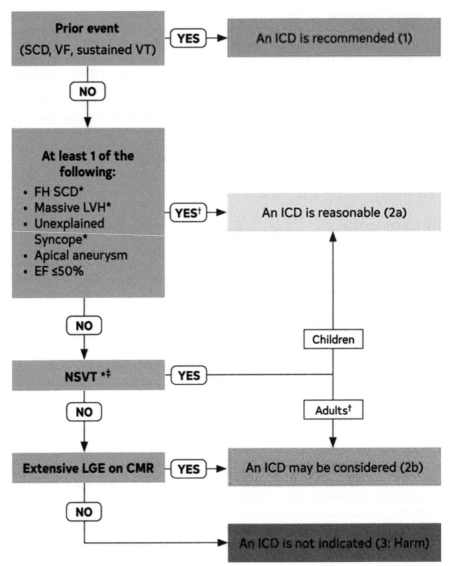

Fig. 1. The ACC/AHA 2020 guidelines algorithm of how to best utilize SCA risk factors to determine ICD recommendations. *ICD decisions in pediatric patients with HCM are based on ≥1 of these major risk factors: family history of HCM SCD, NSVT on ambulatory monitor, massive LVH, and unexplained syncope. ‡It would seem most appropriate to place greater weight on frequent, longer, and faster runs of NSVT. (*From* 2020 AHA/ACC Guideline for the Diagnosis and Treatment of Patients With Hypertrophic Cardiomyopathy. Writing Committee Members, Steve R. Ommen, MD, FACC, FAHA, Chair, Seema Mital, MD, FACC, FAHA, FRCPC, Vice Chair, Michael A. Burke, MD, Sharlene M. Day, MD, Anita Deswal, MD, MPH, FACC, FAHA, Perry Elliott, MD, FRCP, FACC, Lauren L. Evanovich, PhD, Judy Hung, MD, FACC, José A. Joglar, MD, FACC, FAHA, Paul Kantor, MBBCh, MSc, FRCPC, Carey Kimmelstiel, MD, FACC, FSCAI, Michelle Kittleson, MD, PhD, FACC, Mark S. Link, MD, FACC, Martin S. Maron, MD, Matthew W. Martinez, MD, FACC, Christina Y. Miyake, MD, MS, Hartzell V. Schaff, MD, FACC, Christopher Semsarian, MBBS, PhD, MPH, FAHA, Paul Sorajja, MD, FACC, FAHA, FSCAI.)

implantation. Repeated risk assessment for SCA is recommended every 1 to 2 years and for those participating in rigorous activity or competitive sports, it should be annual. Individuals with HCM and their physicians must make decisions together regarding an individual's SCA risk and need for ICD implantation in the context of evolving data and individual HCM patient findings. HCM risk is not the same for all. Current guidelines have focused on shared decision making between patients and physicians for all aspects of HCM care (genetic testing, surgical reduction therapies, ICD indications, anticoagulation choice, and exercise recommendation) to individualize decisions.[1,51] Physicians should discuss that HCM risk varies based on age, race, specific sport, and phenotypic details and the absolute risk is often unquantifiable.[51] An individualized risk assessment is necessary for all HCM patients and provides important findings to help guide an exercise plan through shared decision making (**Fig. 2**). Although risk stratification in HCM has matured to determine those who may be at risk, physicians should reiterate that SCA is possible even in the absence of all major risk factors.[52]

Exercise Prescription for Hypertrophic Cardiomyopathy

Although the optimum exercise prescription remains yet to be determined, the marked benefits of regular exercise may outweigh the risks of inactivity. In addition, many HCM patients want to continue to exercise. In those HCM athletes who have continued participation in competitive sports, in a survey of their health behaviors, 63% had participated in competitive athletics in their lifetime and 10% were still competing in at least one sport and 60% believed that exercise restriction negatively affected their emotional well-being.[30]

As discussed earlier, much of the exercise discussion with patients involves restriction and the possible harms of exercise, regardless of risk stratification including age. This ignores the known harms caused by exercise restriction related to increased comorbid CAD risk factors, loss of autonomy and self-identity, loss of educational

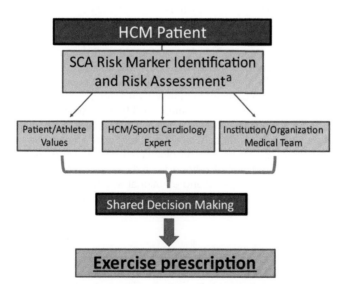

Fig. 2. Illustration of how to approach the discussion with HCM patients about their SCA risk markers and risk assessment to determine a plan for fitness level that is acceptable to all parties involved. [a]Annual assessment.

scholarship/potential income, and the risk of depression or mental health issues. HCM is a heterogeneous disease with variable phenotypic expression as wide as the patient population affected by HCM. As a result, exercise recommendations cannot be a one-size-fits-all approach and should be customized to the individual, including shared decision making in the same way we approach other aspects of HCM. Individualized advice should be provided by those with HCM expertise and take it account age, sex (there appears to be a lower risk of sudden death in women compared with men), severity of disease, presence of symptoms, type and intensity of sport/exercise, and the athlete expectations/risk tolerance (see **Fig. 2**). This approach requires time for assessment and time for the athlete to provide their own input. The 2020 AHA/ACC HCM guidelines specifically advocate for all HCM patients who engage in exercise at any level to undergo a comprehensive evaluation and shared making discussion including potential risks of sports participation conducted by an HCM expert provider.[1]

The comprehensive expert assessment should be before participation in sports and provide a comprehensive clinical evaluation, optimized pharmacologic therapy, and complete risk stratification with cardiac imaging.[1] This should include a maximal effort, symptom-limited exercise test that simulates the level he/she will attain during their training and competition. Exercise-induced rhythm abnormalities and hypotension can be a concerning finding that warrants further consideration before an exercise program can be safely recommended. A well-designed exercise program should include guidance regarding aerobic conditioning, weight training, and include nutrition and hydration recommendations. HCM exercise prescriptions should provide recommendations for frequency, intensity, duration, mode, and rate of progression. The athlete should be made aware of concerning symptoms (dizziness/syncope, shortness of breath, or chest pressure, racing heart rate), which should prompt the athlete to cease practice/competition until further evaluation. This approach allows for individualized exercise prescriptions for recreational exercise and competitive athletes and those who elect to abstain from competitive sports after their diagnosis and risk stratification. Most HCM patients do not have an indication for ICD implantation, so the exercise prescription should include a plan to handle a cardiac emergencies with an EAP/AED with emergency medical services call-to-shock time of under 5 minutes more than 90% of the time.[53,54] Appropriate education and training that is venue specific informs all coaches, families, fellow athletes, and staff to be aware of the risk and have a plan to handle it. We often advocate athletes to consider purchasing their own AED and be an active participant in their own safety.

After risk stratification, some HCM patients will have sufficient risk to warrant ICD implantation. In those who have elected to have an ICD implantation, given there is evidence that it may be safe for those with ICDs to exercise, an exercise prescription is appropriate for them as well.[45,55–57] As discussed earlier, cardiorespiratory fitness level is an important predictor of outcomes, aids in reduction in CAD risk factors and obesity, and improves physical and emotional well-being, therefore all HCM patients require an individualized exercise plan to maximize outcomes and safety.

SUMMARY

HCM is a heterogeneous disease with variable phenotypic expression. Only a small subset of patients with HCM will experience SCA. Cardiorespiratory fitness reduces all-cause and cardiovascular mortality with exercise being the standard of care for most patients with cardiovascular disease to improve functional capacity and reduce morbidity and mortality.

There remains uncertainty as to whether moderate-intensity exercise confers any greater risk for SCA or if withdrawal from sport participation lowers the risk of SCA in HCM-related death. Therefore, I endorse an approach that engages a risk-stratified HCM athlete, his or her family members, the athletic team (overarching institution when applicable) in a balanced discussion regarding the risk that incorporates all available data to determine a safe exercise plan.

CLINICS CARE POINTS

- all patients with HCM require risk stratification prior to exercise.
- all patients with HCM require an exercise prescription as part of their cardiovascular care.
- HCM patients with ICDs will benefit from an exercise prescription that fits their risk profile.

DISCLOSURE

The author has nothing to disclose.

REFERENCES

1. Ommen SR, Mital S, Burke MA, et al. 2020 AHA/ACC Guideline for the Diagnosis and treatment of patients with hypertrophic cardiomyopathy: a report of the American College of Cardiology/American Heart Association joint committee on clinical practice guidelines. J Am Coll Cardiol 2020;76(25):e159–240.
2. Geske JB, Ommen SR, Gersh BJ. Hypertrophic cardiomyopathy: clinical update. JACC Heart Fail 2018;6(5):364–75.
3. Maron BJ, Zipes DP. Introduction: eligibility recommendations for competitive athletes with cardiovascular abnormalities-general considerations. J Am Coll Cardiol 2005;45(8):1318–21.
4. Pelliccia A, Fagard R, Bjørnstad HH, et al. Recommendations for competitive sports participation in athletes with cardiovascular disease: a consensus document from the Study Group of sports cardiology of the working group of cardiac rehabilitation and exercise physiology and the working group of myocardial and pericardial diseases of the european society of cardiology. Eur Heart J 2005; 26(14):1422–45.
5. Ullal AJ, Abdelfattah RS, Ashley EA, et al. Hypertrophic cardiomyopathy as a cause of sudden cardiac death in the young: a meta-analysis. Am J Med 2016; 129(5):486–96.e482.
6. Harmon KG, Asif IM, Maleszewski JJ, et al. Incidence, cause, and comparative frequency of sudden cardiac death in national collegiate athletic association athletes: a decade in review. Circulation 2015;132(1):10–9.
7. Maron BJ, Udelson JE, Bonow RO, et al. Eligibility and disqualification recommendations for competitive athletes with cardiovascular abnormalities: task force 3: hypertrophic cardiomyopathy, arrhythmogenic right ventricular cardiomyopathy and other cardiomyopathies, and myocarditis: a scientific statement from the American heart association and american college of cardiology. Circulation 2015;132(22):e273–80.
8. Marijon E, Tafflet M, Celermajer DS, et al. Sports-related sudden death in the general population. Circulation 2011;124(6):672–81.

9. Holst AG, Winkel BG, Theilade J, et al. Incidence and etiology of sports-related sudden cardiac death in Denmark—Implications for preparticipation screening. Heart Rhythm 2010;7(10):1365–71.

10. Dias KA, Link MS, Levine BD. Exercise training for patients with hypertrophic cardiomyopathy: JACC review topic of the week. J Am Coll Cardiol 2018;72(10): 1157–65.

11. Maron BJ, Carney KP, Lever HM, et al. Relationship of race to sudden cardiac death in competitive athletes with hypertrophic cardiomyopathy. J Am Coll Cardiol 2003;41(6):974–80.

12. Maron BJ, Roberts WC, McAllister HA, et al. Sudden death in young athletes. Circulation 1980;62(2):218–29.

13. Maron BJ, Shirani J, Poliac LC, et al. Sudden death in young competitive athletes. Clinical, demographic, and pathological profiles. JAMA 1996;276(3):199–204.

14. Castelletti S, Gati S. The female athlete's heart: overview and management of cardiovascular diseases. Eur Cardiol 2021;16:e47.

15. Maron BJ, Doerer JJ, Haas TS, et al. Sudden deaths in young competitive athletes: analysis of 1866 deaths in the United States, 1980-2006. Circulation 2009;119:1085–92.

16. Maron BJ, Haas TS, Ahluwalia A, et al. Demographics and epidemiology of sudden deaths in young competitive athletes: from the United States National Registry. Am J Med 2016;129(11):1170–7.

17. Lander BS, Phelan DM, Martinez MW, et al. Hypertrophic cardiomyopathy: updates through the lens of sports cardiology. Curr Treat Options Cardiovasc Med 2021;23(8):53.

18. Warburton DE, Nicol CW, Bredin SS. Health benefits of physical activity: the evidence. CMAJ 2006;174(6):801–9.

19. Aro AL, Nair SG, Reinier K, et al. Population burden of sudden death associated with hypertrophic cardiomyopathy. Circulation 2017;136(17):1665–7.

20. Bagnall RD, Weintraub RG, Ingles J, et al. A prospective study of sudden cardiac death among children and young adults. N Engl J Med 2016;374(25):2441–52.

21. Finocchiaro G, Papadakis M, Robertus JL, et al. Etiology of sudden death in sports: insights from a united kingdom regional registry. J Am Coll Cardiol 2016;67(18):2108–15.

22. Weissler-Snir A, Allan K, Cunningham K, et al. Hypertrophic Cardiomyopathy-Related Sudden Cardiac Death in Young People in Ontario. Circulation 2019; 140(21):1706–16.

23. Landry CH, Allan KS, Connelly KA, et al. Sudden cardiac arrest during participation in competitive sports. N Engl J Med 2017;377(20):1943–53.

24. Myers J, Prakash M, Froelicher V, et al. Exercise capacity and mortality among men referred for exercise testing. N Engl J Med 2002;346(11):793–801.

25. Gulati M, Pandey DK, Arnsdorf MF, et al. Exercise capacity and the risk of death in women: the St James Women Take Heart Project. Circulation 2003;108(13): 1554–9.

26. Maron BJ, Rowin EJ, Casey SA, et al. Hypertrophic cardiomyopathy in children, adolescents, and young adults associated with low cardiovascular mortality with contemporary management strategies. Circulation 2016;133(1):62–73.

27. Maron BJ, Rowin EJ, Casey SA, et al. What do patients with hypertrophic cardiomyopathy die from? Am J Cardiol 2016;117(3):434–5.

28. Desai MY, Bhonsale A, Patel P, et al. Exercise echocardiography in asymptomatic HCM: exercise capacity, and not LV outflow tract gradient predicts long-term outcomes. JACC Cardiovasc Imaging 2014;7(1):26–36.

29. Luiten RC, Ormond K, Post L, et al. Exercise restrictions trigger psychological difficulty in active and athletic adults with hypertrophic cardiomyopathy. Open Heart 2016;3(2):e000488.

30. Reineck E, Rolston B, Bragg-Gresham JL, et al. Physical activity and other health behaviors in adults with hypertrophic cardiomyopathy. Am J Cardiol 2013;111(7): 1034–9.

31. Sweeting J, Ingles J, Timperio A, et al. Physical activity in hypertrophic cardiomyopathy: prevalence of inactivity and perceived barriers. Open Heart 2016;3(2): e000484.

32. Asif IM, Price D, Fisher LA, et al. Stages of psychological impact after diagnosis with serious or potentially lethal cardiac disease in young competitive athletes: a new model. J Electrocardiol 2015;48(3):298–310.

33. Berg AE, Meyers LL, Dent KM, et al. Psychological impact of sports restriction in asymptomatic adolescents with hypertrophic cardiomyopathy, dilated cardiomyopathy, and long QT syndrome. Prog Pediatr Cardiol 2018;49:57–62.

34. Coats CJ, Rantell K, Bartnik A, et al. Cardiopulmonary Exercise Testing and Prognosis in Hypertrophic Cardiomyopathy. Circ Heart Fail 2015;8(6):1022–31.

35. Snir AW, Connelly KA, Goodman JM, et al. Exercise in hypertrophic cardiomyopathy: restrict or rethink. Am J Physiol Heart Circulatory Physiol 2021;320(5): H2101–11.

36. Sharma S, Elliott PM, Whyte G, et al. Utility of metabolic exercise testing in distinguishing hypertrophic cardiomyopathy from physiologic left ventricular hypertrophy in athletes. J Am Coll Cardiol 2000;36(3):864–70.

37. Lele SS, Thomson HL, Seo H, et al. Exercise capacity in hypertrophic cardiomyopathy. Role of stroke volume limitation, heart rate, and diastolic filling characteristics. Circulation 1995;92(10):2886–94.

38. Sheikh N, Papadakis M, Schnell F, et al. Clinical profile of athletes with hypertrophic cardiomyopathy. Circ Cardiovasc Imaging 2015;8(7):e003454.

39. Lear SA, Hu W, Rangarajan S, et al. The effect of physical activity on mortality and cardiovascular disease in 130 000 people from 17 high-income, middle-income, and low-income countries: the PURE study. Lancet 2017;390(10113):2643–54.

40. Klempfner R, Kamerman T, Schwammenthal E, et al. Efficacy of exercise training in symptomatic patients with hypertrophic cardiomyopathy: results of a structured exercise training program in a cardiac rehabilitation center. Eur J Prev Cardiol 2015;22(1):13–9.

41. Dejgaard LA, Haland TF, Lie OH, et al. Vigorous exercise in patients with hypertrophic cardiomyopathy. Int J Cardiol 2018;250:157–63.

42. Saberi S, Wheeler M, Bragg-Gresham J, et al. Effect of moderate-intensity exercise training on peak oxygen consumption in patients with hypertrophic cardiomyopathy: a randomized clinical trial. JAMA 2017;317(13):1349–57.

43. Pelliccia A, Lemme E, Maestrini V, et al. Does sport participation worsen the clinical course of hypertrophic cardiomyopathy? Clinical outcome of hypertrophic cardiomyopathy in athletes. Circulation 2018;137(5):531–3.

44. Pelliccia A, Caselli S, Pelliccia M, et al. Clinical outcomes in adult athletes with hypertrophic cardiomyopathy: a 7-year follow-up study. Br J Sports Med 2020; 54(16):1008–12.

45. Lampert R, Olshansky B, Heidbuchel H, et al. Safety of sports for athletes with implantable cardioverter-defibrillators: long-term results of a prospective multinational registry. Circulation 2017;135(23):2310–2.

46. Fiuza-Luces C, Santos-Lozano A, Joyner M, et al. Exercise benefits in cardiovascular disease: beyond attenuation of traditional risk factors. Nat Rev Cardiol 2018;15(12):731–43.

47. Maron MS, Rowin EJ, Wessler BS, et al. Enhanced American College Of Cardiology/American Heart Association Strategy for prevention of sudden cardiac death in high-risk patients with hypertrophic cardiomyopathy. JAMA Cardiol 2019;4(7): 644–57.

48. Maron BJ, Casey SA, Chan RH, et al. Independent assessment of the European Society of Cardiology sudden death risk model for hypertrophic cardiomyopathy. Am J Cardiol 2015;116(5):757–64.

49. Leong KMW, Chow JJ, Ng FS, et al. Comparison of the prognostic usefulness of the European society of cardiology and American Heart Association/American college of cardiology foundation risk stratification systems for patients with hypertrophic cardiomyopathy. Am J Cardiol 2018;121(3):349–55.

50. Maron BJ, Rowin EJ, Casey SA, et al. Risk stratification and outcome of patients with hypertrophic cardiomyopathy >=60 years of age. Circulation 2013;127(5): 585–93.

51. Pelliccia A, Sharma S, Gati S, et al. 2020 ESC Guidelines on sports cardiology and exercise in patients with cardiovascular disease. Eur Heart J 2021;42(1): 17–96.

52. Spirito P, Autore C, Formisano F, et al. Risk of sudden death and outcome in patients with hypertrophic cardiomyopathy with benign presentation and without risk factors. Am J Cardiol 2014;113(9):1550–5.

53. Travers AH, Rea TD, Bobrow BJ, et al. Part 4: CPR overview: 2010 American heart association guidelines for cardiopulmonary resuscitation and emergency cardiovascular care. Circulation 2010;122(18_suppl_3):S676–84.

54. Hainline B, Drezner J, Baggish A, et al. Interassociation consensus statement on cardiovascular care of college student-athletes. J Am Coll Cardiol 2016;67: 2981–95.

55. Belardinelli R, Capestro F, Misiani A, et al. Moderate exercise training improves functional capacity, quality of life, and endothelium-dependent vasodilation in chronic heart failure patients with implantable cardioverter defibrillators and cardiac resynchronization therapy. Eur J Cardiovasc Prev Rehabil 2006;13(5): 818–25.

56. Lampert R, Olshansky B, Heidbuchel H, et al. Safety of sports for athletes with implantable cardioverter-defibrillators: results of a prospective, multinational registry. Circulation 2013;127(20):2021–30.

57. Saarel EV, Law I, Berul CI, et al. Safety of sports for young patients with implantable cardioverter-defibrillators: long-term results of the multinational ICD sports registry. Circ Arrhythm Electrophysiol 2018;11(11):e006305.

Exercise in the Genetic Arrhythmia Syndromes – A Review

Chinmaya Mareddy, MBBS MBA[a], Matthew Thomas ScM[b],
George McDaniel, MD[c], Oliver Monfredi, MD PhD[a],*

KEYWORDS

- Arrhythmia • Genetic • QT • Brugada • CPVT • LQTS • SQTS • Exercise

KEY POINTS

- Genetic arrhythmia syndromes are rare
- They can be associated with paradoxical arrhythmia and sudden death
- These events can occur preferentially during sports and exercise participation
- Guidelines to help care teams advise patients and their families of the best approach to sports and exercise participation are summarized in this article; historically abundantly cautious disqualifications are giving way to important shared decision making approaches to ongoing participation

Do you know what my favorite part of the game is? The opportunity to play.
Mike Singletary, former linebacker for the Chicago Bears 1981 to 1992

INTRODUCTION

Rates of sudden cardiac arrest and death in athletes are low, less than 1 in 50,000, yet such events are uniformly devastating.[1] A significant proportion of these events are accounted for by patients with a genetic arrhythmia syndrome—congenital long QT syndrome (LQTS), Brugada syndrome (BrS), catecholaminergic polymorphic ventricular tachycardia (CPVT), and short QT syndrome (SQTS). Making decisions regarding restricting exercise in any cardiac patient is highly complex and challenging for both patient and physician, and is even more difficult in athletes. The

[a] Division of Cardiovascular Medicine, Department of Medicine, University of Virginia, 1215 Lee St, Charlottesville, VA 22908, USA; [b] Department of Pediatrics, P.O. Box 800386, Charlottesville, VA 22908, USA; [c] Department of Pediatric Cardiology, Battle Building 6th Floor, 1204 W. Main St, Charlottesville, VA 22903, USA
* Corresponding author.
E-mail address: OJM9W@HSCMAIL.MCC.VIRGINIA.EDU
Twitter: @oLIVERmONFREDI (O.M.)

Clin Sports Med 41 (2022) 485–510
https://doi.org/10.1016/j.csm.2022.02.008
0278-5919/22/© 2022 Elsevier Inc. All rights reserved.

physical and psychological benefits of regular exercise are undoubted, almost regardless of type, duration and dose, and span the entire human life cycle. However, exercise in patients with certain cardiac conditions, for example, arrhythmogenic cardiomyopathy, is undoubtedly detrimental, hastening the progression of disease, and making sentinel events such as heart failure, ventricular arrhythmias, and sudden death more likely. Because of this, historical guidelines have tended to favor nonparticipation in athletes with cardiac conditions, including the genetic arrhythmia syndromes,[2–8] limiting them to so-called class 1A sports (billiards, bowling, cricket, curling, golf, riflery).[7]

In this article, we focus on the genetic arrhythmia syndromes, to giving a brief review and contemporary update on current exercise guidelines to assist treating physicians make recommendations in the process of shared decision making with individual patients and their families.

The genetic arrhythmia syndromes arise because of pathogenic variants (previously referred to as mutations) in genes that encode important cellular electrophysiological characteristics, including ion channels or proteins involved in cellular depolarization

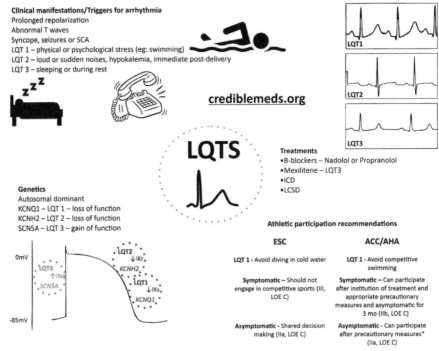

Fig. 1. Illustrative summary of LQTS, including clinical manifestations, genetics, treatments, and recommendations regarding sport and exercise participation. (*From* 2020 AHA/ACC Guideline for the Diagnosis and Treatment of Patients With Hypertrophic Cardiomyopathy Writing Committee Members, Steve R. Ommen, MD, FACC, FAHA, Chair, Seema Mital, MD, FACC, FAHA, FRCPC, Vice Chair, Michael A. Burke, MD, Sharlene M. Day, MD, Anita Deswal, MD, MPH, FACC, FAHA, Perry Elliott, MD, FRCP, FACC, Lauren L. Evanovich, PhD, Judy Hung, MD, FACC, José A. Joglar, MD, FACC, FAHA, Paul Kantor, MBBCh, MSc, FRCPC, Carey Kimmelstiel, MD, FACC, FSCAI, Michelle Kittleson, MD, PhD, FACC, Mark S. Link, MD, FACC, Martin S. Maron, MD, Matthew W. Martinez, MD, FACC, Christina Y. Miyake, MD, MS, Hartzell V. Schaff, MD, FACC, Christopher Semsarian, MBBS, PhD, MPH, FAHA, Paul Sorajja, MD, FACC, FAHA, FSCAI. Reprinted with permission Circulation.2020;142:e558-e631 ©2020 American Heart Association, Inc.)

and repolarization, leading to changes in action potential characteristics that may frequently be recognized on the resting electrocardiogram.

CONGENITAL LONG QT SYNDROME - FIG 1

Congenital LQTS affects 1 in 2000 people,[2] manifesting as the prolongation of repolarization on the ECG, associated with symptoms of syncope, seizures, and sudden cardiac death (SCD).

It is most commonly inherited as an autosomal dominant disorder due to defects in cardiac ion channels that control cardiomyocyte repolarization. Pathogenic variants in 3 genes account for 75% to 80%[9] of genotype positive cases of the condition— KCNQ1 which causes LQT1 (30%–35% of cases),[10–12] KCNH2 which causes LQT2 (25%–40% of cases),[13] and SCN5A which causes LQT3 (5%–10% of cases).[14,15] Abnormalities in multiple other genes encoding ion channel subunits and regulatory proteins are associated with rarer forms of LQTS.[9] Currently, 15% to 20% of patients who are definitively phenotype positive remain genotype negative after testing for causative variants.[16] The detailed genetics of congenital LQTS are extensively reviewed elsewhere,[17] but all manifest as the prolongation of the QT interval on ECG[2,18–20] due to a reduction in net repolarizing current in cardiomyocytes. There is often a characteristic associated abnormality of T wave morphology on the surface ECG.[21,22] A great deal of phenotypic variability exists in patients with LQTS who carry the same gene variant, including variation in penetrance, expressivity, pleiotropy, QT prolongation, and arrhythmia/sudden death risk, suggesting the critical involvement of genetic and potentially nongenetic (age, gender, presence of myocardial fibrosis) modifiers.[23,24]

The prevalence of prolonged QT in elite athletes is estimated at 0.4%.[25] SCD risk in LQTS is both variant[11] and gene specific.[26,27] Individuals with LQT1 have the highest risk of SCD risk during exercise,[5,28] and the substrate for arrhythmia (increasingly recognized to be an increase in the spatial dispersion of repolarization[29]) is exacerbated by the higher sympathetic tone typical of athletic endeavor. Swimming, in particular, imparts an especially high risk in LQT1,[28,30] while in LQT2 arrhythmia is more likely to be triggered by loud or sudden noises (classically alarm clocks or telephones ringing), during transient hypokalemia, or in women in the immediate postpartum period.[31] Contrastingly, arrhythmic events in LQT3 are more likely when sleeping or during periods of quiescence or rest. The first arrhythmic episode in these patients typically occurs before the age of 20, being earlier in patients with LQT1 than LQT2 or 3[28]. Moss and colleagues[32] performed a prospective longitudinal study of 328 probands that showed an annual rate of syncope and probable LQTS-related death of 5% and 0.9%, respectively. Elsewhere, the annual risk of SCD in untreated LQTS1, 2, and 3 patients is estimated to be between 0.3% and 0.6%.[27]

The diagnosis of LQTS is made using a combination of ECG interpretation, exercise ECG (including features such as the response of the QT to dynamic change in heart rate, T wave change in early recovery,[33] and the rate of heart rate recovery after stopping exercise[34]) and genetic analysis. LQTS is diagnosed in the presence of a confirmed pathogenic variant irrespective of the measured QT.[35] Increasingly, detectable abnormalities of ventricular function on cardiac imaging are being associated with LQTS,[36] though this area mandates further study. Even in the absence of overt pathologic prolongation of the QT interval on ECG, consideration should always be given to the Schwartz score when considering a diagnosis of LQTS.[37]

The cornerstone of management of LQTS is beta-blockade in all phenotype positive patients, and the most proven members of this drug group are nadolol[38] and propranolol,[39] while metoprolol and atenolol are not helpful and should not be used in LQTS.[40,41] Beta-blockade should also be considered in patients who carry a clearly pathogenic gene variant, but who are phenotype negative, especially if they are considering sports/athletic participation. Mexiletine is useful in LQT3 and in some patients with LQT2 because of its ability to act as a sodium channel blocker.[42,43] Newer therapeutic approaches exist.[44] Patients with LQTS who experience arrhythmia despite beta-blockade should be considered for left cardiac sympathetic denervation (LCSD)[45–48] to prevent noradrenaline directly interacting with ventricular myocytes. Implantable cardiac defibrillators (ICDs) are typically recommended in secondary prevention, in response to documented ventricular arrhythmia or SCD events.

Sports and Exercise Recommendations in Long QT Syndrome

Recommendations regarding sports participation in LQTS have been debated extensively and have evolved significantly over the past 2 decades.[3–5,49,50] Historical exercise prohibitions are waning, with accumulating data that the risk may not be as high as previously feared. Exercise-induced QT prolongation,[51] vagal predominance,[52] and bradycardia (making correction of actual QT less accurate) further complexify the issue of diagnosis and management of LQTS in athletes. Extensive discussion regarding correct measurement and interpretation of QT interval in athletes can be found elsewhere.[35] Risk stratification of athletes follows similar lines to the normal population—higher risk can be assumed whereby there is QTc $\geq$500 ms, male sex in childhood, female sex in adulthood, and a history of symptoms consistent with arrhythmia. Genotype is important as alluded to above—exercise (especially swimming) is the trigger for arrhythmia in 62% of cardiac events (and 68% of *lethal* cardiac events) in LQTS1, but only 13% of the events seen in both LQTS 2 and 3[28].

Tobert and colleagues[53] recently reviewed outcomes in 494 confirmed patients with LQTS who were given return-to-play approval, 79 of who had previously been symptomatic, and 58 of whom had an ICD. There were zero mortalities in 2056 combined years of follow-up, while 29 patients had $\geq$1 nonlethal cardiac event. Of these 29, only 15 were athletes at the time of the event, and only 3 experienced the event immediately related to sporting participation. Overall, there were 1.16 nonlethal events per 100 years of follow-up. Historically, the same group of researchers[5] reviewed events in 353 LQTS athletes, 130 of whom continued to participate in competitive sports after their diagnosis. Of these, the 70 who were genotype-positive/phenotype-negative did not experience any sport-related event. Of the 60 who were genotype-positive/phenotype-positive, only one had a sporting-related SCD event, leading to an appropriate ICD shock over a combined 650 athlete-years of follow-up. Furthermore, the one patient having the SCD event had it during admitted noncompliance with β-blocker medication.

Aziz and colleagues[54] reported no cardiac events during sports participation in their study of 103 genotype positive patients (58% LQT1, 35% LQT2, 6% LQT3, and 2% multiple pathogenic variants; 67 were asymptomatic, 23 had non-LQTS symptoms, 11 had exertional syncope and 2 had aborted cardiac arrest) over 755 patient-years follow-up. There were ICD shocks in 2 patients (1 during a febrile illness, and the other following noncompliance with beta-blocker). Chambers and colleagues[55] studied 172 genotype positive patients with LQTS (59% LQT1, 29% LQT2, 5% LQT3, and 6% multiple pathogenic variants; 136 were asymptomatic, 33 had syncope and 4 had cardiac arrest) over 1203 patients-years, and found no cardiac events in competitive athletes and no deaths. There were 13 cardiac events in 9 previously symptomatic patients during either recreational exercise or activities of daily living. Turkowski and colleagues[56] reviewed events in 366 athletes with

Table 1
Summary of major European and North American guidelines concerning participation in sports and exercise for patients with genetic arrhythmia syndromes

Genetic Syndrome		ESC Guidelines	ACC/AHA Guidelines
LQTS	A. Symptomatic (Prior CA/Arrhythmic syncope) or individual with QIc>500 ms or genetically confirmed LQTS with a QTc of ≥470 ms in men or ≥ 480 ms in women	Should not engage (III, LOC C)	3 mo restriction until complete evaluation is conducted (I, LOC C) Once complete evaluation is conducted they can be participated after the institution of treatment and appropriate precautionary measures and asymptomatic for 3 mo (IIb LOE C)
	B. LQT1	Avoid swimming	Avoid competitive swimming
	C. Asymptomatic genotype + ve/ phenotype -ve	Shared decision making (IIa LOF C)	Can participate after precautionary measures* (IIa, LOF C)
BrS	A. Symptomatic or ECG + ve	Shared decision making following ICD once they are asymptomatic for 3 mo (IIa, LOE c)	Can participate after the institution of treatment and appropriate precautionary measures and asymptomatic for 3 mo (IIb, LOE C)
	B. Asymptomatic genotype + ve/ phenotype -ve	Can participate in sports that do not increase in core temperature to >39c (IIb, LOE C)	Can participate after precautionary measures*(IIa, LOE C)
CPVT	A. Symptomatic	Should not engage (I, LOE C)	Not recommended except for class IA sports(III LOE C)
	B. Asymptomatic genotype + ve/ phenotype -ve	N.A	Can participate after precautionary measures (IIa, LOC C)
SQTS	A. Symptomatic	N.A	Can participate after the institution of treatment and appropriate precautionary measures and asymptomatic for 3 mo (IIb, LOC C)
	B. Asymptomatic genotype + ve/ phenotype -ve	N.A	Can participate after precautionary measures (LLa LOC C)

(continued on next page)

Table 1
(continued)

Genetic Syndrome		ESC Guidelines	ACC/AHA Guidelines
Idiopathic VF	A. Asymptomatic genotype + ve/ phenotype -ve	N.A	Can participate after precautionary measures (LLa LOE C)
Athletes with pacemakers		May participate in the absence of structural or other heart diseases (IIa, LOE C)	N.A
Athletes with ICDs		Shared decision making taking into account the effects of sports on the underlying substrate, risk of appropriate/inappropriate shocks, psychological impact of shocks and potential risk, for third parties (IIa, LOE C)	• Can participate in sports classified as IA if they are free of VF requiring device therapy for 3 mo (IIa LOE c) • May consider participating in sports with high peak static and dynamic components than class IA if they are free of VF requiring device therapy for 3 mo taking into account risk of appropriate/inappropriate shocks on device-related trauma in high impact sports (IIb LOC C)

genetic heart disease (81% LQTS, 10% CPVT), out of which 44 choose to self-disqualify from athletic activity. After establishing their comprehensive treatment program, only 9/322 athletes (3%) experienced a nonlethal breakthrough cardiac event (4 of which occurred outside of sports) in 961 combined athlete-years of follow-up (0.9 events per 100 athlete-years) compared with 6 of 44 former athletes (14%) in 261 combined follow-up years (2.3 events, all nonlethal, per 100 follow-up years). These 4 important studies concerning the risk of SCD during athletic participation in LQTS are summarized in **Table 1**.

Exercise Guidelines in Symptomatic Long QT Syndrome

ESC guidelines,[50] which are more restrictive than American guidelines, state that patients with congenital LQTS who are phenotype positive or symptomatic (cardiac arrest or cardiac syncope) with or without ICD, should not participate in competitive sports. Individuals with QTc greater than 500 ms or genetically confirmed LQTS with a QTc of $\geq$ 470 ms in men or $\geq$ 480 ms in women even on beta-blockers are recommended to avoid high-intensity recreational and competitive sports. Patients with LQT1 are specifically recommended to avoid sports involving diving into cold water.

Contrastingly, and some may consider more in line with recent research, AHA/ACC guidelines[57] are more lenient regarding sports participation in LQTS. For symptomatic LQTS (except for competitive swimming in previously symptomatic LQTS1) or individuals with confirmed LQTS (QTc $\geq$ 470 ms in men or $\geq$ 480 ms in women), guidelines state that participation in competitive sports may continue after the institution of treatment (beta-blockers) and appropriate precautionary measures (to include avoidance of QT-prolonging drugs, electrolyte replenishment, avoidance of dehydration, avoidance or treatment of hyperthermia, access to or acquisition of a personal AED, and to have an emergency action plan), assuming the athlete has been asymptomatic on treatment of at least 3 months.

Exercise Guidelines in Asymptomatic Long QT Syndrome

For asymptomatic genotype positive/phenotype negative patients with LQTS, current ESC guidelines[50] recommend using shared decision making, depending on both the type and setting of the proposed sport, type of pathogenic variant(s), and extent of precautionary measures undertaken when deciding on allowing sports participation. This represents a shift from prior European guidelines,[3] whereby they suggested nonparticipation in such asymptomatic patients. The AHA/ACC guidelines state that it is reasonable for such patients to participate in competitive sports with appropriate precautionary measures (avoidance of QT-prolonging drugs—www.crediblemeds.org, electrolyte replenishment, avoidance of dehydration, avoidance or treatment of hyperthermia, access to or acquisition of a personal AED, and to have an emergency action plan with appropriate school or team officials). There is plentiful evidence that AEDs are beneficial in the management of sports-related arrhythmias in athletes with LQTS.[58,59] The importance of undertaking all decisions regarding ongoing participation using a shared-decision making approach is emphasised.[60]

BRUGADA SYNDROME - FIG 2

BrS is an autosomal dominant[61] cardiac ion channelopathy. Originally thought to be a purely electrical disease, caused by either early repolarization or delayed depolarization or both,[62–64] it is now known to also be associated with RV structural abnormalities.[65–68] More than 250 associated variants have been reported in 20 different genes, which primarily encode sodium, potassium, and calcium channels.[61] However, the

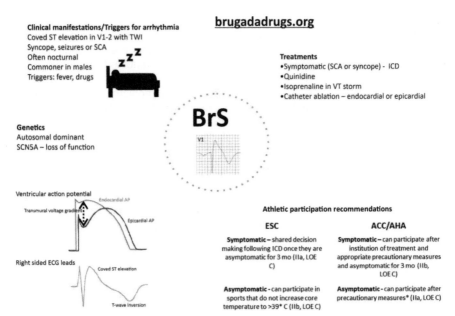

Fig. 2. Illustrative summary of BrS, including clinical manifestations, genetics, treatments, and recommendations regarding sport and exercise participation.

only gene unequivocally linked to BrS is *SCN5A*[69–71] found in around 20% of probands, and encoding the fast sodium channel, responsible for phase 0 rapid upstroke of the cardiac action potential in working atrial and ventricular myocytes. It is notable that pathogenic variants in *SCN5A* causing BrS are loss-of-function, unlike the *SCN5A* pathogenic variants discussed above and associated with LQTS3. The complex inheritance in BrS remains the focus of much research.[72,73]

The prevalence of the Brugada ECG pattern (BrEP) worldwide is 0.1%–0.9%,[74–78] and is highest in Asia (0.9%) and lowest in North America (0.2%).[78] The prevalence of BrEP in the US in 2 single-center studies is 0.012% and 0.43%.[79,80] Other studies have shown that BrS in Asians was nine times more common than in Caucasians and 36 times more common than in Hispanics.[74] BrS and BrEP are more common in men than women, by between 2 and 10 times based on various studies.[74–78]

The characteristic ECG in BrS is reviewed below and extensively elsewhere.[17] It exhibits prominent J waves (the J wave being a distinct deflection at the J point, the junction between the QRS complex and the ST segment). This is thought to reflect the disparity in transient outward K^+ current (I_{to}, carried by $K_v4.3$ channels) from epi-(more) to endocardial (less) surfaces,[81] causing a transmural voltage gradient. This gradient occurs to a higher degree in the right ventricular outflow tract > right ventricle > left ventricle,[82] hence why BrS is viewed predominantly as a right ventricular disease. The resultant repolarization abnormalities lead to the development of reentry during phase 2 of the action potential, and consequently closely coupled premature beats, with the attendant risk of polymorphic VT (the so-called "repolarization hypothesis").[64,83] The competing, but not mutually exclusive, "depolarization hypothesis" suggests that conduction slowing due to a lack of fast sodium current and gap junction protein connexin 43 along with fibrosis in the RVOT are the causes of the electrophysiologic phenomena associated with BrS.[64]

Symptomatically, patients with BrS typically present either with the incidental discovery of the classic BrEP or from symptoms related to arrhythmia,[84] often occurring nocturnally,[85] ranging from transient palpitations to syncope to sudden death. Adverse cardiac events in asymptomatic BrS occur at a rate of 0.5% to 1.2% per year.[86–88] First symptoms usually manifest in the patients 20s and 30s.[17,89] Common triggers include fever, electrolyte abnormality and drugs (see https://www.brugadadrugs.org/).[90] Patients with BrS also exhibit generalized conduction slowing on their ECG, especially if there is an underlying pathologic *SCN5A* variant,[91] and they also have a much higher than expected incidence and prevalence of atrial fibrillation.[84,92]

The diagnosis of BrS revolves around the presence of a type 1 ECG pattern[93]—this can be spontaneous or can result from the conversion of a less diagnostic type 2 ECG pattern, for example, in response to provocative drug testing with intravenous administration of sodium-channel blockers (such as procainamide, ajmaline, flecainide, or pilsicainide).[94] Leads V1-2 can be positioned anywhere from the 2nd to the 4th intercostal space to make the diagnosis.[95] The 2 main categories of ECG abnormality[96] in BrS, referred to as type 1 ("coved") or type 2 ("saddle-back"), have the following distinct characteristics:

1. Type 1 BrEP: coved ST-segment elevation ≥2 mm in 1 right precordial lead (V1 to V3), followed by an r′-wave and a concave or straight ST segment. The descending ST-segment crosses the isoelectric line and is followed by a negative and symmetric T-wave.

2. Type 2 BrEP: saddle-back ST-segment elevation ≥0.5 mm (generally ≥2 mm in V2) in ≥1 right precordial lead (V1 to V3), followed by a convex ST segment. The r′-wave may or may not overlap the J point, but it has a slow downward slope. The ST segment is followed by a positive T-wave in V2, while being of variable morphology in V1.

To facilitate the differentiation of type 2 ECGs highly indicative of BrS from other Brugada-like patterns (such as common patterns seen in athletic training, pectus excavatum, and arrhythmogenic cardiomyopathy), several additional criteria have been suggested and are discussed elsewhere.[97–99]

There are no clear guidelines for risk stratification of patients with asymptomatic BrEP, but a history of syncope, the presence of a spontaneous type 1 ECG, ventricular effective refractory period less than 200 ms, and the presence of QRS fragmentation on ECG are felt to represent significant risk factors for predicting future cardiac events.[100–103] The role of electrophysiological study (EPS) for risk stratification has been controversial.[88,104–108] Pooled analysis[88] of 1312 patients from multiple studies who do not have a prior history of SCD and who underwent programmed ventricular stimulation with up to triple extra stimuli showed that arrhythmia induction during the study was associated with a 2- to 3-fold increased risk of sudden cardiac arrest or defibrillator shock for ventricular tachyarrhythmias over a median follow-up of 38 months. It is also noted that there is decreased specificity of programmed stimulation for assessing risk when triple extra stimuli are included in the protocol. The risk of events appeared greatest among individuals induced with single or double extra-stimuli. Individuals who were not induced exhibited a ~1% annual risk for the development of ventricular arrhythmias, although risk varied substantially according to clinical features such as a history of syncope and spontaneous type 1 ECG pattern. Note that EPS is unnecessary in patients with symptomatic BrS as ICD is already indicated based on current guidelines.[109]

The risk of adverse cardiac events, especially SCD, in BrS/BrEP is relatively low.[105,107,110–113] Probst and colleagues[107] studied 1029 patients with a type 1 ECG (72% men, median age 45 years, 6% SCD, 20% syncope, 64% asymptomatic) with a median follow-up of 31.9 months. The cardiac event rate per year was 7.7% in patients with prior aborted SCD, 1.9% in patients with prior syncope, and 0.5% in asymptomatic patients. Delise and colleagues[113] studied 2176 patients with BrEP across multiple studies,[105,107,110–112] one-third of whom had an ICD. The event rates per 1000 patient-years of follow-up were 31.3 (25–39) and 6.5 (4–10) in patients with and without an ICD, respectively.[113] Total events (including both fast ventricular arrhythmias in patients with ICD and SCD) in these studies ranged from 2.6% to 8.2%. The incidence of SCD (whereby no ICD was implanted) ranged from 0% to 1%, with the exception of a study from Brugada and colleagues[110] which showed a 2.9% incidence of SCD.

Symptomatic patients with BrS (syncope or SCA) have a class 1 indication for ICD implantation.[50,104,109] Medical therapy is limited in BrS. The sodium channel blocker quinidine is the main medicine of choice, and is typically used alongside an ICD to prevent therapies—it has been shown to normalize ST segments in patients with a type 1 ECG.[114–119] The other main drug used in BrS is isoprenaline,[17] which is reserved for VT storm, whereby it may be life-saving. Catheter ablation, for refractory VA or arrhythmia requiring multiple ICD shocks, in BrS can be performed via the endocardial[120–122] or preferentially the epicardial approach.[123–129]

Sports and Exercise Recommendations in Brugada Syndrome

Because of the association between exercise and increased vagal tone during periods of rest, there has historically been concern that exercise and sports participation in BrS may increase the preponderance for arrhythmia, leading to recommendations to restrict participation in competitive sports.[3] However, because of the relatively low incidence of adverse cardiac events in BrS or BrEP[105,107,110–113] discussed above, contemporary exercise recommendations in BrS athletes have become more lenient over time.

Per the recent 2020 ESC guideline statement,[50] following the implantation of an ICD, resumption of leisure or competitive sports may be considered after shared decision making in individuals who have not experienced recurrent arrhythmia for 3 months. In asymptomatic individuals with only the Brugada pattern ECG, asymptomatic pathogenic variant carriers, and asymptomatic athletes with only an inducible ECG pattern, participation in sports activities that are not associated with an increase in core temperature greater than 39 C (eg, endurance events under extremely hot and/or humid conditions) may be considered. Participation is still discouraged for patients with a history of arrhythmic syncope or a family history of SCD with a spontaneous or a drug-induced type 1 ECG.

Per AHA/ACC guidelines,[57] competitive sports participation may be considered for an athlete with either previously symptomatic or electrocardiographically evident BrS assuming appropriate precautionary measures and disease-specific treatments are in place (avoidance of drugs that exacerbate BrS—https://www.brugadadrugs.org/, electrolyte replenishment, avoid dehydration, avoidance or treatment of hyperthermia, personal AED and to have emergency action plan), and that the athlete has been asymptomatic and established on treatment of at least 3 months. Asymptomatic genotype positive/phenotype negative patients may reasonably participate in competitive sports with appropriate precautionary measures (avoidance of drugs that exacerbate BrS, electrolyte replenishment, avoidance of dehydration, avoidance of

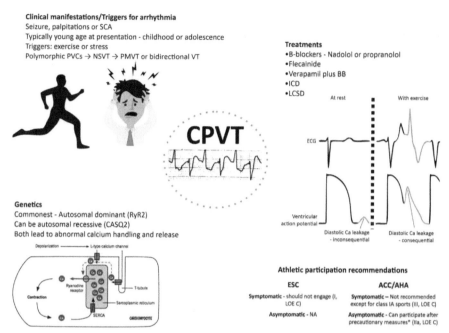

Fig. 3. Illustrative summary of CPVT, including clinical manifestations, genetics, treatments, and recommendations regarding sport and exercise participation.

or treatment of hyperthermia, personal AED, and to have an emergency action plan the appropriate school or team officials).

CATECHOLAMINERGIC POLYMORPHIC VENTRICULAR TACHYCARDIA - FIG 3

CPVT is a familial cardiac ion channelopathy, which presents with polymorphic ventricular arrhythmias induced by either physical or emotional stress, in the absence of any structural heart disease[130] and with a typically normal resting ECG.[17,131,132]

Pathogenic variants in genes encoding cardiac ryanodine receptor 2 (*RYR2*)[133–136] are the most common cause of CPVT (identified in 65% of CPVT probands), with a typically autosomal dominant mode of inheritance. The ryanodine receptor is the calcium release channel of the major intracellular store of Ca2+, the sarcoplasmic reticulum (SR). Pathogenic variants in *CASQ2*, which encodes calsequestrin 2 (an SR Ca2+ binding protein) are rarer and have been associated with autosomal recessive forms of CPVT.[137,138] There are several rarer pathogenic variants that lead to clinical CPVT, including in genes encoding calmodulin and triadin;[17] however, there remain around one-third of patients with clinical CPVT in whom a causative or contributory gene defect cannot be identified.[17] CPVT-associated pathogenic variants lead to abnormal handling of intracellular calcium,[139] with SR Ca2+ overload leading to spontaneous and poorly regulated Ca2+ release. This calcium in turn facilitates transient inward current and delayed after-depolarizations, which lead to ventricular arrhythmia in a process that is greatly amplified by sympathetic tone (exercise, emotion).[140]

Similar to BrS, CPVT is not only genetically but also clinically diverse, with variable penetrance. Clinically, it is associated with premature ventricular contractions (often consistent with an origin from the RVOT, though sometimes polymorphic), nonsustained ventricular tachycardia, polymorphic ventricular tachycardia (PMVT) or the pathognomonic but rarely seen bidirectional VT,[6,141] all occurring at times when catecholamine levels in plasma are elevated. CPVT typically becomes manifest during childhood or adolescence,[141] with symptoms including syncope, seizures, or sudden cardiac arrest. About one-third of patients experience life-threatening cardiac events before the diagnosis or before treatment initiation.[130,132,133,142,143] One of the largest studies to date[142] involving 226 patients with CPVT diagnosed before the age of 19 years from 27 pediatric centers, showed that syncope and cardiac arrest occurred in 54% and 38% of the patients, respectively. The diagnosis requires a high index of suspicion in any individual with arrhythmia, syncope, or seizure occurring in the context of exercise or highly expressed negative or positive emotion. The resting ECG and echocardiogram are typically normal, with the diagnosis being made at stress testing during which a patient typically progresses from having increasing numbers of single RVOT-morphology PVCs, through bigeminy, then couplets, triplets, nonsustained VT then polymorphic VT or bidirectional VT (the latter is rare, though highly specific). These arrhythmias dissipate when exercise ceases.

There are limited data concerning predictors for adverse cardiac events in CPVT: diagnosis at a young age, absence of beta-blockers, proband status, and history of aborted cardiac arrest before diagnosis[132,142,144] are high-risk markers. Given that catecholamine release triggers ventricular arrhythmia in this condition, it is recommended to avoid competitive sports, stressful environments, and strenuous exercise. Beta-blocker medicines without intrinsic sympathomimetic activity (eg, nadolol (when available) or propranolol) are the drugs of choice in CPVT and should be titrated to their maximum tolerated dose. This pharmacotherapy can significantly reduce cardiac events in CPVT.[132,141,145] Flecainide may also be used if patients develop breakthrough symptoms on beta-blockade,[146,147] through an effect on stabilizing "leaky" RyR2s.[146–148] The addition of verapamil to BB can also provide some benefit in reducing ventricular arrhythmias.[149–151] An ICD is indicated in those who survived cardiac arrest or in those who continue to be symptomatic despite medical therapy.[104] Reports of ICD failures to treat VA have been noted in patients with CASQ2 pathogenic variants.[152,153] LCSD is increasingly preferred to ICD (in a triple therapy approach— nadolol, flecainide, and LCSD),[154] as shocks can provoke catecholamine release, leading to worsening and refractory or recurrent arrhythmia, and as such ICD programming to absolutely minimize shocks is paramount yet challenging in these patients.[46,48,155,156] Because of this, ICD monotherapy should never be recommended in CPVT. The ultimate goal of therapy in CPVT is the normalization of the stress test, with the addition of higher doses or additional medications if the stress test remains abnormal, and ultimately the consideration of ICD/LCSD if it proves impossible to normalize the stress.[147]

Sports and Exercise Recommendations in Catecholaminergic Polymorphic Ventricular Tachycardia

There is a high risk of cardiac events in CPVT related to exertion or physical activity and consequently, both ESC and AHA/ACC guidelines are very restrictive when it comes to sports participation.

Ostby and colleagues[6] studied a CPVT cohort of 63 athletes from the Mayo Clinic. 21 of those athletes chose to continue to participate in athletic endeavors (19/21 involved in either high static—class III or high dynamic component class C sports[157]). During follow-up, 9 of the original 63 patients with CPVT (3/21 from athletes and 6/42 from nonathletes) experienced a CPVT-associated cardiac event (syncope or ICD shock) despite medical therapy. There was, however, no difference in events or event rates between the 2 groups. These observational data suggest the importance of shared decision-making once the diagnosis is established, and in the presence of a comprehensive treatment plan, it *may* be acceptable to take the risk of continued sports participation as the event rates, something that historically would have been highly discouraged.

Nonetheless, ESC guidelines[158] recommend complete avoidance of competitive sports, strenuous exercise, and stressful environments. AHA/ACC guidelines[57] state that for patients with symptomatic CPVT or asymptomatic CPVT with exercise-induced premature ventricular contractions in bigeminy, couplets, or nonsustained ventricular tachycardia, participation in competitive sports is not recommended except for class IA sports.[157] Exceptions to this rule "should be made only after consultation with a CPVT specialist", and usually after the institution of therapy and exercise testing documenting an absence of arrhythmia. When it comes to asymptomatic genotype positive/phenotype negative CPVT, it is reasonable to participate in competitive sports with appropriate precautionary measures (compliance with medication regime, personal AED and to have emergency action plan).

SHORT QT-SYNDROME - FIG 4

SQTS is a rare (total reported cases <1000), autosomal dominant cardiac ion channel-opathy characterized by accelerated repolarization exemplified by an abnormally short QT interval on the ECG. It is associated with an increased risk of atrial and ventricular arrhythmias in patients without structural heart disease.[159,160]

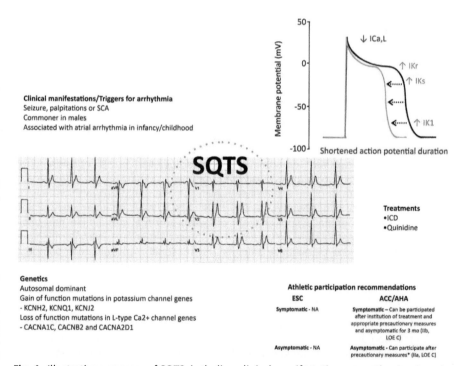

Fig. 4. Illustrative summary of SQTS, including clinical manifestations, genetics, treatments, and recommendations regarding sport and exercise participation.

SQTS is usually defined as QTc ≤ 340 ms, or QTc interval ≤ 360 ms and one or more of the following: confirmed pathogenic variant, family history of SQTS, family history of sudden death at age less than 40 or younger, or survival from a VT/VF episode in the absence of heart disease.[161] Pathogenic variants in potassium channel genes (*KCNH2*, *KCNQ1*, *KCNJ2*) lead to gain of function (compared with the loss-of-function variants in LQTS). Pathogenic variants in L-type Ca2+ channel genes (*CACNA1C*, *CACNB2*, and *CACNA2D1*) have been implicated in an overlap syndrome incorporating features of SQTS with BrS[162–167]; these are loss-of-function variants and lead to shortening of the action potential. Causative pathogenic variants are only found in 20% of patients with clinical SQTS, however.[17] As alluded to above, SQTS is very rare, with a prevalence of around 0.02% to 0.1%, being more common in men[168–171]. Arrhythmias in SQTS are associated with exaggerated dispersal of repolarization from epi-to endocardium, favoring the development of highly lethal ventricular arrhythmias.[172,173] Arrhythmia occurs across all age groups, and the incidence of cardiac arrest by age 40 is greater than 40%.[160,174] Atrial arrhythmias, especially atrial fibrillation and flutter, are also common and can present with palpitations in infants and even newborn children.[175] Other ECG features that can give a clue to the presence of SQTS include PR segment depression, tall symmetric T waves with very little discrete ST segment, U waves, and failure of the QT interval to change in response to exercise.[176–179]

The finding of a short QTc in the range of 300 to 360 ms warrants monitoring and follow-up without any prophylactic treatment.[17,171,180] More markedly shortened QTc values of ≤ 300 ms are associated with an increased risk of SCD especially during sleep or at rest.[181,182] The main predictor of arrhythmia in SQTS is a history of prior nonfatal cardiac arrest. Symptomatic patients (documented arrhythmia, cardiac arrest, or syncope) should receive an ICD. Quinidine, which can prolong QTc, can be considered in asymptomatic individuals with very short QT intervals, or a family history of SCD, and in symptomatic patients to reduce the number of ICD shocks.[109,175,181,183,184] Isoprenaline infusion can be helpful in electrical storm episodes but is clearly not a long-term solution in the ambulatory setting.[185]

Sports and Exercise Recommendations in Short QT Syndrome

Because of its rarity, there is a paucity of data backing up any of the exercise recommendations in SQTS. As there are no specific triggers for adverse events in SQTS, no specific guidelines from ESC are available at this time.

Per AHA/ACC guidelines,[57] competitive sports participation may be considered for an athlete with SQTS who was previously symptomatic assuming appropriate precautionary measures are in place (electrolyte replenishment, avoid dehydration, avoidance or treatment of hyperthermia, personal AED and to have an emergency action plan with the appropriate school or team officials), and that the athlete has been asymptomatic and established on treatment of at least 3 months. Asymptomatic genotype positive/phenotype negative patients may reasonably participate in competitive sports with appropriate precautionary measures as mentioned above.

WHY ARE ESC AND AHA/ACC GUIDELINES DIFFERENT?

Although there are many commonalities between the guidelines issued by the major North American and European societies, important differences persist, and the reasons underlying these have been discussed elsewhere.[35] These include human factors (different groups of individuals discussing the same issue are always likely to come up with conclusions that differ in some significant way), alongside societal/

cultural factors. The latter are shaped by experience and, in the case of the European guidelines, more ubiquitous screening, particularly in the Italian medical system, may have led to the more conservative approach.[8] It has also been suggested that ideological differences related to personal freedom versus society's paternalistic responsibility plays a role in the observed differences.[35,49] There is undoubtedly significant evolution, however, in the concept of return to play after diagnosis and appropriate management in a number of the genetic arrhythmia syndromes,[57,186] driven in large part by the studies of Ackerman and colleagues, most recently,[53] along with the importance of shared-decision making in any final verdict on returning to sports or not.[187] While more progress needs to be made, the evolution of our understanding of these issues over the past 2 decades has increasingly allowed ongoing safe participation with minimal necessary exclusions, and this can only be viewed as being good for both the hearts and heads of athletes and their families. The tennis player Andre Agassi once said "What makes something special is not just what you have to gain, but what you feel there is to lose". There is much to be lost in patients with genetic arrhythmia syndromes when they are poorly managed, and the goal of this review, and many of the excellent papers in the bibliography is to ensure that, whereby possible, the special relationship between athletes and sports is retained, even in the face of these complex conditions.

DISCLOSURE

The authors have nothing to disclose

CLINICS CARE POINTS

- Risk of arrhythmia and sudden death can be higher during exercise in genetic arrhythmia syndromes
- Guidelines exist to help treating teams advise patients and families regarding this risk, and how best to manage it
- The focus of treating teams needs to be on encouraging and facilitating participation in sports and exercise whereby safe to do so, in appropriately disqualifying patients whereby sports and exercise participation is clearly not safe, and in participating in shared-decision making whereby the risk:benefit balance remains unclear

REFERENCES

1. Semsarian C, Sweeting J, Ackerman MJ. Sudden cardiac death in athletes. BMJ 2015;350:h1218. https://doi.org/10.1136/bmj.h1218.
2. Ackerman MJ. Cardiac channelopathies: it's in the genes. Nat Med 2004;10(5): 463–4.
3. Pelliccia A, Fagard R, Bjørnstad HH, et al. Recommendations for competitive sports participation in athletes with cardiovascular disease: A consensus document from the Study Group of Sports Cardiology of the Working Group of Cardiac Rehabilitation and Exercise Physiology and the Working Group of Myocardial and Pericardial Diseases of the European Society of Cardiology. Eur Heart J 2005;26(14):1422–45.
4. Johnson JN, Ackerman MJ. Competitive Sports Participation in Athletes With Congenital Long QT Syndrome. JAMA 2012;308(8):764–5.

5. Johnson JN, Ackerman MJ. Return to play? Athletes with congenital long QT syndrome. Br J Sports Med 2013;47(1):28–33.

6. Ostby SA, Bos JM, Owen HJ, et al. Competitive Sports Participation in Patients With Catecholaminergic Polymorphic Ventricular Tachycardia. JACC Clin Electrophysiol 2016;2(3):253–62.

7. Maron BJ, Zipes DP. Introduction: eligibility recommendations for competitive athletes with cardiovascular abnormalities-general considerations. J Am Coll Cardiol 2005;45(8):1318–21.

8. Pelliccia A, Zipes DP, Maron BJ. Bethesda Conference #36 and the European Society of Cardiology Consensus Recommendations revisited a comparison of U.S. and European criteria for eligibility and disqualification of competitive athletes with cardiovascular abnormalities. J Am Coll Cardiol 2008;52(24): 1990–6.

9. Giudicessi JR, Wilde AAM, Ackerman MJ. The genetic architecture of long QT syndrome: A critical reappraisal. Trends Cardiovasc Med 2018;28(7):453–64.

10. Wang Q, Curran ME, Splawski I, et al. Positional cloning of a novel potassium channel gene: KVLQT1 mutations cause cardiac arrhythmias. Nat Genet 1996;12(1):17–23.

11. Moss AJ, Shimizu W, Wilde AAM, et al. Clinical aspects of type-1 long-QT syndrome by location, coding type, and biophysical function of mutations involving the KCNQ1 gene. Circulation 2007;115(19):2481–9.

12. Chen S, Zhang L, Bryant R, et al. KCNQ1 mutations in patients with a family history of lethal cardiac arrhythmias and sudden death. Clin Genet 2003;63(4): 273–82.

13. Curran ME, Splawski I, Timothy KW, et al. A molecular basis for cardiac arrhythmia: HERG mutations cause long QT syndrome. Cell 1995;80(5): 795–803.

14. Wang Q, Shen J, Li Z, et al. Cardiac sodium channel mutations in patients with long QT syndrome, an inherited cardiac arrhythmia. Hum Mol Genet 1995;4(9): 1603–7.

15. Wang Q, Shen J, Splawski I, et al. SCN5A mutations associated with an inherited cardiac arrhythmia, long QT syndrome. Cell 1995;80(5):805–11.

16. Ackerman MJ, Priori SG, Willems S, et al. HRS/EHRA expert consensus statement on the state of genetic testing for the channelopathies and cardiomyopathies this document was developed as a partnership between the Heart Rhythm Society (HRS) and the European Heart Rhythm Association (EHRA). Heart Rhythm 2011;8(8):1308–39.

17. Schwartz PJ, Ackerman MJ, Antzelevitch C, et al. Inherited cardiac arrhythmias. Nat Rev Dis Primer 2020;6(1):58.

18. Jervell A, Lange-Nielsen F. Congenital deaf-mutism, functional heart disease with prolongation of the Q-T interval, and sudden death. Am Heart J 1957; 54(1):59–68.

19. Romano C, Gemme G, Pongiglione R. [RARE CARDIAC ARRYTHMIAS OF THE PEDIATRIC AGE. II. SYNCOPAL ATTACKS DUE TO PAROXYSMAL VENTRICULAR FIBRILLATION. (PRESENTATION OF 1ST CASE IN ITALIAN PEDIATRIC LITERATURE)]. Clin Pediatr (Bologna) 1963;45:656–83.

20. Ward OC. A NEW FAMILIAL CARDIAC SYNDROME IN CHILDREN. J Ir Med Assoc 1964;54:103–6.

21. Antzelevitch C. Ionic, molecular, and cellular bases of QT-interval prolongation and torsade de pointes. Eur Eur Pacing Arrhythm Card Electrophysiol J Work

Groups Card Pacing Arrhythm Card Cell Electrophysiol Eur Soc Cardiol 2007; 9(Suppl 4):iv4–15.

22. Bohnen MS, Peng G, Robey SH, et al. Molecular Pathophysiology of Congenital Long QT Syndrome. Physiol Rev 2017;97(1):89–134.

23. Schwartz PJ, Crotti L, George AL. Modifier genes for sudden cardiac death. Eur Heart J 2018;39(44):3925–31.

24. Lee YK, Sala L, Mura M, et al. MTMR4 SNVs modulate ion channel degradation and clinical severity in congenital long QT syndrome: insights in the mechanism of action of protective modifier genes. Cardiovasc Res 2021;117(3):767–79.

25. Basavarajaiah S, Wilson M, Whyte G, et al. Prevalence and significance of an isolated long QT interval in elite athletes. Eur Heart J 2007;28(23):2944–9.

26. Zareba W, Moss AJ, Schwartz PJ, et al. Influence of the genotype on the clinical Course of the long-QT syndrome. N Engl J Med 1998;339:960–5. https://doi.org/10.1056/NEJM199810013391404.

27. Priori SG, Schwartz PJ, Napolitano C, et al. Risk stratification in the long-QT syndrome. N Engl J Med 2003;348(19):1866–74.

28. Schwartz PJ, Priori SG, Spazzolini C, et al. Genotype-Phenotype Correlation in the Long-QT Syndrome. Circulation 2001;103(1):89–95.

29. ANTZELEVITCH C, OLIVA A. Amplification of spatial dispersion of repolarization underlies sudden cardiac death associated with catecholaminergic polymorphic VT, long QT, short QT and Brugada syndromes. J Intern Med 2006; 259(1):48–58.

30. Ackerman MJ, Tester DJ, Porter CJ. Swimming, a gene-specific arrhythmogenic trigger for inherited long QT syndrome. Mayo Clin Proc 1999;74(11):1088–94.

31. Khositseth A, Tester DJ, Will ML, et al. Identification of a common genetic substrate underlying postpartum cardiac events in congenital long QT syndrome. Heart Rhythm 2004;1(1):60–4.

32. Moss AJ, Schwartz PJ, Crampton RS, et al. The long QT syndrome. Prospective longitudinal study of 328 families. Circulation 1991;84(3):1136–44.

33. Horner JM, Horner MM, Ackerman MJ. The diagnostic utility of recovery phase QTc during treadmill exercise stress testing in the evaluation of long QT syndrome. Heart Rhythm 2011;8(11):1698–704.

34. Crotti L, Spazzolini C, Porretta AP, et al. Vagal reflexes following an exercise stress test: a simple clinical tool for gene-specific risk stratification in the long QT syndrome. J Am Coll Cardiol 2012;60(24):2515–24.

35. Schnell F, Behar N, Carré F. Long-QT Syndrome and Competitive Sports. Arrhythmia Electrophysiol Rev 2018;7(3):187–92.

36. De Ferrari GM, Schwartz PJ. Long QT syndrome, a purely electrical disease? Not anymore. Eur Heart J 2009;30(3):253–5.

37. Schwartz PJ, Moss AJ, Vincent GM, et al. Diagnostic criteria for the long QT syndrome. An update. Circulation 1993;88(2):782–4.

38. Ackerman MJ, Priori SG, Dubin AM, et al. Beta-blocker therapy for long QT syndrome and catecholaminergic polymorphic ventricular tachycardia: Are all beta-blockers equivalent? Heart Rhythm 2017;14(1):e41–4.

39. Schwartz PJ, Ackerman MJ. The long QT syndrome: a transatlantic clinical approach to diagnosis and therapy. Eur Heart J 2013;34(40):3109–16.

40. Chatrath R, Bell CM, Ackerman MJ. Beta-blocker therapy failures in symptomatic probands with genotyped long-QT syndrome. Pediatr Cardiol 2004;25(5):459–65.

41. Chockalingam P, Crotti L, Girardengo G, et al. Not all beta-blockers are equal in the management of long QT syndrome types 1 and 2: higher recurrence of events under metoprolol. J Am Coll Cardiol 2012;60(20):2092–9.

42. Mazzanti A, Maragna R, Faragli A, et al. Gene-Specific Therapy With Mexiletine Reduces Arrhythmic Events in Patients With Long QT Syndrome Type 3. J Am Coll Cardiol 2016;67(9):1053–8.

43. Bos JM, Crotti L, Rohatgi RK, et al. Mexiletine Shortens the QT Interval in Patients With Potassium Channel-Mediated Type 2 Long QT Syndrome. Circ Arrhythm Electrophysiol 2019;12(5):e007280. https://doi.org/10.1161/CIRCEP.118.007280.

44. Schwartz PJ, Gnecchi M, Dagradi F, et al. From patient-specific induced pluripotent stem cells to clinical translation in long QT syndrome Type 2. Eur Heart J 2019;40(23):1832–6.

45. Schwartz PJ, De Ferrari GM, Pugliese L. Cardiac sympathetic denervation 100years later: Jonnesco would have never believed it. Int J Cardiol 2017;237:25–8.

46. Coleman MA, Bos JM, Johnson JN, et al. Videoscopic left cardiac sympathetic denervation for patients with recurrent ventricular fibrillation/malignant ventricular arrhythmia syndromes besides congenital long-QT syndrome. Circ Arrhythm Electrophysiol 2012;5(4):782–8.

47. Schwartz PJ, Priori SG, Cerrone M, et al. Left cardiac sympathetic denervation in the management of high-risk patients affected by the long-QT syndrome. Circulation 2004;109(15):1826–33.

48. Olde Nordkamp LRA, Driessen AHG, Odero A, et al. Left cardiac sympathetic denervation in the Netherlands for the treatment of inherited arrhythmia syndromes. Neth Heart J 2014;22(4):160–6.

49. Pelliccia A. Long QT syndrome, implantable cardioverter defibrillator (ICD) and competitive sport participation: when science overcomes ethics. Br J Sports Med 2014;48(15):1135–6.

50. Pelliccia A, Sharma S, Gati S, et al. 2020 ESC Guidelines on sports cardiology and exercise in patients with cardiovascular disease: The Task Force on sports cardiology and exercise in patients with cardiovascular disease of the European Society of Cardiology (ESC). Eur Heart J 2021;42(1):17–96.

51. Napolitano C, Bloise R, Priori SG. Long QT syndrome and short QT syndrome: how to make correct diagnosis and what about eligibility for sports activity. J Cardiovasc Med 2006;7(4):250–6.

52. Funck-Brentano C, Jaillon P. Rate-corrected QT interval: techniques and limitations. Am J Cardiol 1993;72(6):17B–22B.

53. Tobert KE, Bos JM, Garmany R, et al. Return-to-Play for Athletes With Long QT Syndrome or Genetic Heart Diseases Predisposing to Sudden Death. J Am Coll Cardiol 2021;78(6):594–604.

54. Aziz PF, Sweeten T, Vogel RL, et al. Sports Participation in Genotype Positive Children With Long QT Syndrome. JACC Clin Electrophysiol 2015;1(1–2):62–70.

55. Chambers KD, Beausejour Ladouceur V, Alexander ME, et al. Cardiac Events During Competitive, Recreational, and Daily Activities in Children and Adolescents With Long QT Syndrome. J Am Heart Assoc 2017;6(9):e005445.

56. Turkowski KL, Bos JM, Ackerman NC, et al. Return-to-Play for Athletes With Genetic Heart Diseases. Circulation 2018;137(10):1086–8.

57. Ackerman MJ, Zipes DP, Kovacs RJ, et al. Eligibility and Disqualification Recommendations for Competitive Athletes With Cardiovascular Abnormalities: Task Force 10: The Cardiac Channelopathies: A Scientific Statement From the

American Heart Association and American College of Cardiology. J Am Coll Cardiol 2015;66(21):2424–8.

58. Pundi KN, Bos JM, Cannon BC, et al. Automated external defibrillator rescues among children with diagnosed and treated long QT syndrome. Heart Rhythm 2015;12(4):776–81.

59. Drezner JA, Toresdahl BG, Rao AL, et al. Outcomes from sudden cardiac arrest in US high schools: a 2-year prospective study from the National Registry for AED Use in Sports. Br J Sports Med 2013;47(18):1179–83.

60. Providencia R, Teixeira C, Segal OR, et al. Empowerment of athletes with cardiac disorders: a new paradigm. EP Eur 2018;20(8):1243–51.

61. Sarquella-Brugada G, Campuzano O, Arbelo E, et al. Brugada syndrome: clinical and genetic findings. Genet Med 2016;18(1):3–12.

62. Haïssaguerre M, Nademanee K, Hocini M, et al. Depolarization versus repolarization abnormality underlying inferolateral J-wave syndromes: New concepts in sudden cardiac death with apparently normal hearts. Heart Rhythm 2019;16(5): 781–90.

63. Morita H, Zipes DP, Wu J. Brugada syndrome: insights of ST elevation, arrhythmogenicity, and risk stratification from experimental observations. Heart Rhythm 2009;6(11 Suppl):S34–43.

64. Wilde AAM, Postema PG, Di Diego JM, et al. The pathophysiological mechanism underlying Brugada syndrome: depolarization versus repolarization. J Mol Cell Cardiol 2010;49(4):543–53.

65. Frustaci A, Priori SG, Pieroni M, et al. Cardiac histological substrate in patients with clinical phenotype of Brugada syndrome. Circulation 2005;112(24):3680–7.

66. Frustaci A, Russo MA, Chimenti C. Structural myocardial abnormalities in asymptomatic family members with Brugada syndrome and SCN5A gene mutation. Eur Heart J 2009;30(14):1763.

67. Catalano O, Antonaci S, Moro G, et al. Magnetic resonance investigations in Brugada syndrome reveal unexpectedly high rate of structural abnormalities. Eur Heart J 2009;30(18):2241–8.

68. van Hoorn F, Campian ME, Spijkerboer A, et al. SCN5A Mutations in Brugada Syndrome Are Associated with Increased Cardiac Dimensions and Reduced Contractility. PLOS ONE 2012;7(8):e42037.

69. Chen Q, Kirsch GE, Zhang D, et al. Genetic basis and molecular mechanism for idiopathic ventricular fibrillation. Nature 1998;392(6673):293–6.

70. Hosseini SM, Kim R, Udupa S, et al. Reappraisal of Reported Genes for Sudden Arrhythmic Death. Circulation 2018;138(12):1195–205.

71. Le Scouarnec S, Karakachoff M, Gourraud JB, et al. Testing the burden of rare variation in arrhythmia-susceptibility genes provides new insights into molecular diagnosis for Brugada syndrome. Hum Mol Genet 2015;24(10):2757–63.

72. Bezzina CR, Barc J, Mizusawa Y, et al. Common variants at SCN5A-SCN10A and HEY2 are associated with Brugada syndrome, a rare disease with high risk of sudden cardiac death. Nat Genet 2013;45(9):1044–9.

73. Probst V, Wilde AAM, Barc J, et al. SCN5A mutations and the role of genetic background in the pathophysiology of Brugada syndrome. Circ Cardiovasc Genet 2009;2(6):552–7.

74. Vutthikraivit W, Rattanawong P, Putthapiban P, et al. Worldwide Prevalence of Brugada Syndrome: A Systematic Review and Meta-Analysis. Acta Cardiol Sin 2018;34(3):267–77.

75. Miyasaka Y, Tsuji H, Yamada K, et al. Prevalence and mortality of the Brugada-type electrocardiogram in one city in Japan. J Am Coll Cardiol 2001;38(3): 771–4.

76. Matsuo K, Akahoshi M, Nakashima E, et al. The prevalence, incidence and prognostic value of the Brugada-type electrocardiogram: A population-based study of four decades. J Am Coll Cardiol 2001;38(3):765–70.

77. Junttila MJ, Raatikainen MJP, Karjalainen J, et al. Prevalence and prognosis of subjects with Brugada-type ECG pattern in a young and middle-aged Finnish population. Eur Heart J 2004;25(10):874–8.

78. Quan XQ, Li S, Liu R, et al. A meta-analytic review of prevalence for Brugada ECG patterns and the risk for death. Medicine (Baltimore) 2016;95(50):e5643.

79. Monroe MH, Littmann L. Two-Year case collection of the brugada syndrome electrocardiogram pattern at a large teaching hospital. Clin Cardiol 2000; 23(11):849–51.

80. Pa TEL SS, Anees SS, Ferrick KJ. Prevalence of a Brugada Pattern Electrocardiogram in an Urban Population in the United States. Pacing Clin Electrophysiol 2009;32(6):704–8.

81. Yan GX, Antzelevitch C. Cellular basis for the electrocardiographic J wave. Circulation 1996;93(2):372–9.

82. Di Diego JM, Sun ZQ, Antzelevitch C. I(to) and action potential notch are smaller in left vs. right canine ventricular epicardium. Am J Phys 1996;271(2 Pt 2): H548–61.

83. Antzelevitch C, Yan GX. J-wave syndromes: Brugada and early repolarization syndromes. Heart Rhythm 2015;12(8):1852–66.

84. Brugada P, Brugada J. Right bundle branch block, persistent ST segment elevation and sudden cardiac death: a distinct clinical and electrocardiographic syndrome. A multicenter report. J Am Coll Cardiol 1992;20(6):1391–6.

85. Matsuo K, Kurita T, Inagaki M, et al. The circadian pattern of the development of ventricular fibrillation in patients with Brugada syndrome. Eur Heart J 1999; 20(6):465–70.

86. Sieira J, Ciconte G, Conte G, et al. Asymptomatic Brugada Syndrome. Circ Arrhythm Electrophysiol 2015;8(5):1144–50.

87. Sieira J, Conte G, Ciconte G, et al. Clinical characterisation and long-term prognosis of women with Brugada syndrome. Heart Br Card Soc 2016;102(6):452–8.

88. Sroubek J, Probst V, Mazzanti A, et al. Programmed Ventricular Stimulation for Risk Stratification in the Brugada Syndrome: A Pooled Analysis. Circulation 2016;133(7):622–30.

89. Milman A, Andorin A, Gourraud JB, et al. Age of First Arrhythmic Event in Brugada Syndrome. Circ Arrhythm Electrophysiol 2017;10(12):e005222.

90. Michowitz Y, Milman A, Sarquella-Brugada G, et al. Fever-related arrhythmic events in the multicenter Survey on Arrhythmic Events in Brugada Syndrome. Heart Rhythm 2018;15(9):1394–401.

91. Smits JPP, Eckardt L, Probst V, et al. Genotype-phenotype relationship in Brugada syndrome: electrocardiographic features differentiate SCN5A-related patients from non-SCN5A-related patients. J Am Coll Cardiol 2002;40(2):350–6.

92. Morita H, Kusano-Fukushima K, Nagase S, et al. Atrial fibrillation and atrial vulnerability in patients with Brugada syndrome. J Am Coll Cardiol 2002;40(8): 1437–44.

93. Wilde AaM, Antzelevitch C, Borggrefe M, et al. Proposed diagnostic criteria for the Brugada syndrome. Eur Heart J 2002;23(21):1648–54.

94. Brugada J, Campuzano O, Arbelo E, et al. Present Status of Brugada Syndrome: JACC State-of-the-Art Review. J Am Coll Cardiol 2018;72(9):1046–59.

95. Antzelevitch C, Yan GX, Ackerman MJ, et al. J-Wave syndromes expert consensus conference report: Emerging concepts and gaps in knowledge. Heart Rhythm 2016;13(10):e295–324.

96. de Luna AB, Brugada J, Baranchuk A, et al. Current electrocardiographic criteria for diagnosis of Brugada pattern: a consensus report. J Electrocardiol 2012;45(5):433–42.

97. Chevallier S, Forclaz A, Tenkorang J, et al. New Electrocardiographic Criteria for Discriminating Between Brugada Types 2 and 3 Patterns and Incomplete Right Bundle Branch Block. J Am Coll Cardiol 2011;58(22):2290–8.

98. Serra G, Baranchuk A, Bayés-De-Luna A, et al. Base of the triangle to determine a Brugada electrocardiogram pattern. EP Eur 2015;17(3):505.

99. New electrocardiographic criteria to differentiate the Type-2 Brugada pattern from electrocardiogram of healthy athletes with r'-wave in leads V1/V2 | EP Europace | Oxford Academic. Available at: https://academic.oup.com/europace/article/16/11/1639/603704. Accessed October 1, 2021.

100. Priori SG, Gasparini M, Napolitano C, et al. Risk stratification in Brugada syndrome: results of the PRELUDE (PRogrammed ELectrical stimUlation preDictive valuE) registry. J Am Coll Cardiol. 2012;;59(1):37-45.

101. Mizusawa Y, Morita H, Adler A, et al. Prognostic significance of fever-induced Brugada syndrome. Heart Rhythm 2016;13(7):1515–20.

102. Morita H, Kusano KF, Miura D, et al. Fragmented QRS as a Marker of Conduction Abnormality and a Predictor of Prognosis of Brugada Syndrome. Circulation 2008;118(17):1697–704.

103. Adler A, Rosso R, Chorin E, et al. Risk stratification in Brugada syndrome: Clinical characteristics, electrocardiographic parameters, and auxiliary testing. Heart Rhythm 2016;13(1):299–310.

104. Priori SG, Wilde AA, Horie M, et al. HRS/EHRA/APHRS expert consensus statement on the diagnosis and management of patients with inherited primary arrhythmia syndromes: document endorsed by HRS, EHRA, and APHRS in May 2013 and by ACCF, AHA, PACES, and AEPC in June 2013. Heart Rhythm 2013;10(12):1932–63.

105. Delise P, Allocca G, Marras E, et al. Risk stratification in individuals with the Brugada type 1 ECG pattern without previous cardiac arrest: usefulness of a combined clinical and electrophysiologic approach. Eur Heart J 2011;32(2):169–76.

106. Priori SG, Napolitano C, Gasparini M, et al. Natural history of Brugada syndrome: insights for risk stratification and management. Circulation 2002;105(11):1342–7.

107. Probst V, Veltmann C, Eckardt L, et al. Long-Term Prognosis of Patients Diagnosed With Brugada Syndrome. Circulation 2010;121(5):635–43.

108. Gehi AK, Duong TD, Metz LD, et al. Risk stratification of individuals with the Brugada electrocardiogram: a meta-analysis. J Cardiovasc Electrophysiol 2006;17(6):577–83.

109. Al-Khatib SM, Stevenson WG, Ackerman MJ, et al. 2017 AHA/ACC/HRS Guideline for Management of Patients With Ventricular Arrhythmias and the Prevention of Sudden Cardiac Death: A Report of the American College of Cardiology/American Heart Association Task Force on Clinical Practice Guidelines and the Heart Rhythm Society. Circulation 2018;138(13):e272–391.

110. Brugada J, Brugada R, Brugada P. Determinants of sudden cardiac death in individuals with the electrocardiographic pattern of Brugada syndrome and no previous cardiac arrest. Circulation 2003;108(25):3092–6.

111. Kamakura S, Ohe T, Nakazawa K, et al. Long-term prognosis of probands with Brugada-pattern ST-elevation in leads V1-V3. Circ Arrhythm Electrophysiol 2009;2(5):495–503.

112. Risk Stratification in Brugada Syndrome: Results of the PRELUDE (PROgrammed ELectrical stimUlation preDictive valuE) Registry - ScienceDirect. Available at: https://www.sciencedirect.com/science/article/pii/S073510971104 530X. Accessed October 6, 2021.

113. Delise P, Allocca G, Sitta N, et al. Event rates and risk factors in patients with Brugada syndrome and no prior cardiac arrest: a cumulative analysis of the largest available studies distinguishing ICD-recorded fast ventricular arrhythmias and sudden death. Heart Rhythm 2014;11(2):252–8.

114. Alings M, Dekker L, Sadée A, et al. Quinidine induced electrocardiographic normalization in two patients with Brugada syndrome. Pacing Clin Electrophysiol PACE 2001;24(9 Pt 1):1420–2.

115. Antzelevitch C, Brugada P, Brugada J, et al. The Brugada syndrome: from Bench to Bedside. Hoboken, NJ: John Wiley & Sons; 2008.

116. Viskin S, Wilde AAM, Tan HL, et al. Empiric quinidine therapy for asymptomatic Brugada syndrome: Time for a prospective registry. Heart Rhythm 2009;6(3): 401–4.

117. Belhassen B, Glick A, Viskin S. Excellent long-term reproducibility of the electrophysiologic efficacy of quinidine in patients with idiopathic ventricular fibrillation and Brugada syndrome. Pacing Clin Electrophysiol PACE 2009;32(3):294–301.

118. Pellegrino PL, Di Biase M, Brunetti ND. Quinidine for the management of electrical storm in an old patient with Brugada syndrome and syncope. Acta Cardiol 2013;68(2):201–3.

119. Márquez MF, Bonny A, Hernández-Castillo E, et al. Long-term efficacy of low doses of quinidine on malignant arrhythmias in Brugada syndrome with an implantable cardioverter-defibrillator: A case series and literature review. Heart Rhythm 2012;9(12):1995–2000.

120. Shah AJ, Hocini M, Lamaison D, et al. Regional substrate ablation abolishes Brugada syndrome. J Cardiovasc Electrophysiol 2011;22(11):1290–1.

121. Nakagawa E, Takagi M, Tatsumi H, et al. Successful radiofrequency catheter ablation for electrical storm of ventricular fibrillation in a patient with Brugada syndrome. Circ J Off J Jpn Circ Soc 2008;72(6):1025–9.

122. Sunsaneewitayakul B, Yao Y, Thamaree S, et al. Endocardial mapping and catheter ablation for ventricular fibrillation prevention in Brugada syndrome. J Cardiovasc Electrophysiol 2012;23(Suppl 1):S10–6.

123. Cortez-Dias N, Plácido R, Marta L, et al. Epicardial ablation for prevention of ventricular fibrillation in a patient with Brugada syndrome. Rev Port Cardiol Orgao Of Soc Port Cardiol Port J Cardiol Off J Port Soc Cardiol 2014;33(5): 305.e1–7.

124. Brugada J, Pappone C, Berruezo A, et al. Brugada Syndrome Phenotype Elimination by Epicardial Substrate Ablation. Circ Arrhythm Electrophysiol 2015;8(6): 1373–81.

125. Nademanee K, Veerakul G, Chandanamattha P, et al. Prevention of ventricular fibrillation episodes in Brugada syndrome by catheter ablation over the anterior right ventricular outflow tract epicardium. Circulation 2011;123(12):1270–9.

126. Zhang P, Tung R, Zhang Z, et al. Characterization of the epicardial substrate for catheter ablation of Brugada syndrome. Heart Rhythm 2016;13(11):2151–8.
127. Rodríguez-Mañero M, Sacher F, de Asmundis C, et al. Monomorphic ventricular tachycardia in patients with Brugada syndrome: A multicenter retrospective study. Heart Rhythm 2016;13(3):669–82.
128. Sacher F, Jesel L, Jais P, et al. Insight into the mechanism of Brugada syndrome: epicardial substrate and modification during ajmaline testing. Heart Rhythm 2014;11(4):732–4.
129. Rizzo A, de Asmundis C, Brugada P, et al. Ablation for the treatment of Brugada syndrome: current status and future prospects. Expert Rev Med Devices 2020; 17(2):123–30.
130. Leenhardt A, Lucet V, Denjoy I, et al. Catecholaminergic Polymorphic Ventricular Tachycardia in Children. Circulation 1995;91(5):1512–9.
131. Postma AV, Denjoy I, Kamblock J, et al. Catecholaminergic polymorphic ventricular tachycardia: RYR2 mutations, bradycardia, and follow up of the patients. J Med Genet 2005;42(11):863–70.
132. Hayashi M, Denjoy I, Extramiana F, et al. Incidence and Risk Factors of Arrhythmic Events in Catecholaminergic Polymorphic Ventricular Tachycardia. Circulation 2009;119(18):2426–34.
133. Laitinen PJ, Brown KM, Piippo K, et al. Mutations of the cardiac ryanodine receptor (RyR2) gene in familial polymorphic ventricular tachycardia. Circulation 2001;103(4):485–90.
134. Priori SG, Napolitano C, Tiso N, et al. Mutations in the cardiac ryanodine receptor gene (hRyR2) underlie catecholaminergic polymorphic ventricular tachycardia. Circulation 2001;103(2):196–200.
135. Lieve KV, van der Werf C, Wilde AA. Catecholaminergic Polymorphic Ventricular Tachycardia. Circ J Off J Jpn Circ Soc 2016;80(6):1285–91.
136. Tester DJ, Spoon DB, Valdivia HH, et al. Targeted Mutational Analysis of the RyR2-Encoded Cardiac Ryanodine Receptor in Sudden Unexplained Death: A Molecular Autopsy of 49 Medical Examiner/Coroner's Cases. Mayo Clin Proc 2004;79(11):1380–4.
137. Lahat H, Pras E, Olender T, et al. A missense mutation in a highly conserved region of CASQ2 is associated with autosomal recessive catecholamine-induced polymorphic ventricular tachycardia in Bedouin families from Israel. Am J Hum Genet 2001;69(6):1378–84.
138. Postma AV, Denjoy I, Hoorntje TM, et al. Absence of calsequestrin 2 causes severe forms of catecholaminergic polymorphic ventricular tachycardia. Circ Res 2002;91(8):e21–6.
139. Cerrone M, Napolitano C, Priori SG. Catecholaminergic polymorphic ventricular tachycardia: A paradigm to understand mechanisms of arrhythmias associated to impaired Ca(2+) regulation. Heart Rhythm 2009;6(11):1652–9.
140. Baltogiannis GG, Lysitsas DN, di Giovanni G, et al. CPVT: Arrhythmogenesis, Therapeutic Management, and Future Perspectives. A Brief Review of the Literature. Front Cardiovasc Med 2019;6:92. https://doi.org/10.3389/fcvm.2019.00092.
141. Priori SG, Napolitano C, Memmi M, et al. Clinical and Molecular Characterization of Patients With Catecholaminergic Polymorphic Ventricular TachycardiaCirculation 2002;106:69–74.
142. Roston TM, Vinocur JM, Maginot KR, et al. Catecholaminergic Polymorphic Ventricular Tachycardia in Children. Circ Arrhythm Electrophysiol 2015;8(3):633–42.

143. Swan H, Piippo K, Viitasalo M, et al. Arrhythmic disorder mapped to chromosome 1q42-q43 causes malignant polymorphic ventricular tachycardia in structurally normal hearts. J Am Coll Cardiol 1999;34(7):2035–42.

144. Lieve K, Van Der Werf C, Bos J, et al. Risk stratification in patients with catecholaminergic polymorphic ventricular tachycardia. Heart Rhythm 2017;14:122–3. Available at: https://lirias.kuleuven.be/1905126. Accessed October 8, 2021.

145. Nadolol decreases the incidence and severity of ventricular arrhythmias during exercise stress testing compared with β1-selective β-blockers in patients with catecholaminergic polymorphic ventricular tachycardia | Elsevier Enhanced Reader. doi:10.1016/j.hrthm.2015.09.029

146. van der Werf C, Kannankeril PJ, Sacher F, et al. Flecainide therapy reduces exercise-induced ventricular arrhythmias in patients with catecholaminergic polymorphic ventricular tachycardia. J Am Coll Cardiol 2011;57(22):2244–54.

147. Watanabe H, van der Werf C, Roses-Noguer F, et al. Effects of flecainide on exercise-induced ventricular arrhythmias and recurrences in genotype-negative patients with catecholaminergic polymorphic ventricular tachycardia. Heart Rhythm 2013;10(4):542–7.

148. Kannankeril PJ, Moore JP, Cerrone M, et al. Efficacy of Flecainide in the Treatment of Catecholaminergic Polymorphic Ventricular Tachycardia: A Randomized Clinical Trial. JAMA Cardiol 2017;2(7):759–66.

149. Swan H, Laitinen P, Kontula K, et al. Calcium channel antagonism reduces exercise-induced ventricular arrhythmias in catecholaminergic polymorphic ventricular tachycardia patients with RyR2 mutations. J Cardiovasc Electrophysiol 2005;16(2):162–6.

150. Rosso R, Kalman JM, Rogowski O, et al. Calcium channel blockers and beta-blockers versus beta-blockers alone for preventing exercise-induced arrhythmias in catecholaminergic polymorphic ventricular tachycardia. Heart Rhythm 2007;4(9):1149–54.

151. Katz G, Khoury A, Kurtzwald E, et al. Optimizing catecholaminergic polymorphic ventricular tachycardia therapy in calsequestrin-mutant mice. Heart Rhythm 2010;7(11):1676–82.

152. Mohamed U, Gollob MH, Gow RM, et al. Sudden cardiac death despite an implantable cardioverter-defibrillator in a young female with catecholaminergic ventricular tachycardia. Heart Rhythm 2006;3(12):1486–9.

153. Marai I, Khoury A, Suleiman M, et al. Importance of ventricular tachycardia storms not terminated by implantable cardioverter defibrillators shocks in patients with CASQ2 associated catecholaminergic polymorphic ventricular tachycardia. Am J Cardiol 2012;110(1):72–6.

154. van der Werf C, Lieve KV, Bos JM, et al. Implantable cardioverter-defibrillators in previously undiagnosed patients with catecholaminergic polymorphic ventricular tachycardia resuscitated from sudden cardiac arrest. Eur Heart J 2019; 40(35):2953–61.

155. De Ferrari GM, Dusi V, Spazzolini C, et al. Clinical Management of Catecholaminergic Polymorphic Ventricular Tachycardia: The Role of Left Cardiac Sympathetic Denervation. Circulation 2015;131(25):2185–93.

156. Roses-Noguer F, Jarman JWE, Clague JR, et al. Outcomes of defibrillator therapy in catecholaminergic polymorphic ventricular tachycardia. Heart Rhythm 2014;11(1):58–66.

157. Mitchell JH, Haskell W, Snell P, et al. Task Force 8: Classification of sports. J Am Coll Cardiol 2005;45(8):1364–7.

158. ESC Guidelines on sports cardiology and exercise in patients with cardiovascular disease. European Heart Journal | Oxford Academic 2020. Available at: https://academic.oup.com/eurheartj/article/42/1/17/5898937. Accessed September 18, 2021.

159. Gussak I, Brugada P, Brugada J, et al. Idiopathic short QT interval: a new clinical syndrome? Cardiology 2000;94(2):99–102.

160. Gaita F, Giustetto C, Bianchi F, et al. Short QT Syndrome: a familial cause of sudden death. Circulation 2003;108(8):965–70.

161. Priori SG, Blomström-Lundqvist C, Mazzanti A, et al. ESC Guidelines for the management of patients with ventricular arrhythmias and the prevention of sudden cardiac death: The Task Force for the Management of Patients with Ventricular Arrhythmias and the Prevention of Sudden Cardiac Death of the European Society of Cardiology (ESC)Endorsed by: Association for European Paediatric and Congenital Cardiology (AEPC). Eur Heart J 2015;36(41):2793–867.

162. Brugada R, Hong K, Dumaine R, et al. Sudden death associated with short-QT syndrome linked to mutations in HERG. Circulation 2004;109(1):30–5.

163. Bellocq C, van Ginneken ACG, Bezzina CR, et al. Mutation in the KCNQ1 gene leading to the short QT-interval syndrome. Circulation 2004;109(20):2394–7.

164. Priori SG, Pandit SV, Rivolta I, et al. A novel form of short QT syndrome (SQT3) is caused by a mutation in the KCNJ2 gene. Circ Res 2005;96(7):800–7.

165. Antzelevitch C, Pollevick GD, Cordeiro JM, et al. Loss-of-function mutations in the cardiac calcium channel underlie a new clinical entity characterized by ST-segment elevation, short QT intervals, and sudden cardiac death. Circulation 2007;115(4):442–9.

166. Templin C, Ghadri JR, Rougier JS, et al. Identification of a novel loss-of-function calcium channel gene mutation in short QT syndrome (SQTS6). Eur Heart J 2011;32(9):1077–88.

167. Hong K, Piper DR, Diaz-Valdecantos A, et al. De novo KCNQ1 mutation responsible for atrial fibrillation and short QT syndrome in utero. Cardiovasc Res 2005; 68(3):433–40.

168. Kobza R, Roos M, Niggli B, et al. Prevalence of long and short QT in a young population of 41,767 predominantly male Swiss conscripts. Heart Rhythm 2009;6(5):652–7.

169. Anttonen O, Junttila MJ, Rissanen H, et al. Prevalence and prognostic significance of short QT interval in a middle-aged Finnish population. Circulation 2007;116(7):714–20.

170. Guerrier K, Kwiatkowski D, Czosek RJ, et al. Short QT Interval Prevalence and Clinical Outcomes in a Pediatric Population. Circ Arrhythm Electrophysiol 2015;8(6):1460–4.

171. Dhutia H, Malhotra A, Parpia S, et al. The prevalence and significance of a short QT interval in 18,825 low-risk individuals including athletes. Br J Sports Med 2016;50(2):124–9.

172. Odening KE, Bodi I, Franke G, et al. Transgenic short-QT syndrome 1 rabbits mimic the human disease phenotype with QT/action potential duration shortening in the atria and ventricles and increased ventricular tachycardia/ventricular fibrillation inducibility. Eur Heart J 2019;40(10):842–53.

173. Shinnawi R, Shaheen N, Huber I, et al. Modeling Reentry in the Short QT Syndrome With Human-Induced Pluripotent Stem Cell-Derived Cardiac Cell Sheets. J Am Coll Cardiol 2019;73(18):2310–24.

174. Mazzanti A, Kanthan A, Monteforte N, et al. Novel insight into the natural history of short QT syndrome. J Am Coll Cardiol 2014;63(13):1300–8.

175. Giustetto C, Schimpf R, Mazzanti A, et al. Long-term follow-up of patients with short QT syndrome. J Am Coll Cardiol 2011;58(6):587–95.
176. Tülümen E, Giustetto C, Wolpert C, et al. PQ segment depression in patients with short QT syndrome: a novel marker for diagnosing short QT syndrome? Heart Rhythm 2014;11(6):1024–30.
177. Schimpf R, Antzelevitch C, Haghi D, et al. Electromechanical coupling in patients with the short QT syndrome: further insights into the mechanoelectrical hypothesis of the U wave. Heart Rhythm 2008;5(2):241–5.
178. Anttonen O, Junttila MJ, Maury P, et al. Differences in twelve-lead electrocardiogram between symptomatic and asymptomatic subjects with short QT interval. Heart Rhythm 2009;6(2):267–71.
179. Wolpert C, Schimpf R, Giustetto C, et al. Further insights into the effect of quinidine in short QT syndrome caused by a mutation in HERG. J Cardiovasc Electrophysiol 2005;16(1):54–8.
180. Gollob MH, Redpath CJ, Roberts JD. The short QT syndrome: proposed diagnostic criteria. J Am Coll Cardiol 2011;57(7):802–12.
181. Villafañe J, Atallah J, Gollob MH, et al. Long-term follow-up of a pediatric cohort with short QT syndrome. J Am Coll Cardiol 2013;61(11):1183–91.
182. Iribarren C, Round AD, Peng JA, et al. Short QT in a cohort of 1.7 million persons: prevalence, correlates, and prognosis. Ann Noninvasive Electrocardiol Off J Int Soc Holter Noninvasive Electrocardiol Inc 2014;19(5):490–500.
183. ESC Guidelines for the management of patients with ventricular arrhythmias and the prevention of sudden cardiac death. European Heart Journal | Oxford Academic 2015. Available at: https://academic.oup.com/eurheartj/article/36/41/2793/2293363. Accessed October 6, 2021.
184. Gaita F, Giustetto C, Bianchi F, et al. Short QT syndrome: pharmacological treatment. J Am Coll Cardiol 2004;43(8):1494–9.
185. Nador F, Beria G, De Ferrari GM, et al. Unsuspected echocardiographic abnormality in the long QT syndrome. Diagnostic, prognostic, and pathogenetic implications. Circulation 1991;84(4):1530–42.
186. Maron BJ, Udelson JE, Bonow RO, et al. Eligibility and Disqualification Recommendations for Competitive Athletes With Cardiovascular Abnormalities: Task Force 3: Hypertrophic Cardiomyopathy, Arrhythmogenic Right Ventricular Cardiomyopathy and Other Cardiomyopathies, and Myocarditis: A Scientific Statement From the American Heart Association and American College of Cardiology. J Am Coll Cardiol 2015;66(21):2362–71.
187. Etheridge SP, Saarel EV. Toward a Long and Happy Life of a Patient With Genetic Heart Disease. J Am Coll Cardiol 2021;78(6):605–7.

Sports Participation and Physical Activity in Individuals with Heritable Thoracic Aortic Disease and Aortopathy Conditions

Mary B. Sheppard, MD[a,b,c], Alan C. Braverman, MD[d],*

KEYWORDS

• Marfan • Aortopathy • Aortic aneurysm • Exercise • Physical activity • Sports

KEY POINTS

• Individuals with underlying aortopathy conditions require multidisciplinary evaluation to establish the correct diagnosis, image the aorta, and provide appropriate exercise recommendations.

• Recreational exercise and physical activities performed at a low-to-moderate aerobic pace are generally low-risk for most individuals with genetic aortopathies and heritable thoracic aortic disease (HTAD).

• Individuals with genetic aortopathies and HTADs are advised to avoid intense physical exertion, contact sports, and intense weightlifting or isometric exercise involving straining and reaching muscle fatigue.

INTRODUCTION

The presence of underlying aortic disease, whether due to a genetic mutation or degenerative disease, increases the risk for aneurysm formation and complications of aortic dissection and rupture. Due to this concern, low-impact physical activities

[a] Department of Family and Community Medicine, Saha Aortic Center, University of Kentucky College of Medicine, 741 South Limestone Biomedical Biological Sciences Research Building Room B247, Lexington, KY 40536, USA; [b] Department of Surgery, Saha Aortic Center, University of Kentucky College of Medicine, 741 South Limestone Biomedical Biological Sciences Research Building Room B247, Lexington, KY 40536, USA; [c] Department of Physiology, Saha Aortic Center, University of Kentucky College of Medicine, 741 South Limestone Biomedical Biological Sciences Research Building Room B247, Lexington, KY 40536, USA; [d] Marfan Syndrome and Aortopathy Clinic, Aortopathy and Master Clinician Fellowship Program, Cardiovascular Division, John T. Milliken Department of Medicine, Washington University School of Medicine, 660 South Euclid Avenue, Box 8086, St. Louis, MO 63110, USA
* Corresponding author.
E-mail address: abraverm@wustl.edu
Twitter: @MaryBShep (M.B.S.); @AlanBraverman7 (A.C.B.)

Clin Sports Med 41 (2022) 511–527
https://doi.org/10.1016/j.csm.2022.02.009
0278-5919/22/© 2022 Elsevier Inc. All rights reserved.

Abbreviations	
HTAD	heritable thoracic aortic disease
MFS	Marfan syndrome
BSA	body surface area
LDS	Loeys-Dietz syndrome
vEDS	vascular Ehlers-Danlos syndrome
TS	Turner syndrome
BAV	bicuspid aortic valve
BP	blood pressure
MET	metabolic equivalent of task
NFL	National Football League
CBS	combined benefit score
BAPN	beta-aminoproprionotrile
ATAAD	acute type A aortic dissection
AHA	American Heart Association
ACC	American College of Cardiology
ESC	European Society of Cardiology

and safe levels of exercise are recommended for people with heritable thoracic aortic disease (HTAD) and aortopathy conditions. The guiding principle has historically been to avoid the increased load placed on the aorta during more intense training, exercise, and athletic competition.[1] Recent information from clinical studies of individuals without underlying aortopathy suggests that there may be adaptive remodeling of the aorta that accompanies years of endurance exercise among master athletes.[2] Mouse models of Marfan syndrome (MFS) have demonstrated the benefit of moderate physical activity to aortic health.[3,4] These data inform us that while the aorta serves as a mechanical conduit of blood, it is also a living organ, with important roles in mechanotransduction and propagation of pulsatile blood flow and has the ability to alter gene expression in response to variations in aortic load.

Myocardial cells respond to exercise by generating a higher contractile force and stroke volume. When faced with an increase in metabolic demand, the conditioned heart responds more effectively that the unconditioned heart. It is possible that smooth muscle cells of the aorta behave similarly. If exposed to progressive increases in load over time, it is possible the conditioned aorta may potentially respond to stresses more effectively than an unconditioned aorta. However, it is not yet established in people with an underlying aortopathy condition that regular exercise has a beneficial effect on the aorta. More research is needed in this area.

HERITABLE THORACIC AORTIC DISEASE AND AORTOPATHY OVERVIEW

Aortopathy refers to any disease of the aorta and is often used in describing the underlying conditions at risk for aortic aneurysm or dissection. Genetic aortopathies exhibit defects in the aortic media due to abnormalities in extracellular matrix proteins, vascular smooth muscle cells, or contractile proteins, which lead to abnormal mechanotransduction. Histologically, genetic aortic disease is characterized by decreased deposition of extracellular matrix, degradation of structural components such as elastin, and apoptosis of smooth muscle cells.[5] This medial degeneration leads to progressive disruption of the integrity of the aortic wall and alters its elastic properties, impairing the aorta's ability to respond to an increased load and placing it at risk for aneurysm and aortic dissection.[5] Due to the force of pulsatile flow of blood, the aortic root and ascending thoracic aorta are significantly impacted by the hemodynamic effects of exercise. In aortopathy conditions, physical activity must be adjusted to account for the aorta's altered susceptibility to complications, such as progressive dilation, rupture, or dissection.

When evaluating the athlete for underlying aortic disease, adherence to standardized measurement conventions is essential. The normal aortic root is about 30 to 35 mm in diameter,[6] although this varies based on age, sex, height, and body surface area (BSA). In elite athletes aged 9 to 59 years (mean age 25), the aortic diameter is rarely greater than 36 mm in women and rarely greater than 40 mm in men.[6] Nomograms can determine the expected aortic size for a person's age, sex, and BSA.[7] A z-score calculation enables comparison of the individual's aortic diameter relative to the population and a determination of how many standard deviations the aortic diameter is from the expected diameter based on their age, BSA, and sex.[1] A z-score greater than 2 signifies that the aortic diameter is greater than 97.5% of the population and is considered enlarged. A z-score greater than 3 indicates that the aortic diameter is larger than 99.9% of the population. Mild aortic dilatation is defined by a z-score of 2.0 to 3.0; moderate dilatation by a z-score of 3.01 to 4.0; and severe aortic dilation by a z-score greater than 4.[7]

AORTOPATHY CONDITIONS

Pathogenic variants can cause isolated thoracic aortic aneurysm (nonsyndromic HTAD) or have pleiotropic effects (syndromic HTAD).[8,9] Nonsyndromic HTAD conditions are also referred to as familial thoracic aortic aneurysms (FTAAs). Syndromic HTADs may have extra-aortic features that can increase a clinician's suspicion of an underlying aortic disease.[9] Therefore, athletes should undergo a preparticipation history and physical examination that includes evaluation for features of MFS and related disorders and a detailed family history of thoracic aortic aneurysm disease, cerebral aneurysm, or unexplained sudden death at a young age.[9] If features concerning for an underlying genetic aortopathy are present, then further evaluation including an echocardiogram, slit-lamp eye examination (to evaluate for ectopia lentis), and medical genetic consultation (as appropriate) are recommended. When sharing decisions about physical activity in individuals with aortopathy, the underlying condition, aortic diameter, the individual's age, family history, type of exercise, and level of exertion need to be considered. Genetic variants and clinical features of some of the conditions associated with HTAD and aortopathy are listed in **Table 1**.[9]

MFS is due to pathogenic variants in the *FBN1* gene, which encodes fibrillin-1 protein.[10] Because of long-bone overgrowth, individuals with MFS are typically tall for their family. This tall stature may prompt undiagnosed individuals to play competitive sports, such as basketball and volleyball. Extra-aortic manifestations that can affect exercise guidance include ocular disease (retinal detachment, lens dislocation), orthopedic concerns (back, hip, and feet), pneumothorax, restrictive lung disease, cardiomyopathy, valvular disease, and arrhythmias.[11]

Loeys-Dietz syndrome (LDS) is caused by pathogenic variants in one of several genes affecting the TGF-beta signaling pathway (*TGFBR1*, *TGFBR2*, *SMAD3*, *TGFB2*, and *TGFB3*).[12] People with LDS may have a more aggressive arterial disease than in MFS and may have an increased risk of cervical spine complications due to atlanto-axial instability.[13]

Vascular Ehlers-Danlos syndrome (vEDS) is caused by pathogenic variants in the *COL3A1* gene, which leads to vascular fragility and risk of dissection or rupture of medium-sized arteries without prior aneurysm formation.[14] Abnormal bruising and varicose veins are common and affected individuals are at risk for hollow organ and uterine rupture.

Table 1
Heritable thoracic aortic aneurysm conditions.[9]

Condition	Gene	Clinical Features
[a]Syndromic HTAD		
MFS	FBN1	Aortic root aneurysm, AD, TAA, MVP, arachnodactyly, scoliosis, pectus deformities, ectopia lentis, myopia, tall stature, PTX, dural ectasia, dolichocephaly, malar hypoplasia, retrognathia, downslanting palpebral fissures
LDS	TGFBR1, TGFBR2, *SMAD3, TGFB2, TGFB3	TAA, branch vessel aneurysms, AD, arterial tortuosity, MVP, craniosynostosis, hypertelorism, bluish sclera, bifid uvula, translucent skin, visible veins, clubfoot, dural ectasia, *premature osteoarthritis
vEDS	COL3A1	TAA, AAA, arterial rupture, AD, MVP, bowel and uterine rupture, PTX, translucent skin, facial features, atrophic scars, small joint hypermobility, easy bruising, clubfoot, carotid-cavernous fistula
Nonsyndromic HTAD (Familial TAAD)		
FTAA	ACTA2	TAA, AD, BAV, Moya-Moya, premature CAD and CVD, livedo reticularis, iris flocculi
FTAA	MYH11	TAA, AD, PDA
FTAA	MYLK	AD at relatively small aortic size
FTAA	PRKG1	Aortic root aneurysm and AD
FTAA	FOXE3	TAA, AD
FTAA	THSD4	TAA, AD
BAV associated Ascending Aortic Aneurysm		
Familial BAV/AS and TAA	NOTCH1	Aortic stenosis, TAA
BAV with TAA	TGFBR1, TGFBR2, TGFB2, TGFB3, ACTA2, MAT2A, GATA5, SMAD6, LOX, ROBO4, TBX20	Syndromic and nonsyndromic FTAA with an increased frequency of BAV

AD, aortic dissection; TAA, thoracic aortic aneurysm; MVP, mitral valve prolapse; PTX, pneumothorax; FTAAD, familial thoracic aortic aneurysm (and dissection) syndrome; AAA, abdominal aortic aneurysm; PDA, patent ductus arteriosus; CAD, coronary artery disease; CVD, cerebrovascular disease; BAV, bicuspid aortic valve.

[a] Some individuals with pathogenic variants in a gene that can lead to syndromic HTAD have very few or no syndromic features and variants in some genes causing syndromic HTAD may also lead to nonsyndromic HTAD.

From Thakker PD, Braverman AC. Cardiogenetics: genetic testing in the diagnosis and management of patients with aortic disease. Heart 2021;107:619-626.

Nonsyndromic HTAD is due to pathogenic variations in multiple genes including *ACTA2, MYH11, MYLK, PRKG1*, and others.[8] These autosomal dominant conditions are often diagnosed after an aortic dissection occurs or a thoracic aortic aneurysm is discovered in the patient or a relative.

Turner syndrome (TS), due to partial or complete absence of the second X-chromosome, associates with bicuspid aortic valve (BAV), aortic dilation, and risk of aortic dissection.[15] Because of short stature, aortic size indexed to body size should be used in girls aged greater than 15 years and women with TS to determine exercise recommendations.[15] Evidence is lacking on the aortic risks for competitive athletics with TS, but guidelines apply based on their specific valvular, congenital heart, or aortic disease.[15]

BAV, affecting 1% of the population, commonly associates with aortic aneurysm in the ascending aorta and/or aortic root, which is a risk factor for aortic dissection.[16] Although pathogenic variants are not identified in most patients with BAV and aortic aneurysm, certain genetic variants may associate with this condition (see **Table 1**). Additional exercise restrictions may apply if there is significant valvular dysfunction.[7]

If an individual with aortopathy undergoes mechanical heart valve replacement, lifelong anticoagulation is required. Because of bleeding risk, those on anticoagulants must avoid contact sports and activities that increase risk of fall or trauma.

EXERCISE PHYSIOLOGY AND CLINICAL RELEVANCE
The Impact of Dynamic Versus Static Exercise on Blood Pressure

Exercise can be broadly categorized depending on its static and/or dynamic components. In static (isometric) exercise, the length of muscle fibers do not change during contraction, resulting in sustained compression of blood vessels. Blood vessels in muscle are compressed throughout muscle contraction. In dynamic (isotonic) exercise, changes in sarcomere length results in blood vessel compression that is intermittent. Blood movement creates a sheer force, stimulating nitric oxide release, which induces vasodilation of muscular arteries.[17] Therefore, peripheral blood vessels dilate during dynamic exercise, but not during static exercise.

Mean arterial blood pressure (BP) increases during static and dynamic exercise. However, the increase in systolic BP occurring during dynamic exercise is accompanied by a decrease in diastolic BP due to the dilation of peripheral blood vessels.[1] Because static exercise does not cause dilation of peripheral blood vessels, static exercise causes a higher increase in the mean arterial BP compared with dynamic exercise.

A distinction between types of exercise based on their effect on BP is important because BP directly affects aortic wall stress. With an increase in BP, the aortic wall must generate a higher counterforce to propel blood. The structural and cellular changes that occur in aortopathy compromise the aortic wall's ability to accommodate the increased aortic load generated by physical activity.

In addition to static and dynamic considerations, the intensity of exercise significantly affects the BP and heart rate response to exercise. The metabolic equivalent of task (MET) is a physiologic measure expressing the energy cost (or calories) of physical activities. While exercising, the MET equivalent is the energy expended compared with rest, so MET values indicate intensity. An activity with a MET value of 5 means you are expending 5 times the energy (number of calories) than you would at rest.[18] Systolic BP may increase by 8 to 12 mm Hg per MET of aerobic activity with only minimal effect on diastolic BP. Physical activities have previously been classified according to an estimate of the METs required to perform the activity[18] (**Table 2**).

CLASSIFICATION OF SPORTS/EXERCISE

Recreational athletics are generally considered to involve a light-to-moderate level of intensity. In competitive athletics, participants typically push their bodies to their

Table 2
Level of intensity of physical activities and exercise (in METS)

Light (<3 METS)	Moderate (3–6 METS)	High (>6 METS)
Walking—slowly	Walking—briskly (4 mph)	Jogging at 6 mph
Standing—light	Hiking level terrain	Shoveling snow or dirt
work (cooking,	Bicycling—light effort (5–10 mph)	Carrying heavy loads
washing dishes)	Badminton—recreational	Bicycling fast (14–16 mph)
Fishing—sitting	Archery	Backpacking up hills
Playing most	Recreational Frisbee	Calisthenics at vigorous effort
musical	Tennis—doubles	Most competitive sports
instruments	Leisurely swimming	(basketball, soccer, field hockey,
	Table tennis	lacrosse, ice hockey, swimming).
	Yoga	Running
	Pilates	Rock climbing
	Water aerobics	Heavy farming (bailing hay)
	Golf (walking, pulling cart)	
	Light calisthenics	
	Ballroom dancing	
	Basketball-shooting baskets	
	Moderate gardening, yardwork	
	Moderate housework	
	(washing windows,	
	vacuuming, mopping)	
	Mowing lawn (power mower)	

highest physical limits in an effort to excel.[19] However, this type of classification can be misleading as very competitive activities can be done at a low level of metabolic intensity (ie, golf or bowling). Moreover, high-intensity activities are often done recreationally (ie, body-building), domestically (ie, shoveling snow), professionally (ie, bailing hay), or even emergently (ie, sprinting to catch a plane). Therefore, shared decisions about physical activities and sports participation are informed by the intensity of the static and dynamic components[19] (**Fig. 1**).

Measurements of exercise intensity can be difficult to collect. Heart rate is easy to measure, but is not always reflective of intensity (such as in a well-conditioned athlete). Other metrics, such as the integral of absolute acceleration, can be inaccurate when activities involve periods of sedentary activity.[20] Measures of VO_2, or the rate of oxygen consumption measured during incremental exercise,[10] can be used to determine the intensity of dynamic exercise. VO_2 max is an individual's maximal oxygen uptake.[10] Although a specific VO_2 max can be calculated for an individual, the peak VO_2 max generally achieved during competition is used to classify the intensity of dynamic exercise along the x-axis of **Fig. 1**.[21]

Because static exercise places more stress on the aorta than dynamic exercise, a person with underlying aortic disease is advised to avoid physical activities with high static components. Wearable technology that tracks VO_2 consumption during dynamic exercise is being developed.[22] Broad categorization of activities into low (<50% VO_2 max), moderate (50%–75% VO_2 max), and high (>75% VO_2 max) intensity levels offers a general guide based on the peak VO_2 max generally achieved during training and competition.

EFFECTS OF EXERCISE ON THE THORACIC AORTA: CLINICAL STUDIES

Rowing and cycling are 2 activities with a very high static component. Previous studies demonstrate systolic BP can exceed 200 mm Hg during competitive rowing and

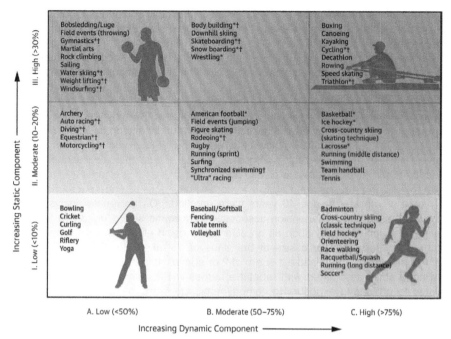

Fig. 1. Classification of Sports. This classification is based on peak static and dynamic components achieved during competition; however, higher values may be reached during training. The increasing dynamic component is defined in terms of the estimated percentage of maximal oxygen uptake (VO_2 max) achieved and results in an increasing cardiac output. The increasing static component is related to the estimated percentage of maximal voluntary contraction reached and results in an increasing BP load. The lowest total cardiovascular demands (cardiac output and BP) are shown in the palest color, with increasing dynamic load depicted by increasing blue intensity and increasing static load by increasing red intensity. Note the graded transition between categories, which should be individualized from player position and style of play. *Danger of bodily collision. †Increased risk if syncope occurs. (Reproduced with permission from: Levine BD, Baggish AL, Kovacs RJ, et al. Eligibility and Disqualification Recommendations for Competitive Athletes with Cardiovascular Abnormalities: Task Force 1: Classification of Sports: Dynamic, Static, and Impact: A Scientific Statement from the AHA and ACC. J Am Coll Cardiol. 2015;66:2350-2355.)

cycling.[17,23] During maximal weightlifting, systolic BP > 300 mm Hg has been recorded.[24] Multiple studies have evaluated aortic diameter in elite strength-trained athletes (without underlying aortic disease) to assess aortic size and outcomes. Babaee Bigi and colleagues evaluated strength-trained, men athletes comparing them to healthy age-matched and height-matched subjects. Aortic diameters at the sinuses of Valsalva and proximal ascending aorta were significantly larger in elite strength-trained athletes and the duration of high-intensity training correlated with larger aortic diameters.[25]

A meta-analysis of 5580 elite athletes reported a small, but significantly larger aortic root diameter compared with 727 nonathletic controls.[26] Few studies in the meta-analysis controlled for BSA and height, so differences in aortic root size may have related to the larger body size of athletes. Even so, the authors concluded that the small increase in aortic root size is clinically insignificant, cautioning that any marked increase in aortic root diameter should not be attributed to athlete's heart.[26]

Using Mitchell classification of sports based on the static and dynamic components of exercise,[21] Boraita and colleagues reported aortic size related to prolonged and intense exercise training in 3281 elite athletes.[27] Although aortic measurements at the sinuses and ascending aorta were statistically larger in those participating in sports with a high dynamic component, the aortic root diameters remained within established limits for the general population.[27]

Pellicia and colleagues[6] and Gentry and colleagues[28] also found that men athletes (cyclists/swimmers and former National Football League (NFL) players, respectively) have slightly larger aortas at the sinuses of Valsalva or ascending aorta than nonathletic controls[6,28] (**Fig. 2**). It is not known whether the larger aortic size in former NFL players will lead to negative aortic outcomes. In 2020, Churchill and colleagues examined the effect of long-term exercise in endurance athletes.[2] A total of 442 masters-level rowers and runners aged 50 to 75 years who performed endurance training for 10 years or more after age 40 years were enrolled.[2] On univariate analysis, age, sex, body size, and hypertension associated with aortic size. Cumulative years of training as well as designation as an elite rower or an elite marathon runner were both associated with aortic size at the sinus of Valsalva (**Fig. 3**). Overall, almost 25% of study individuals had a z-score of 2 or above.[2] It is theorized that endurance rowing, a sport associated with repetitive surges in BP, may lead to aortic dilation related to prolonged exposure to hemodynamic stressors, particular at the level of the sinuses of Valsalva.[2] The clinical significance of the aortic dilation is unknown and follow-up is essential to determine whether this is adaptive or predictive of future risk.

EFFECTS OF EXERCISE IN AORTOPATHY CONDITIONS

Acute aortic events leading to sudden death in athletes are rare, comprising only 1% to 2% of all sudden cardiac death in athletes.[29] However, underrecognition of underlying aortic disease and HTAD increases the risk of acute aortic events in competitive athletes.[30] In the US National Registry of Sudden Death in Athletes, 12 of the 23 people who died of aortic dissection or rupture were suspected to have MFS but many were ultimately cleared to return to competition.[30] There are high profile cases of acute aortic dissection in elite athletes causing sudden death, such as in Chris Patton and

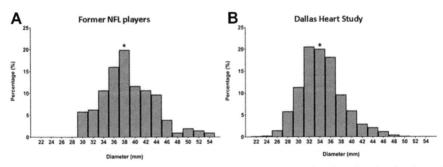

Fig. 2. Distribution of ascending aortic diameters. Histograms showing the distribution of ascending aortic diameters in former NFL athletes (*A*) compared with the Dallas Heart Study (*B*). Mean ascending aortic diameter in the former NFL athletes were 38 ± 5 mm compared with 34 ± 4 mm in the Dallas Heart Study (*P* < .0001). *Mean ascending aortic diameter. (Reproduced with permission from: Gentry JL, Carruthers D, Joshi PH, et al. Ascending Aortic Dimensions in Former National Football League Athletes. Circ Cardiovasc Imaging 2017;10:e006852. https://doi.org/10.1161/CIRCIMAGING.117.006852.)

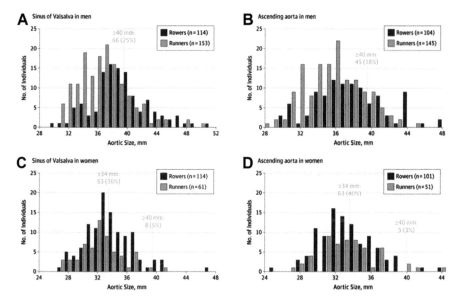

Fig. 3. Distributions of aortic size at both the sinuses of Valsalva and the ascending aorta, measured leading edge–to–leading edge, are shown for men and women, with separate distributions presented for rowers and runners. Among men, 25% (66 of 267) measured 40 mm or larger at the sinuses of Valsalva and 18% (45 of 249) in the ascending aorta. Aortic sizes among rowers exhibited a rightward shift compared with that of runners ($P < .01$) in all cases except the ascending aorta in women, where the distribution was similar. (Reproduced with permission from: Churchill TW, Groezinger E, Kim JH, et al. Association of Ascending Aortic Dilatation and Long-term Endurance Exercise Among Older Masters-Level Athletes. JAMA Cardiol. 2020;5:522-531.)

Flo Hyman, who were unaware they had MFS. Because of the concern about potential for aortic events during high-impact sports and many competitive sports, individuals with MFS and other genetic aortopathies are generally prohibited from participation. However, the effects of various levels of exercise on aortic growth and integrity in people with aortopathy conditions is unknown. To evaluate the effects of exercise on aortic wall structure, diameter, and function in aortopathy conditions, animal models of aortic disease have been used.[3,4,31,32]

Animal Models of Exercise in Aortopathy Conditions

Marfan models

Two studies have demonstrated that dynamic exercise improves aortic disease in a mouse model of MFS.[3,4] In the $Fbn1^{C1041G/+}$ mouse, moderate intensity dynamic exercise (starting at 4 months of age) decreased the rate of aortic root dilation compared with sedentary controls.[4] Exercised Marfan mice did not have any statistically significant difference in aortic root stiffness, medial fibrosis, or elastic lamina ruptures compared with sedentary Marfan mice.[4] In this study, moderate exercise normalized aortic growth to values seen in wild type animals.

In a study evaluating dynamic exercise in the $Fbn1^{C1041G/+}$ mouse, 1-month-old Marfan mice and wild type controls were subjected to voluntary cage-wheel exercise, forced treadmill exercise for 30 minutes 5 days a week (at 55% VO_2 max), or a sedentary lifestyle for 5 months.[3] Among Marfan mice, aortic wall strength was increased and the aortic diameter was significantly smaller in mice who underwent 5 months of voluntary or forced exercise compared with sedentary mice[3] (**Fig. 4**).

Gibson and colleagues compared sedentary Marfan mice to those reaching maximum exercise speeds selected to represent 55%, 65%, 75%, and 85% VO_2 max. A combined benefit score (CBS) was a composite measure of the effects of exercise on elastin fiber length, elastin fragmentation, and wall elasticity. Among Marfan mice, the CBS was lowest among sedentary mice, highest at 55% VO_2 max, and then progressively declined as exercise intensity increased.[3] Tran and colleagues found that a running intensity up to 65% VO_2 max protected against elastin fiber fragmentation within the aortic wall of $Fbn1^{mgR/mgR}$ mice.[31]

Acquired aortopathy

Beta-Aminopropionitrile (BAPN), a lysyl oxidase inhibitor, disrupts aortic architecture leading to aortic aneurysm and aortic dissection in animal models.[33] Aicher and colleagues administered BAPN versus control to mice at 3 to 4 weeks of age for 5 to 6 months. Mice were subjected to forced exercise 5 days a week an intensity at 65% to 75% VO_2 max. Mortality after 26 weeks was 0% in mice in the forced exercise cohort, and 24% in the sedentary BAPN-administered mice. Exercise increased elastin expression in BAPN-treated animals and decreased BAPN-induced wall thickening, wall tension, and lumen diameter.[33] Multiple BAPN-induced genes normalized with exercise, including TGF-beta pathway genes, inflammation-related genes, and vascular-injury and response-related genes.

AORTIC DISSECTION RELATED TO EXERCISE

Although aortic dissection related to exercise is a concern for individuals with aortopathy and their health care providers, the literature describing this phenomenon is limited. A review of 26 articles and 12 case reports published between 1987 to 2016

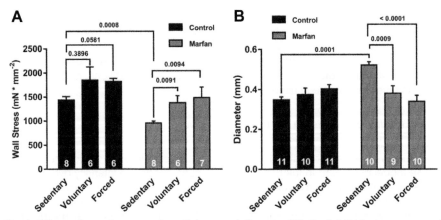

Fig. 4. Effects of exercise on aortic wall stress and diameter (dilation). (*A*) Maximum amount of wall stress of aortas of sedentary, voluntary, and forced exercise control and MFS mice. Both voluntary and forced exercise routines significantly increased aortic wall strength in MFS aorta. (*B*) Estimated dilation of aortas of sedentary, voluntary, and forced exercise control and MFS mice, demonstrating a significant decrease in diameter of MFS aortic rings. Values are means ± SE, *n* as indicated on each bar, *P* as indicated. (Reproduced with permission from: Gibson C et al. J Appl Physiol Bethesda Md 1985 2017;123:147-160.)

described a total of 49 patients who experienced aortic dissection during exercise.[34] Of these 49 patients, 42 had a Stanford type A and 7 had a Stanford type B dissection. Weightlifting was the sport associated with aortic dissection in 26/49 patients. Four of the 49 patients had MFS and 1 had an unspecified connective tissue disorder; only 2 of the patients were women.

A study of 615 patients (mean age 64 years) with acute type A aortic dissection (ATAAD) evaluated whether the ATAAD was associated with a sporting activity.[35] A total of 590 patients of the 615 (96%) of the ATAADs were not associated with a sporting activity. Of the 25 ATAADs that were associated with a sporting activity, 8 were associated with golf, 4 with swimming, 4 with cycling, and only 3 with weightlifting.[35] A study from the International Registry of Acute Aortic Dissection reported physical activity and emotional state at the time of aortic dissection in a subset of participants. Although activities (including weightlifting or intense emotional stressors) were reported at symptom onset in some individuals, most participants did not describe such precipitating factors at dissection onset.[36]

RECOMMENDATIONS
Competitive Sports

Guidelines regarding competitive sports and exercise in athletes with aortopathy outline concerns about aortic dilation and risk of aortic dissection and rupture in susceptible individuals.[7,15,37] There are no randomized or controlled data detailing aortic outcomes in individuals with aortopathy who continue to participate in competitive athletics. The guidelines and recommendations are by nature restrictive and conservative, emphasize safety and risk minimization, and rely on expert consensus (**Table 3**). The underlying condition, aortic diameter, family history, and other factors inform recommendations about exercise. Regular, serial aortic imaging follow-up is important to evaluate for any aortic growth.

The 2015 American College of Cardiology/American Heart Association (ACC/AHA) guidelines on eligibility and disqualification may have been too restrictive for some individuals with BAV.[7] It is understood that many adolescents and adults with BAV have mildly dilated aortas, yet have aortic diameters in a range (ie, 4.0–4.5 cm) that associates with a low risk of acute aortic dissection. In these cases, after an informed and shared decision-making discussion, many experts agree to allow continued participation in competitive sports with serial imaging follow-up of aortic dimensions. In these instances, it is important to exclude cases of underlying genetic aortopathy (ie, those associated with HTAD) and TS because these conditions have higher risks of aortic complications. Avoidance of intense weight training is recommended for athletes with BAV and significant aortic dilation.

Recreational Sports and Physical Activities

The Marfan Foundation guidelines for recreational exercise and physical activity (*www.Marfan.org/physical activity guidelines*) recommend people with MFS and other aortopathy conditions perform low-to-moderate aerobic exercise and physical activity at a level that does not exceed approximately 50% of capacity. The European Society of Cardiology (ESC) guidelines also emphasize the importance of physical fitness and low-risk recreational activities in individuals with aortopathy conditions.[37] Noncompetitive, dynamic exercise including walking, jogging, leisure bicycling, and other low-intensity aerobic exercise are favored. Avoidance of contact sports, intense exercise to the point of exhaustion and strenuous lifting is recommended.

Table 3
Sports and Exercise Recommendations for Competitive Athletes with Aortopathy (high school and older)

Guideline	Condition	Recommendation
2015 ACC/AHA[7]	MFS	Low and moderate static/low dynamic sports if: no evidence of aortic dilation (z-score >2 or >40 mm); no more than mild MR; LVEF >40%; no FH of aortic dissection at aortic diameter <50 mm
	LDS, vEDS, nonsyndromic HTAD	Low static, low dynamic sports if: no evidence of aortic dilation (z-score >2) or dissection; no more than mild MR; no extra-aortic features that make participation hazardous
	BAV	All competitive sports if: aortic root and ascending aorta not dilated (function of BAV also important)
		Low and moderate static and dynamic sports when the aorta is moderately dilated (z-score 2–3.5; aortic root/ascending aorta 40–42 mm in men or 36–39 mm in women)
		Low-intensity competitive sports when the aorta measures 43–45 mm.
		Should not participate in competitive sports if aorta >45 mm
	Unexplained aortic dilation	All competitive athletics may be considered in athletes with unexplained mild aortic dilation (z-score 2–2.5 or aortic size 40–41 mm in tall men or 35–37 mm in tall women) after evaluation for underling genetic aortopathy, which may include genetic testing and family screening
2018 TS Scientific Statement[15]	TS (>15 y old)	All competitive sports if ASI <2.0 cm/m²
		Low and moderate static and dynamic sports if ASI 2–2.3 cm/m²
		Should not participate in competitive sports if ASI >2.3 cm/m²
2020 ESC[37]	MFS and other HTAD;	Avoid high and very high intensity exercise, contact and power sport and preference for

(continued on next page)

Table 3 (continued)		
Guideline	Condition	Recommendation
		endurance over power sports
		When aorta dilated >40 mm, only skill sports or mixed or endurance sports at low intensity
		When aorta >45 mm, sports are contraindicated
	TS	Aortic size not dilated: all sports permitted with preference for endurance over power sports
		ASI 2.0–2.5 cm/m²: only skill sports or mixed or endurance sports at low intensity
		ASI >2.5 cm/m²: sports are contraindicated
	BAV	Aortic size <40 mm: all sports permitted with preference for endurance over power sports
		Aortic size 40–45 mm: avoid high and very high intensity exercise, contact and power sport and preference for endurance over power sports
		Aortic size 45–50 mm: only skill sports or mixed or endurance sports at low intensity
		Aortic size >50 mm: sports are contraindicated
	Unexplained aortic dilation	Aortic size 40–45 mm: avoid high and very high intensity exercise, contact and power sport and preference for endurance over power sports
		Aortic size 45–50 mm: only skill sports or mixed or endurance sports at low intensity
		Aortic size >50 mm: sports are contraindicated

Abbreviations: ACC, American College of Cardiology; AHA, American Heart Association; MFS, Marfan syndrome; MR, mitral regurgitation; LVEF, left ventricular ejection fraction; FH, family history; LDS, Loeys-Dietz syndrome; vEDS, vascular Ehlers-Danlos syndrome; BAV, bicuspid aortic valve; ASI, aortic size index; ESC, European Society Of Cardiology; HTAD, heritable thoracic aortic disease.

EXERCISE AFTER AORTIC SURGERY IN GENETIC AORTOPATHY CONDITIONS

Physical activity recommendations after elective aneurysm surgery are to remain active with aerobic activities performed in moderation.[7,37] In many HTAD conditions, the remaining aortic segments are at risk for future dilation and dissection, which informs exercise recommendations.[7] Noncompetitive, dynamic, and leisurely exercises are favored. Competitive contact sports and strenuous activities involving heavy lifting or intense straining that require the Valsalva maneuver are to be avoided. Individual exercise prescriptions should be tailored to a patient's specific condition and hemodynamic response to exercise. More data are needed about safety and long-term effects of high-intensity, endurance, and competitive exercise following thoracic aortic aneurysm repair. BAV aortopathy, a condition in which the disease is limited to the proximal aorta, represents a special subgroup. A return to many types of physical activity is probably low risk for many patients after BAV-related aneurysm resection, and this shared decision is also informed by valve function.[37]

EXERCISE AFTER AORTIC DISSECTION

Very little data exists on the effects of exercise following aortic dissection. Mental health concerns are common in this population with anxiety, depression, and post-traumatic stress are commonly reported.[36] In a survey of 314 individuals after surviving acute aortic dissection, 24% no longer engaged in any exercise, 27% stopped being sexually active, 32% had new-onset depression, and 32% had new-onset anxiety.[36] Those who exercised routinely had lower BP and less depression.[36] Mild-to-moderate aerobic exercise of 3 to 5 METS in stable patients postaortic dissection is considered low-risk.[36] Exercise recommendations must consider patient-specific features, such as aortic size and BP response to exercise.

In carefully selected patients who have undergone repair of aortic dissection, cardiac rehabilitation has been shown to be low-risk.[38,39] Although upcoming aortic disease guidelines may inform participation in cardiac rehabilitation, many individuals are currently not receiving cardiac rehabilitation following recovery from aortic dissection or thoracic aortic aneurysm resection.

FUTURE DIRECTIONS

Exercise and physical activity are important components of health and well-being for all people, including those with HTAD and other aortopathy conditions. Because of concern about aortic risks, restrictions are placed on high-intensity competitive sports that are predicted to associate with increased aortic wall stress or aortic events. However, this guidance is based on a paucity of clinical data. In too many cases, individuals with genetic aortopathy or after aortic dissection are counseled to avoid all exercise. This misinformation has led to an increase in anxiety, depression, and posttraumatic stress and a lower quality of life. Guidelines from the AHA, ESC, and the Marfan Foundation emphasize the importance of regular low-to-moderate, recreational aerobic physical activity to maintain health. In mouse models of aortopathy, moderate exercise has been found to be protective and improves aortic ultrastructure and function. If this research holds true for people with aortopathy conditions, aortic conditioning through safe levels of physical activity and recreational exercise could potentially have favorable effects on the aorta and have the potential to "buffer" the hemodynamic effects from the inevitable stressors and circumstances of life. Outcome studies of exercise and physical activity in people with HTAD and aortopathy conditions will inform guidance in the future.

CLINICS CARE POINTS

- Preparticipation history and physical examination of athletes should include evaluation for features suggesting MFS, LDS, and vEDS and a careful family history for thoracic aortic aneurysm and dissection, cerebral aneurysm, or unexplained sudden death at a young age.

- Physical activity in individuals with thoracic aortic disease should be modified to account for the aorta's increased susceptibility to complications.

- Physical activity in individuals with aortopathy needs to be considered according to the intensity of its static and dynamic components.

- Underrecognition of aortic disease increases the risk of sudden death in competitive athletes.
- Nomograms based on age, sex, and body size are used when measuring the aorta to determine whether the aorta is enlarged and how the diameter compares to the expected size.
- Although strength-trained and endurance athletes may have a slight increase in aortic root diameter, significant dilation of the aortic root and/or ascending aorta should not be attributed to an "athlete's heart."
- If aortopathy is suspected, further evaluation with an echocardiogram, slit-lamp eye examination (to evaluate for ectopia lentis), and medical genetic consultation (as appropriate) is recommended.
- In an individual with aortopathy, the underlying cause, aortic diameter, individual's age, and family history are important variables to discuss in shared decision-making about physical activity.
- Guidelines emphasize the importance of regular low-to-moderate, recreational aerobic physical activity as appropriate in individuals with HTAD to maintain health.
- Individuals with HTAD and aortopathy conditions are prohibited from participation in high-intensity exercise, contact sports, intense weightlifting, and most competitive athletics.
- Following surgical repair of the aorta, individuals with HTAD remain at risk for dilation and dissection of the remaining segments of the aorta, an important consideration in shared-decision making about physical activity.
- Long-term elite endurance master rowers and runners have an increased prevalence of proximal aortic dilation, but its clinical significance is not known.

DISCLOSURE

The authors have nothing to disclose.

RESEARCH SUPPORT

Mary Sheppard's research is supported by NIH KO1 HL149984. Alan Braverman's research is supported by the Pam and Ron Rubin Fund and the Noemi and Michael Neidorff Aortopathy and Master Clinician Fellowship at Washington University School of Medicine.

REFERENCES

1. Cheng A, Owens D. Marfan syndrome, inherited aortopathies and exercise: What is the right answer? Br J Sports Med 2016;50(2):100–4.
2. Churchill TW, Groezinger E, Kim JH, et al. Association of Ascending Aortic Dilatation and Long-term Endurance Exercise Among Older Masters-Level Athletes. JAMA Cardiol 2020;5(5):522–31.
3. Gibson C, Nielsen C, Alex R, et al. Mild aerobic exercise blocks elastin fiber fragmentation and aortic dilatation in a mouse model of Marfan syndrome associated aortic aneurysm. J Appl Physiol Bethesda Md 1985 2017;123(1):147–60.
4. Mas-Stachurska A, Siegert A-M, Batlle M, et al. Cardiovascular Benefits of Moderate Exercise Training in Marfan Syndrome: Insights From an Animal Model. J Am Heart Assoc 2017;6(9):e006438.
5. Nataatmadja M, West M, West J, et al. Abnormal Extracellular Matrix Protein Transport Associated With Increased Apoptosis of Vascular Smooth Muscle Cells in Marfan Syndrome and Bicuspid Aortic Valve Thoracic Aortic Aneurysm. Circulation 2003;108(10_suppl_1):II–329.

6. Pelliccia A, Di Paolo FM, De Blasiis E, et al. Prevalence and clinical significance of aortic root dilation in highly trained competitive athletes. Circulation 2010; 122(7):698–706, 3 p following 706.

7. Braverman AC, Harris KM, Kovacs RJ, et al. American Heart Association Electro-cardiography and Arrhythmias Committee of Council on Clinical Cardiology, Council on Cardiovascular Disease in Young, Council on Cardiovascular and Stroke Nursing, Council on Functional Genomics and Translational Biology, and American College of Cardiology. Eligibility and Disqualification Recommenda-tions for Competitive Athletes With Cardiovascular Abnormalities: Task Force 7: Aortic Diseases, Including Marfan Syndrome: A Scientific Statement From the American Heart Association and American College of Cardiology. Circulation 2015;132(22):e303–9.

8. Pinard A, Jones GT, Milewicz DM. Genetics of Thoracic and Abdominal Aortic Diseases. Circ Res 2019;124(4):588–606.

9. Thakker PD, Braverman AC. Cardiogenetics: genetic testing in the diagnosis and management of patients with aortic disease. Heart Br Card Soc 2021;107(8): 619–26.

10. Dietz HC, Cutting CR, Pyeritz RE, et al. Marfan syndrome caused by a recurrent de novo missense mutation in the fibrillin gene. Nature 1991;352(6333):337–9.

11. Loeys BL, Dietz HC, Braverman AC, et al. The revised Ghent nosology for the Marfan syndrome. J Med Genet 2010;47(7):476–85.

12. Schepers D, Tortora G, Morisaki H, et al. A mutation update on the LDS-associated genes TGFB2/3 and SMAD2/3. Hum Mutat 2018;39(5):621–34.

13. MacCarrick G, Black JH, Bowdin S, et al. Loeys-Dietz syndrome: a primer for diagnosis and management. Genet Med Off J Am Coll Med Genet 2014;16(8): 576–87.

14. Shalhub S, Byers PH, Hicks KL, et al. A multi-institutional experience in vascular Ehlers-Danlos syndrome diagnosis. J Vasc Surg 2020;71(1):149–57.

15. Silberbach M, Roos-Hesselink JW, Andersen NH, et al. Cardiovascular Health in Turner Syndrome: A Scientific Statement From the American Heart Association. Circ Genomic Precis Med 2018;11(10):e000048.

16. Braverman AC. Aortic replacement for bicuspid aortic valve aortopathy: When and why? J Thorac Cardiovasc Surg 2019;157(2):520–5.

17. Joannides R, Haefeli WE, Linder L, et al. Nitric oxide is responsible for flow-dependent dilatation of human peripheral conduit arteries in vivo. Circulation 1995;91(5):1314–9.

18. Ainsworth BE, Haskell WL, Whitt MC, et al. Compendium of physical activities: an update of activity codes and MET intensities. Med Sci Sports Exerc 2000;32(9 Suppl):S498–504.

19. Levine BD, Baggish AL, Kovacs RJ, et al. Eligibility and Disqualification Recom-mendations for Competitive Athletes With Cardiovascular Abnormalities: Task Force 1: Classification of Sports: Dynamic, Static, and Impact: A Scientific State-ment From the American Heart Association and American College of Cardiology. J Am Coll Cardiol 2015;66(21):2350–5.

20. Bouten CV, Westerterp KR, Verduin M, et al. Assessment of energy expenditure for physical activity using a triaxial accelerometer. Med Sci Sports Exerc 1994; 26(12):1516–23.

21. Mitchell JH, Haskell W, Snell P, et al. Task Force 8: classification of sports. J Am Coll Cardiol 2005;45(8):1364–7.

22. Cook AJ, Ng B, Gargiulo GD, et al. Instantaneous VO2 from a wearable device. Med Eng Phys 2018;52:41–8.

23. Clifford PS, Hanel B, Secher NH. Arterial blood pressure response to rowing. Med Sci Sports Exerc 1994;26(6):715–9.
24. MacDougall JD, Tuxen D, Sale DG, et al. Arterial blood pressure response to heavy resistance exercise. J Appl Physiol Bethesda Md 1985 1985;58(3):785–90.
25. Babaee Bigi MA, Aslani A. Aortic root size and prevalence of aortic regurgitation in elite strength trained athletes. Am J Cardiol 2007;100(3):528–30.
26. Iskandar A, Thompson PD. A meta-analysis of aortic root size in elite athletes. Circulation 2013;127(7):791–8.
27. Boraita A, Heras M-E, Morales F, et al. Reference Values of Aortic Root in Male and Female White Elite Athletes According to Sport. Circ Cardiovasc Imaging 2016;9(10):e005292.
28. Gentry JL, Carruthers D, Joshi PH, et al. Ascending Aortic Dimensions in Former National Football League Athletes. Circ Cardiovasc Imaging 2017;10(11):e006852.
29. Maron BJ, Thompson PD, Ackerman MJ, et al. Recommendations and considerations related to preparticipation screening for cardiovascular abnormalities in competitive athletes: 2007 update: a scientific statement from the American Heart Association Council on Nutrition, Physical Activity, and Metabolism: endorsed by the American College of Cardiology Foundation. Circulation 2007;115(12):1455–643.
30. Harris KM, Tung M, Haas TS, et al. Under-recognition of aortic and aortic valve disease and the risk for sudden death in competitive athletes. J Am Coll Cardiol 2015;65(8):860–2.
31. Tran PHT, Skrba T, Wondimu E, et al. The influence of fibrillin-1 and physical activity upon tendon tissue morphology and mechanical properties in mice. Physiol Rep 2019;7(21):e14267.
32. Lalich JJ, Barnett BD, Bird HR. Production of aortic rupture in turkey poults fed beta-aminopropionitrile. AMA Arch Pathol 1957;64(6):643–8.
33. Aicher BO, Zhang J, Muratoglu SC, et al. Moderate aerobic exercise prevents matrix degradation and death in a mouse model of aortic dissection and aneurysm. Am J Physiol Heart Circ Physiol 2021;320(5):H1786–801.
34. Thijssen CGE, Bons LR, Gökalp AL, et al. Exercise and sports participation in patients with thoracic aortic disease: a review. Expert Rev Cardiovasc Ther 2019;17(4):251–66.
35. Itagaki R, Kimura N, Itoh S, et al. Acute type a aortic dissection associated with a sporting activity. Surg Today 2017;47(9):1163–71.
36. Chaddha A, Kline-Rogers E, Braverman AC, et al. Survivors of Aortic Dissection: Activity, Mental Health, and Sexual Function. Clin Cardiol 2015;38(11):652–9.
37. Pelliccia A, Sharma S, Gati S, et al. 2020 ESC Guidelines on sports cardiology and exercise in patients with cardiovascular disease. Eur Heart J 2021;42(1):17–96.
38. Corone S, Iliou M-C, Pierre B, et al. French registry of cases of type I acute aortic dissection admitted to a cardiac rehabilitation center after surgery. Eur J Cardiovasc Prev Rehabil Off J Eur Soc Cardiol Work Groups Epidemiol Prev Card Rehabil Exerc Physiol 2009;16(1):91–5.
39. Fuglsang S, Heiberg J, Hjortdal VE, et al. Exercise-based cardiac rehabilitation in surgically treated type-A aortic dissection patients. Scand Cardiovasc J SCJ 2017;51(2):99–105.

Cardiac Concerns in the Pediatric Athlete

Jamie N. Colombo, DO[a], Christine N. Sawda, MD[b], Shelby C. White, MD[c],*

KEYWORDS

- Congenital heart disease • Sports participation • Young Athlete

KEY POINTS

- Acquired heart disease can be attributed to lack of physical activity in the American population.
- Pediatric athletes must be assessed by providers familiar with cardiovascular changes occurring around puberty to avoid unnecessary concern for heart disease.
- Most patients with congenital heart disease should be encouraged to engage in unrestricted physical activity and sports participation.
- Activity limitations are specific to the cardiac lesion and should be put into place after complete cardiovascular evaluation by a pediatric cardiologist.

INTRODUCTION

Cardiovascular disease remains the number one cause of death in Americans; it is no secret that exercise mitigates this risk.[1] Exercise and regular physical activity are beneficial for physical health including aerobic conditioning, endurance, strength, mental health, and overall improved quality of life (QoL).[2,3] Unfortunately, today many children and adolescents are sedentary, lacking the recommended daily amount of physical activity leading to higher rates of obesity, cardiovascular disease, stroke, diabetes, anxiety, and depression.[1,4,5] Given this rising concern, the World Health Organization (WHO) launched a 12-year plan to improve physical activity in children and adolescents by reducing the inactivity rate by 15% in the world.[4] How does this apply to children and adolescents with acquired or congenital heart disease (CHD)?

One in 100 children will be born with CHD, making it the most common congenital malformation.[6,7] Many of these children are living until adulthood, some with a normal life expectancy.[8,9] In fact, today, there are more than 1,000,000 adults living with CHD,

---

[a] Department of Pediatrics, Division of Cardiology, Washington University School of Medicine/ St. Louis Children's Hospital, 1 Childrens Place, St. Louis, MO 63110, USA; [b] Department of Pediatrics, Division of Cardiology, Children's National Medical Center, 111 Michigan Avenue Northwest, Washington, DC 20010, USA; [c] Department of Pediatrics, Division of Cardiology, University of Virginia, PO Box 800386, Charlottesville, VA 22908, USA
* Corresponding author.
E-mail address: sw2bd@virginia.edu

Clin Sports Med 41 (2022) 529–548
https://doi.org/10.1016/j.csm.2022.02.010
0278-5919/22/Published by Elsevier Inc.

sportsmed.theclinics.com

and that number is expected to increase by 5% per year.[8] Children with CHD are traditionally thought of as medically fragile and at risk for sudden cardiac arrest, as a result they have long been sheltered from engaging in various forms of physical activity including both competitive sport and recreational exercise. This has led to a problem with greater than 54% of adults and 26% of children with CHD being obese or over weight.[10,11] Additionally, their risk of psychological disorders including anxiety, depression, and reduced self-esteem are high.[12,13] Regular physical activity can mitigate these comorbidities. Emerging research demonstrates that regular exercise is safe and beneficial for children and adolescents with CHD when paired with exercise testing to assess functional capacity, exercise training regimens, and frequent counseling during follow-up appointments.[14–16]

Most children and adolescents with CHD should follow the same recommendations as described below by the WHO. In 2019, the WHO released new guidelines for physical activity starting in infancy, recommending those aged less than 1 year engage in floor-based play for at least 1 hour per day.[17] Children aged older than 5 years should participate in at least 60 minutes of moderate to vigorous physical activity per day with resistance training at least 3 days per week. According to the Journal of American Medical Association, even a single episode of physical activity can improve cognitive function, memory, attention and decrease daytime fatigue.[18]

CONSIDERATIONS FOR THE PERIPUBERTAL ATHLETE

The interaction between growth, training, and maturity must be considered when assessing the cardiovascular system of pediatric athletes. Physiologic changes associated with athletic training have been well documented in adults with regard to increased left ventricular chamber size and wall thickness depending on the form of athletic activity undertaken, endurance versus strength training.[19] Understanding these adaptations to exercise is important because the changes seen on cardiovascular testing may mimic those of heart disease. Much less is known about athletic remodeling that occurs in children, particularly in the preadolescent and early-adolescent age range.

Studies attempting to define the "athlete's heart" phenotype in children have described low resting heart rates and increased left ventricular chamber size when compared with control groups.[20–22] The extent that the anatomic findings in young athletes are a result of training versus genetic preselection is unknown; those children with increased left ventricular diameter could be more likely to perform at a higher level of athletic competition. The degree of ventricular dilation in peripubertal athletes seems to be less conspicuous than that observed in adult athletes, generally at the upper limits of normal range for age.[23] As such, if there is a finding of significant left ventricular enlargement or hypertrophy in a prepubertal or early-pubertal athlete, heart disease such as cardiomyopathy must be considered.

ELECTROCARDIOGRAM DIFFERENCES IN PEDIATRIC PATIENTS

The basic principles of electrocardiogram (ECG) interpretation between pediatric and adult athletes are the same; however, there are features of the pediatric ECG, which differ significantly from the normal adult pattern and vary according to the age of the child.

Marked changes occur between infancy and adolescence due to the transition in anatomy and physiology, most notably related to the right ventricular dominance seen in young children, which is represented by increased R wave amplitude in the right precordial leads (V1) and decreases with age. There is an associated increase in R wave amplitude in left precordial leads (V6) as the left ventricle becomes dominant. Generally, the R/s ratio in V1 remains greater than 1 up to 3 years of age, but this may persist; there are multiple datasets that describe the normal ECG standards in pediatrics according to age and these should be referenced when considering ventricular hypertrophy in a pediatric patient.[24–26]

It is also valuable to be aware of the expected changes seen in T-wave morphology throughout childhood and adolescence. Anterior (V1–V3) T-waves are normally inverted after the first week of life until adolescence and may remain inverted until physical maturity is complete (the "juvenile" ECG pattern, **Fig. 1**). This is in contrast to adult ECG findings, in which inverted T-waves in anterior leads can represent right heart strain or myocardial infarction.[27] Isolated T-wave inversion in anterior leads in athletes aged less than 16 years should not be considered abnormal.[28,29]

PHYSICAL ACTIVITY IN PATIENTS WITH CONGENITAL HEART DISEASE

Distinction must be made between physical activity, leisure or recreational sport and competitive sport participation. Physical activity is defined as any movements resulting from muscle contraction that increases the metabolic rate above the resting level. Recreational sport is informal or organized physical activity without pressure to play, continue to play, or play at a higher intensity than is desired by the participant. In general, children and adolescents with CHD are encouraged to participate in physical activity or recreational sport as outlined by the WHO above.

In contrast, competitive sport is an organized form of physical activity that requires fixed rules and commitment; involving pressure or continuation to train and play at a high intensity regardless of whether that intensity is desired by the participant.[15] Specific sport classifications by the 36th Bethesda Conference based on dynamic and static activities are used to determine the safety of competitive sport for patients with CHD based on guidelines from the American Heart Association (AHA) and American College of Cardiology (ACC).[30] Despite growing recommendations to encourage physical activity in youth populations with CHD, there remain several obstructive factors aside from formal exercise restrictions including exercise capacity, parental anxiety, and perceived self-efficacy.[13,14]

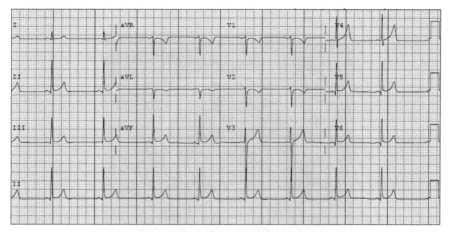

Fig. 1. ECG from 16-year-old man demonstrating T wave inversion in anterior precordial leads (V1, V2); patient is without cardiovascular disease; and this represents "juvenile" ECG pattern.

Advances in medical and surgical care have improved the life expectancy of children with CHD resulting in an increased survival into adulthood and an estimated 1 million Americans with CHD are alive today. As such, QoL is emerging as an important health outcome for these patients. It is well documented that children with CHD perceive a lower physical and psychosocial QoL than healthy children across all age groups.[31] In patients with CHD, competitive sports participation was found to be associated with improved QoL when adjusting for disease severity.[32] Competitive sports participation can protect against depression and SI by boosting self-esteem and increasing social support.[33] Additionally, physical activity when performed on a sports team is associated with improved academic outcomes.[34] Competitive sports participation is found to be associated with improved exercise capacity and lower BMI. Studies have shown that decreased oxygen consumption during cardiopulmonary exercise testing (CPET) as well as a decreased anaerobic threshold are significantly correlated with decreased subject perception of physical well-being.[35] Similarly, patients who have had a Fontan procedure with higher levels of exercise capacity, as determined by CPET, report an improved perception of their physical and psychosocial well-being.[12]

ACYANOTIC CONGENITAL HEART DISEASE

CHD is a wide spectrum ranging from simple to complex. Left to right shunting lesions are common; including simple shunt lesions such as atrial septal defect (ASD) and ventricular septal defects (VSD). Many simple defects will resolve spontaneously without the need for surgery. Should intervention be required, outcomes are typically excellent.[36]

Atrial Septal Defect

ASD describes a shunting lesion between the top 2 chambers of the heart (**Figs. 2 and 3**). Severity ranges from a small patent foramen ovale to larger, hemodynamically significant lesions that require closure. The incidence ranges from 6% to 10% of all forms of CHD or ∼1 in 1500 children.[36] Most patients are asymptomatic and may not present to cardiology care until the third or fourth decade of life. Hemodynamic significance is determined by right ventricular dilation and the presence of pulmonary hypertension.

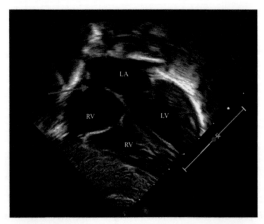

Fig. 2. Transthoracic echocardiogram with a subcostal coronal image depicting a secundum ASD in 2D (*red arrow*). LA, left atrium; LV, left ventricle; RA, right atrium; RV, right ventricle.

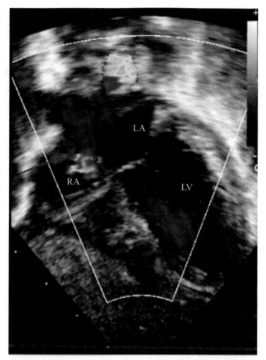

Fig. 3. Transthoracic echocardiogram with a subcostal coronal image depicting a secundum ASD with color demonstrating a left to right shunt (*red arrow*). LA, left atrium; LV, left ventricle; RA, right atrium.

In patients with unrepaired ASDs exercise capabilities are determined by ventricular volume overload and pulmonary hypertension. As most lesions are small, exercise limitations are usually not necessary. Studies have shown that in adult patients with unrepaired ASDs maximal oxygen uptake (VO_{2max}) may be impaired compared with healthy peers; however, this is not traditionally seen in pediatric populations.[37] Competitive sports participation is dictated by the presence of pulmonary hypertension (pulmonary artery systolic pressure >40 mm Hg or mean gradient >25 mm Hg).[37,38] If pulmonary hypertension is present, patients should be restricted to Class 1A sports or low dynamic and static activity.[38] Regular exercise or recreational play should be encouraged with the exception of scuba diving due to the risk of paradoxic air embolism.

Ventricular Septal Defects

VSDs make up 20% to 30% of all CHD or up to 3.9 in 1000 live birth percentage.[36] VSDs typically present early in life compared with ASDs. Small lesions create a pressure gradient between the 2 ventricles leading to a murmur that can be heard on physical examination. Larger lesions in infants will present with signs of heart failure such as tachypnea and poor growth (**Figs. 4 and 5**). Although up to 85% of small lesions will close within the first year of life, large lesions require surgical closure early in life due to risk for pulmonary hypertension.[7]

As with ASDs, sports restriction is determined by the presence of pulmonary hypertension. Children with small defects or who have undergone surgical repair are typically asymptomatic and have normal exercise capabilities.[38,39] As the aging CHD population grows, long-term effects both after VSD closure and on small unrepaired

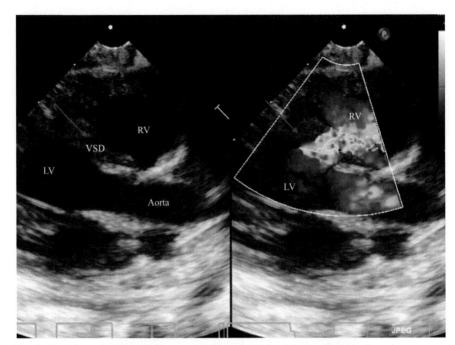

Fig. 4. Transthoracic echocardiogram with a parasternal long axis view in color compare showing a moderate high muscular ventricular septal defect with a left to right shunt (*red arrow*). LV, left ventricle; VSD, ventricular septal defect; RV, right ventricle.

lesions demonstrate mild ventricular dysfunction leading to lower exercise capacity in this population compared with healthy peers.[40,41]

OBSTRUCTIVE CONGENITAL HEART DISEASE
Bicuspid Aortic Valve

Bicuspid aortic valve (BAV) is the most common congenital heart defect, with an estimated prevalence between 0.5% and 2% of the population[7,42] (**Fig. 6**). There is a male predominance of approximately 3 to 1. BAV is often associated with left heart obstructive lesions; more than half of patients with coarctation of the aorta (CoA) have been

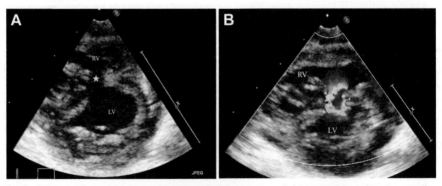

Fig. 5. (*A*) Transthoracic echocardiogram with a parasternal short axis view showing moderate muscular VSD (*yellow star*). (*B*) Same image with color shows bidirectional flow. LV, left ventricle; VSD, ventricular septal defect; RV, right ventricle.

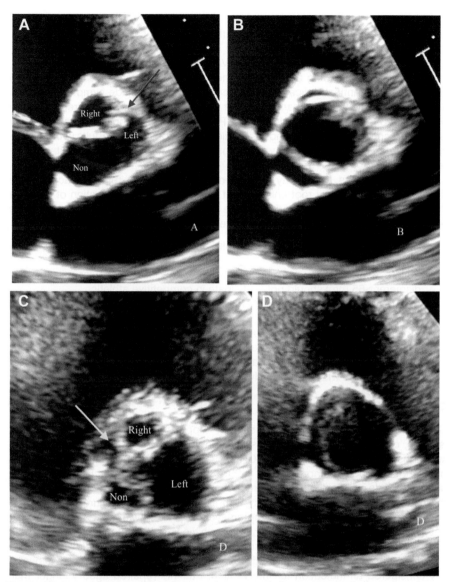

Fig. 6. (*A*) Transthoracic echocardiogram (parasternal short axis view) demonstrating a closed BAV with left and right coronary cusp fusion as depicted by the red arrow. (*B*) BAV in systole demonstrating the characteristic fish-mouth appearance of an open valve. (*C*) Transthoracic echocardiogram (parasternal short axis view) demonstrating a closed BAV with right and non-coronary cusp fusion as depicted by the yellow arrow. (*D*) BAV in systole demonstrating again the characteristic fish-mouth appearance.

found to have BAV.[43] BAV is also commonly accompanied by dilation of the sinuses of Valsalva, the tubular ascending aorta, or both. Although BAV and its associated aortopathy can lead to dissection in older patients, this complication is very rare in active young athletes.[44] Specific to women athletes, patients with Turner syndrome (chromosome 45 XO) should be sure to undergo cardiovascular evaluation because more than half of these girls will have a cardiovascular abnormality. Of these, BAV and coarctation comprise the majority, and these patients may be especially prone to aortic dissection.[45,46]

Cardiac intervention in patients with BAV can be required for aortic stenosis (AS), insufficiency, or ascending aorta enlargement. Twenty percent of patients with AS will require intervention. Indications for intervention in AS include symptoms, severe aortic valve gradient, ECG changes at rest or with exercise, or in children who may be interested in competitive athletics.[47,48] Percutaneous balloon aortic valvuloplasty is the interventional strategy of choice in children and some young adults with AS. Valvuloplasty can be complicated by aortic insufficiency, which may necessitate valve replacement.[49,50]

Recommendations for activity restriction most commonly relate to aortic valve dysfunction and/or aortic root enlargement. As AS progresses, duration of exercise decreases, delta systolic blood pressure decreases, and ST segment changes occur.[51,52] ACC/AHA guidelines[38] recommend the following:

- Athletes with severe AS (mean Doppler >40 mm Hg) should not participate in competitive athletics.
- Athletes with severe aortic insufficiency with left ventricular dilation (LV diameter >65 mm) should not participate in competitive athletics.
- Athletes with dilated aortic root (>45 mm) should only participate in low-intensity competitive athletics.
- Athletes with BAV and mild or less valve dysfunction and no significant aortic root dilation (<40 mm) do not have restrictions.
- Athletes with mild aortic root dilation may consider avoidance of extreme weight lifting or sports with heavy bodily contact.[38,47,53]

COARCTATION OF THE AORTA

CoA is a narrowing of the blood vessel that happens either discreetly, at the aortic isthmus, or diffusely across the transverse aortic arch. It occurs in 4 out of 10,000 live births, comprising 4% to 8% of CHD.[7,54] The presentation of patients with CoA occurs in a bimodal distribution and is 2 to 3 times more common in men. The first group consists of symptomatic infants who present often in cardiogenic shock in the neonatal period or later in infancy with symptoms of heart failure. Older infants and children most often remain asymptomatic and present with hypertension (classically in the right arm due to typical brachiocephalic vessel arrangement) or a murmur related to the coarctation itself or associated aortic valve disease. In older patients, a blood pressure gradient of 20 mm Hg between upper and lower extremities is generally considered an indication for intervention. Patients repaired aged younger than 5 years have the greatest risk of reintervention, whereas patients repaired aged older than 9 years have a greater prevalence of residual hypertension.[55,56]

Type of intervention for CoA depends on the anatomy of the aortic arch narrowing and the age/weight of the patient at time of diagnosis. Surgical intervention is preferred in younger children with native CoA due to high rates of recurrence with balloon angioplasty. In older children and adults, percutaneous stenting is possible with similar reintervention rates to surgery and fewer complications (**Fig. 7**).[56,57] Lifelong follow-up is warranted for patients with CoA after repair, given risk of recoarctation, other aortic complications (such as aneurysm at the site of repair), systemic hypertension (at rest or exercise-induced), and other associated CHD. There are mixed data regarding the reduced exercise capacity in patients after coarctation repair independent of exercise-induced hypertension.[58–60]

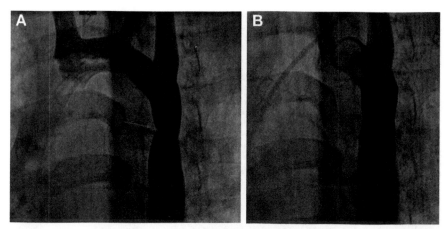

Fig. 7. (*A*) Aortic angiography demonstrating CoA in the juxtaductal region of the descending thoracic aorta as depicted by red arrow. This patient is a 14-year-old competitive soccer player with a preintervention gradient of 20 mm Hg between the upper and lower extremity. (*B*) Following stent placement, the blood pressure gradient was reduced to zero.

Activity restriction in patients with coarctation is determined by other structural heart disease as well as presence of exercise-induced hypertension or resting systemic arm/leg blood pressure gradient. Patients with unrepaired coarctation do not require restriction if they have the following:

- Normal exercise test
- Resting arm/leg systolic blood pressure gradient less than 20 mm Hg
- Peak systolic blood pressure less than 95th percentile of predicted with exercise

Patients following coarctation repair, either surgical or transcatheter, can participate in noncontact sports that do not require high-intensity static exercise after 3 months following procedure if above criteria are met.[38]

TETRALOGY OF FALLOT

Tetralogy of Fallot (TOF) is the most common form of cyanotic CHD accounting for 7% to 10% of all CHD.[61] Four elements make up the diagnosis: right ventricular outflow tract obstruction, VSD, overriding aorta, and right ventricular hypertrophy (**Fig. 8**). Typical repair is completed within the first 6 months of life, which includes VSD closure and reconstruction of the right ventricular outflow tract. As a result, patients are often left with free pulmonary valve insufficiency leading to right ventricular dilation and dysfunction. Although many patients remain asymptomatic in childhood due to false awareness of their functional class, this can lead to exercise intolerance with VO_2 max up to 20% less than age-matched peers.[62,63]

Over time patients with repaired TOF are at risk for arrhythmia, concomitant left ventricular dysfunction and sudden cardiac arrest prompting evaluation for pulmonary valve replacement. Due to these risks patients must observe regular cardiology follow-up and thorough evaluation before sports participation with exercise stress testing. For those with significant ventricular dysfunction, ejection fraction (EF) less than 40%, severe right ventricular outflow tract obstruction, or arrhythmias, high-intensity competitive sports should be avoided.[38]

Physical activity restrictions in TOF patients with severe pulmonary valve regurgitation and RV dilation in absence of the aforementioned risk factors are not well defined

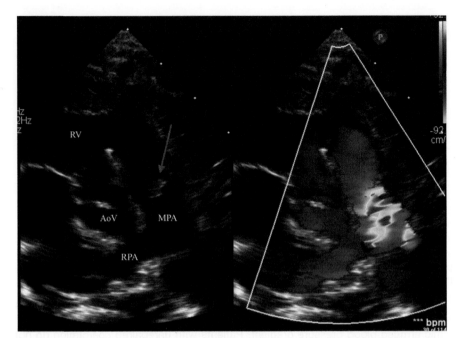

Fig. 8. Transthoracic echocardiogram (parasternal short axis view) in 2D and color comparison of a neonate with TOF with a thickened pulmonary valve (*red arrow*). Color imaging shows aliasing of flow as depicted by yellow speckling indicating high velocity flow across the native valve. AoV, aortic valve; MPA, main pulmonary artery; RPA, right pulmonary artery; RV, right ventricle.

due to lack of evidence. However, studies have shown patients with TOF have a decreased cardiac index and lower stroke volumes due to RV dilation when compared with healthy peers.[63,64] Aly and colleagues demonstrated by MRI that patients with TOF who were obese had higher biventricular volume, great LV mass, lower EF, and decreased exercise capacity compared with normal weight peers.[65] To assess for risk factors, careful evaluation of the patient by the pediatric cardiologist should be conducted at regular intervals. Risks should be discussed and joint decision-making should occur.

FONTAN

The Fontan procedure is the third and final step in surgical palliation for patients with single ventricle CHD. It is aimed at separating oxygenated and deoxygenated blood through anastomosis of the superior and inferior vena cava to the pulmonary arteries (**Fig. 9**). This allows systemic venous return to completely bypass the heart. Today there are more than 70,000 patients with a Fontan, and the 30-year survival is approximately 85%.[66] With the absence of a subpulmonary ventricle, patients with Fontan physiology are known to have a markedly impaired response to physical activity and low oxygen consumption at peak exercise and anaerobic threshold. Chronic elevation of central venous pressure leads to decreased preload and low cardiac output.[66–69] Despite a global reduction in exercise capacity, each patient with Fontan physiology is different, making thorough cardiovascular evaluation of the utmost importance before participation in sports. Restrictions should be based on CPET,

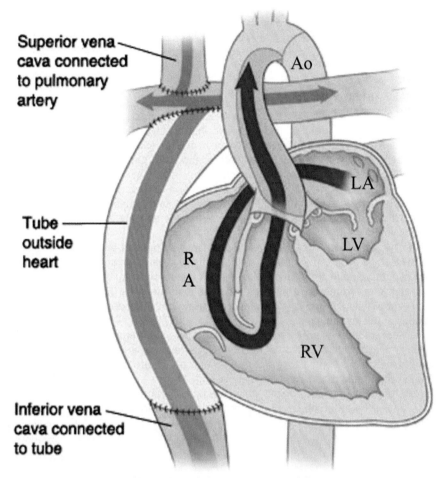

Superior vena cava connected to pulmonary artery

Tube outside heart

Inferior vena cava connected to tube

Fig. 9. Cartoon depiction of hypoplastic left heart syndrome following extracardiac Fontan or stage III palliation. Ao, aorta; LA, left atrium; LV, left ventricle; RA, right atrium, RV, right ventricle.

echocardiogram, and ECG findings to evaluate for arrhythmia, cyanosis, heart failure, or symptomatic limitations.

Exercise capacity declines with age in this population for multiple reasons, including chronotropic and/or inotropic incompetence, decreased muscle mass, restrictive lung disease due to multiple intrathoracic surgeries, and cyanosis.[66,68,70,71] Additionally, patients are often sedentary, obese, and suffer from psychological distress further exacerbating exercise intolerance.[66,72] Due to the perceived risk of adverse cardiovascular events many patients with single ventricle CHD were discouraged from strenuous physical activity and most forms of competitive athletics. According to the AHA and the ACC, patients with Fontan physiology should be limited to 1A, low dynamic, and static athletic competition.[38,73] However, both anaerobic and aerobic exercise rehabilitation have been shown to increase functional capacity, strength, and QoL.[71,74–76] Regimented training with moderate-to-vigorous exercise including weight lifting can improve physical fitness as demonstrated by increased peak oxygen consumption and stroke volume on MRI.[71] Moreover, multiple studies have demonstrated minimal risk for arrhythmia, stroke, or sudden death related to sports practice.[74] Although additional data needs to be collected, some institutions now recommend regular intense exercise programs to promote general health and improved QoL.[75]

CORONARY ARTERY PATHOLOGY
Kawasaki Disease

Kawasaki disease is a self-limited systemic inflammatory reaction presenting as a constellation of symptoms including fever, rash, conjunctivitis, cracking and erythema of the oral mucosa, as well as cervical lymphadenopathy. On a microscopic level, Kawasaki disease causes a primary vasculopathy affecting medium-sized arteries, namely the coronary arteries. It is the most common form of acquired heart disease occurring in ~25 cases per 100,000 children aged younger than 5 years in the United States. Although the cause remains unknown, there is a higher prevalence in individuals of Asian descent.[77]

In the pediatric population, Kawasaki disease may present with a clinical picture consistent with shock, myocarditis, pericarditis, valvulitis, or arrhythmia. However, coronary artery aneurysm formation is the most feared consequence placing the individual at risk for thrombosis and progressive stenosis over time (**Fig. 10**). Treatment is aimed at preventing systemic inflammation by using both high dose aspirin and immunoglobulin until fever subsides.

Long-term outcomes are based on coronary artery involvement with most children demonstrating only mild dilation of the coronary arteries at time of diagnosis with resolution over the following 1 to 2 months. Complications are more commonly seen in patients with medium and giant aneurysms (**Fig. 11**).

Sports participation for pediatric athletes is based on the presence of residual dilation or aneurysm of the coronary arteries and the need for anticoagulation following acute illness. According to the 2017 AHA statement, all patients with Kawasaki disease should be provided with counseling for physical activity.[77] Patients should be

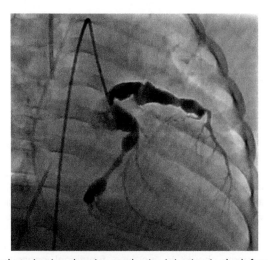

Fig. 10. Cardiac catheterization showing a selective injection in the left coronary artery in a patient with Kawasaki disease. Angiogram shows multiple large aneurysms of the left anterior descending and circumflex artery.

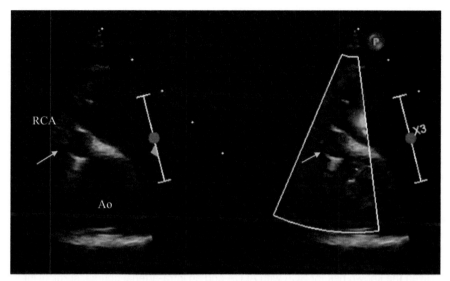

Fig. 11. Transthoracic echocardiogram showing a dilated right coronary artery with small aneurysm in color compare (*yellow arrow*). Ao, aorta; RCA, right coronary artery.

deterred from sport for 8 weeks following initial diagnosis.[78] In patients who require ongoing anticoagulation therapy, contact sport should be restricted. In the presence of medium or greater coronary artery aneurysms (z-score >5), exercise stress testing should be considered assessing for myocardial ischemia or arrhythmia as markers of risk for sudden cardiac arrest before returning to play.[77–79]

Patients with Kawasaki disease and coronary artery aneurysms do not seem to be at a disadvantage with regard to exercise capacity.[77,80] When comparing age-matched peers with history of Kawasaki disease with and without aneurysm, both groups demonstrated an equal endurance and chronotropic response to exercise.[80] However, when comparing patients with history of Kawasaki disease to that of the general population, patients with Kawaski were found to participate less in moderate-to-vigorous physical activity and have a lower exercise self efficacy.[81] They fail to reach the recommended daily amount of exercise leading to a lower exercise capacity over time.[82] This demonstrates the importance of exercise counseling at every encounter to promote optimal long-term outcomes.

ANOMALOUS CORONARY ARTERY ORIGIN

Anomalous aortic origin of the coronary artery (AAOCA) from the inappropriate sinus of Valsalva is a rare finding occurring in 0.1% to 0.7% of the population.[83] Two main types exist: anomalous origin of the left coronary artery off the right sinus of Valsalva (ALCA) and anomalous origin of the right coronary artery off the left sinus of Valsalva (ARCA). Occasionally the anomalous coronary artery may arise from the noncoronary cusp. AAOCA is further broken down by coronary artery course: prepulmonic (anterior), retroaortic (posterior), retrocardiac, intraseptal, or intra-arterial (between the pulmonary artery and the aorta). Finally, AAOCA can travel within the aortic wall (intramural course), this variation is usually found in association with intra-arterial subtypes.

Although many subtypes are not known to be clinically relevant, both ALCA and ARCA can be associated with sudden cardiac arrest (SCA), thought to be secondary to myocardial ischemia and ventricular arrhythmia. Coronary artery anomalies are associated with 17% of sudden cardiac death in competitive athletes in the United States.[38] The risk for SCA is highest if an intra-arterial or intramural course is present **(Fig. 12)**, specifically if there is a slit-like opening at the site of attachment to the aorta.[84] Additionally, ARCA is more common than ALCA, but ALCA carries the higher risk of SCA (Brothers 2017 and Brothers 2016). The true prevalence of SCA from an AAOCA is unknown as data is obtained from autopsied patients; however, it is almost exclusively seen as a disease of the young, less than 35 year old in association with strenuous exercise.[83–85]

The cause of AAOCA is unknown and there is no known genetic link in humans.[83] Most patients with AAOCA are diagnosed incidentally when the patient is seen for an unrelated concern such as a heart murmur. However, some patients will present with palpitations, near-syncope, syncope or cardiac arrest. Initial testing includes echocardiogram and ECG, although computed tomography or magnetic resonance angiography is usually required for confirmatory diagnosis. Functional testing with exercise stress testing or myocardial perfusion imaging should be interpreted with a grain of salt because there is a significant rate of false-positive and false-negative results.[84]

Given the known risk for SCA with ALCA and an intra-arterial course, surgical intervention is recommended especially if symptoms are present. However, guidelines for ARCA are not as clear and often spark significant debate.[83,84] In these cases, the risk and benefit of surgery must be considered.

Because physical activity is noted to be a significant risk factor for both ALCA and ARCA, one must consider restriction from exercise. The 2015 AHA and ACC Guidelines for exercise with ARCA suggest the patient should be evaluated with a stress test before engaging in competitive sport. If the patient is asymptomatic and has a negative stress test, one could consider participation knowing that a negative stress test does not completely eliminate the risk. The physician and the family should engage in meaningful conversations to weigh the risk and benefits of athletics and come up with a mutually agreeable plan. If the patient is symptomatic, demonstrates

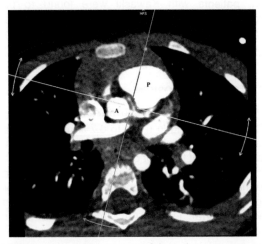

Fig. 12. A 5-year-old girl with anomalous origin of the right coronary artery off the left sinus of Valsalva. An intra-arterial course between the aorta and pulmonary artery is seen with a 4 mm intramural segment (*red arrow*). Ao, aorta; PA, pulmonary artery.

signs of ischemia or arrhythmia, athletics should be restricted, with the exception of Class 1A, and surgery should be highly considered. However, patients with ALCA, intra-arterial subtype, should be restricted from competitive sport regardless of symptoms due to the risk of SCA and surgery should be strongly considered. Athletes can resume sport participation 3 months after appropriate surgical recovery.[38]

SUMMARY

A concerning trend toward a sedentary lifestyle is becoming more evident in pediatric patients with congenital and acquired heart disease leading to an increase in obesity in this population. Although some patients will require frequent evaluations and joint decision-making with the family to facilitate safety before participation in highly static and dynamic forms of competitive physical activity, most of these patients should be allowed to engage in an unrestricted fashion. Patients should be encouraged to lead active lifestyles with close monitoring by their pediatric cardiologist.

DISCLOSURE

The authors have nothing to disclose.

REFERENCES

1. De Ferranti SD, Steinberger J, Ameduri R, et al. Cardiovascular Risk Reduction in High-Risk Pediatric Patients: A Scientific Statement From the American Heart Association. Vol 139.; 2019. doi:10.1161/CIR.0000000000000618
2. Garber CE, Blissmer B, Deschenes MR, et al. Quantity and quality of exercise for developing and maintaining cardiorespiratory, musculoskeletal, and neuromotor fitness in apparently healthy adults: Guidance for prescribing exercise. Med Sci Sports Exerc 2011;43(7):1334–59.
3. Landry BW, Driscoll SW. Physical activity in children and adolescents. PM R 2012; 4(11):826–32.
4. Chaput JP, Willumsen J, Bull F, et al. WHO guidelines on physical activity and sedentary behaviour for children and adolescents aged 5–17 years: summary of the evidence. Int J Behav Nutr Phys Act 2020;17(1):1–9.
5. Pieles GE, Horn R, Williams CA, et al. Paediatric exercise training in prevention and treatment. Arch Dis Child 2014;99(4):380–5.
6. Marelli AJ, Mackie AS, Ionescu-Ittu R, et al. Congenital heart disease in the general population: Changing prevalence and age distribution. Circulation 2007; 115(2):163–72.
7. Hoffman JIE, Kaplan S. The incidence of congenital heart disease. J Am Coll Cardiol 2002;39(12):1890–900.
8. Brickner ME, Hillis LDLR. Congenital heart disease in adults. First of two parts. N Engl J Med 2000;342(4):256–63.
9. Van Der Bom T, Bouma BJ, Meijboom FJ, et al. The prevalence of adult congenital heart disease, results from a systematic review and evidence based calculation. Am Heart J 2012;164(4):568–75.
10. Barbiero SM, D'Azevedo Sica C, Schuh DS, et al. Overweight and obesity in children with congenital heart disease: Combination of risks for the future? BMC Pediatr 2014;14(1):1–6.
11. Pinto NM, Marino BS, Wernovsky G, et al. Obesity is a common comorbidity in children with congenital and acquired heart disease. Pediatrics 2007;120(5): e1157–64.

12. McCrindle BW, Williams RV, Mital S, et al. Physical activity levels in children and adolescents are reduced after the Fontan procedure, independent of exercise capacity, and are associated with lower perceived general health. Arch Dis Child 2007;92(6):509–14.

13. Moola F, Fusco C, Kirsh JA. The perceptions of caregivers toward physical activity and health in youth with congenital heart disease. Qual Health Res 2011;21(2): 278–91.

14. van Deutekom AW, Lewandowski AJ. Physical activity modification in youth with congenital heart disease: a comprehensive narrative review. Pediatr Res 2021; 89(7):1650–8.

15. Takken T, Giardini A, Reybrouck T, et al. Recommendations for physical activity, recreation sport, and exercise training in paediatric patients with congenital heart disease: A report from the Exercise, Basic & Translational Research Section of the European Association of Cardiovascular Preventio. Eur J Prev Cardiol 2012;19(5): 1034–65.

16. Tran D, Maiorana A, Ayer J, et al. Recommendations for exercise in adolescents and adults with congenital heart disease. Prog Cardiovasc Dis 2020;63(3): 350–66.

17. World Health Organization. World Health Organisation Guidleines for Physical Activity, Sedentary Behaviour, and Sleep for Children under 5 Years of Age. 2019. https://www.who.int/publications/i/item/9789241550536%0Ahttps://apps.who.int/iris/bitstream/handle/10665/311664/9789241550536-eng.pdf?sequence=1&isAllowed=y%0Ahttp://www.who.int/iris/handle/10665/311664.

18. Piercy KL, Troiano RP, Ballard RM, et al. The physical activity guidelines for Americans. JAMA - J Am Med Assoc 2018;320(19):2020–8.

19. Pluim BM, Zwinderman AH, Van Der Laarse A, et al. The athlete's heart: A meta-analysis of cardiac structure and function. Circulation 2000;101(3):336–44.

20. Ayabakan C, Akalin F, Mengütay S, et al. Athlete's heart in prepubertal male swimmers. Cardiol Young 2006;16(1):61–6.

21. McClean G, Riding NR, Ardern CL, et al. Electrical and structural adaptations of the paediatric athlete's heart: A systematic review with meta-analysis. Br J Sports Med 2018;52(4):230.

22. Rowland TW, Delaney BC, Siconolfi SF. ' Athlete's Heart ' in Prepubertal Children. Pediatrics 1987;79(5):800–4.

23. Rowland T. Morphologic features of the "athlete's heart" in children: A contemporary review. Pediatr Exerc Sci 2016;28(3):345–52.

24. Rautaharju PM, Davignon A, Soumis F, et al. Evolution of QRS-T relationship from birth to adolescence in Frank-lead orthogonal electrocardiograms of 1492 normal children. Circulation 1979;60(1):196–204.

25. Rijnbeek PR, Witsenburg M, Schrama E, et al. New normal limits for the paediatric electrocardiogram. Eur Heart J 2001;22(8):702–11.

26. Saarel EV, Granger S, Kaltman JR, et al. Electrocardiograms in Healthy North American Children in the Digital Age. Circ Arrhythmia Electrophysiol 2018; 11(7):1–8.

27. Said SA. Cardiac and non-cardiac causes of T-wave inversion in the precordial leads in adult subjects: A Dutch case series and review of the literature. World J Cardiol 2015;7(2):86–100.

28. Dhutia H, Malhotra A, Gabus V, et al. Cost Implications of Using Different ECG Criteria for Screening Young Athletes in the United Kingdom. J Am Coll Cardiol 2016;68(7):702–11.

29. Sharma S, Drezner JA, Baggish A, et al. International Recommendations for Electrocardiographic Interpretation in Athletes. J Am Coll Cardiol 2017;69(8): 1057–75.

30. Levine BD, Baggish AL, Kovacs RJ, et al. Eligibility and Disqualification Recommendations for Competitive Athletes with Cardiovascular Abnormalities: Task Force 1: Classification of Sports: Dynamic, Static, and Impact: A Scientific Statement from the American Heart Association and American College of Cardiology. Circulation 2015;132(22):e262–6.

31. Uzark K, Jones K, Slusher J, et al. Quality of life in children with heart disease as perceived by children and parents. Pediatrics 2008;121(5).

32. Dean PN, Gillespie CW, Greene EA, et al. Sports participation and quality of life in adolescents and young adults with congenital heart disease. Congenit Heart Dis 2015;10(2):169–79.

33. Babiss LA, Gangwisch JE. Sports participation as a protective factor against depression and suicidal ideation in adolescents as mediated by self-esteem and social support. J Dev Behav Pediatr 2009;30(5):376–84.

34. Fox CK, Barr-Anderson D, Neumark-Sztainer D, et al. Physical activity and sports team participation: Associations with academic outcomes in middle school and high school students. J Sch Health 2010;80(1):31–7.

35. Amedro P, Picot MC, Moniotte S, et al. Correlation between cardio-pulmonary exercise test variables and health-related quality of life among children with congenital heart diseases. Int J Cardiol 2016;203:1052–60.

36. Colombo JN, McCulloch MA. Acyanotic congenital heart disease: Left-to-right shunt lesions. Neoreviews 2018;19(7):e375–83.

37. Amedro P, Guillaumont S, Bredy C, et al. Atrial septal defect and exercise capacity: Value of cardio-pulmonary exercise test in assessment and follow-up. J Thorac Dis 2018;10(11):S2864–73.

38. Van Hare GF, Ackerman MJ, Evangelista JAK, et al. Eligibility and Disqualification Recommendations for Competitive Athletes with Cardiovascular Abnormalities: Task Force 4: Congenital Heart Disease: A Scientific Statement from the American Heart Association and American College of Cardiology. Circulation 2015; 132(22):e281–91.

39. Binkhorst M, van de Belt T, de Hoog M, et al. Exercise Capacity and Participation of Children With a Ventricular Septal Defect. Am J Cardiol 2008;102(8):1079–84.

40. Maagaard M, Eckerström F, Redington A, et al. Comparison of Outcomes in Adults With Ventricular Septal Defect Closed Earlier in Life Versus Those in Whom the Defect Was Never Closed. Am J Cardiol 2020;133:139–47.

41. Eckerström F, Rex CE, Maagaard M, et al. Cardiopulmonary dysfunction in adults with a small, unrepaired ventricular septal defect: A long-term follow-up. Int J Cardiol 2020;306:168–74.

42. Basso C, Boschello M, Perrone C, et al. An echocardiographic survey of primary school children for bicuspid aortic valve. Am J Cardiol 2004;93(5):661–3.

43. Roos-Hesselink JW, Schölzel BE, Heijdra RJ, et al. Aortic valve and aortic arch pathology after coarctation repair. Heart 2003;89:1074–7.

44. Larson EW, Edwards WD. Risk factors for aortic dissection: A necropsy study of 161 cases. Am J Cardiol 1984;53(6):849–55.

45. Lin AE, Lippe B, Rosenfeld RG. Further delineation of aortic dilation, dissection, and rupture in patients with Turner syndrome. Pediatrics 1998;102(1):820–6.

46. Sybert VP. Cardiovascular malformations and complications in Turner syndrome. Pediatrics 1998;101(1):E11.

47. Otto CM, Nishimura RA, Bonow RO, et al. 2020 ACC/AHA Guideline for the Management of Patients with Valvular Heart Disease: A Report of the American College of Cardiology/American Heart Association Joint Committee on Clinical Practice Guidelines.; 2021. doi:

48. Siu SC, Silversides CK. Bicuspid Aortic Valve Disease. J Am Coll Cardiol 2010; 55(25):2789–800.

49. Niaz T, Fernandes SM, Sanders SP, et al. Clinical history and management of bicuspid aortic valve in children and adolescents. Prog Cardiovasc Dis 2020; 63(4):425–33.

50. Pedra CAC, Sidhu R, McCrindle BW, et al. Outcomes after balloon dilation of congenital aortic stenosis in children and adolescents. Cardiol Young 2004; 14(3):315–21.

51. Alpert BS, Kartodihardjo W, Harp R, et al. Exercise blood pressure response—a predictor of severity of aortic stenosis in children. J Pediatr 1981;98(5):763–5.

52. Santana S, Gidding SS, Xie S, et al. Correlation of Echocardiogram and Exercise Test Data in Children with Aortic Stenosis. Pediatr Cardiol 2019;40(7):1516–22.

53. Braverman AC, Harris KM, Kovacs RJ, et al. Eligibility and Disqualification Recommendations for Competitive Athletes with Cardiovascular Abnormalities: Task Force 7: Aortic Diseases, Including Marfan Syndrome: A Scientific Statement from the American Heart Association and American College of Cardi. Circulation 2015;132(22):e303–9.

54. Reller MD, Strickland MJ, Riehle-Colarusso T, et al. Prevalence of Congenital Heart Defects in Metropolitan Atlanta, 1998-2005. J Pediatr 2008;153(6):807–13.

55. Brouwer RMHJ, Erasmus ME, Ebels T, et al. Influence of age on survival, late hypertension, and recoarctation in elective aortic coarctation repair: Including longterm results after elective aortic coarctation repair with a follow-up from 25 to 44 years. J Thorac Cardiovasc Surg 1994;108(3):525–31.

56. Brown ML, Burkhart HM, Connolly HM, et al. Coarctation of the aorta: Lifelong surveillance is mandatory following surgical repair. J Am Coll Cardiol 2013;62(11): 1020–5.

57. Joshi G, Skinner G, Shebani SO. Presentation of coarctation of the aorta in the neonates and the infant with short and long term implications. Paediatr Child Heal (United Kingdom) 2017;27(2):83–9.

58. Dijkema EJ, Sieswerda GT, JMPJ Breur, et al. Exercise Capacity in Asymptomatic Adult Patients Treated for Coarctation of the Aorta. Pediatr Cardiol 2019;40(7): 1488–93.

59. Hager A, Kanz S, Kaemmerer H, et al. Exercise Capacity and Exercise Hypertension After Surgical Repair of Isolated Aortic Coarctation. Am J Cardiol 2008; 101(12):1777–80.

60. Morrical BD, Anderson JH, Taggart NW. Exercise Capacity Before and After Stent Placement for Coarctation of the Aorta: A Single-Center Case Series. Pediatr Cardiol 2017;38(6):1143–7.

61. Bailliard F, Anderson RH. Tetralogy of Fallot. Orphanet J Rare Dis 2009;4(1):1–10.

62. Sabate Rotes A, Johnson JN, Burkhart HM, et al. Cardiorespiratory Response to Exercise before and after Pulmonary Valve Replacement in Patients with Repaired Tetralogy of Fallot: A Retrospective Study and Systematic Review of the Literature. Congenit Heart Dis 2015;10(3):263–70.

63. Kipps AK, Graham DA, Harrild DM, et al. Longitudinal exercise capacity of patients with repaired tetralogy of Fallot. Am J Cardiol 2011;108(1):99–105.

64. Marcuccio E, Arora G, Quivers E, et al. Noninvasive measurement of cardiac output during exercise in children with tetralogy of fallot. Pediatr Cardiol 2012; 33(7):1165–70.

65. Aly S, Lizano Santamaria RW, Devlin PJ, et al. Negative Impact of Obesity on Ventricular Size and Function and Exercise Performance in Children and Adolescents With Repaired Tetralogy of Fallot. Can J Cardiol 2020;36(9):1482–90.

66. Rychik J, Atz AM, Celermajer DS, et al. Evaluation and Management of the Child and Adult with Fontan Circulation: A Scientific statement from the American heart association 2019;140.

67. Seckeler MD, Barber BJ, Colombo JN, et al. Exercise Performance in Adolescents With Fontan Physiology (from the Pediatric Heart Network Fontan Public Data Set). Am J Cardiol 2021;149(520):119–25.

68. Rato J, Sousa A, Cordeiro S, et al. Sports practice predicts better functional capacity in children and adults with Fontan circulation. Int J Cardiol 2020;306: 67–72.

69. Weinreb SJ, Dodds KM, Burstein DS, et al. End-organ function and exercise performance in patients with fontan circulation: What characterizes the high performers? J Am Heart Assoc 2020;9(24):1–10.

70. Turquetto ALR, Canêo LF, Agostinho DR, et al. Impaired Pulmonary Function is an Additional Potential Mechanism for the Reduction of Functional Capacity in Clinically Stable Fontan Patients. Pediatr Cardiol 2017;38(5):981–90.

71. Cordina RL, O'Meagher S, Karmali A, et al. Resistance training improves cardiac output, exercise capacity and tolerance to positive airway pressure in Fontan physiology. Int J Cardiol 2013;168(2):780–8.

72. Freud L, Webster G, Costello JM, et al. Growth and Obesity Among Older Single Ventricle Patients Presenting for Fontan Conversion. World J Pediatr Congenit Hear Surg 2015;6(4):514–20.

73. Maron BJ, Harris KM, Thompson PD, et al. Eligibility and Disqualification Recommendations for Competitive Athletes with Cardiovascular Abnormalities: Task Force 14: Sickle Cell Trait: A Scientific Statement from the American Heart Association and American College of Cardiology. J Am Coll Cardiol 2015;66(21): 2444–6.

74. Sutherland N, Jones B, d'Udekem Y. Should We Recommend Exercise after the Fontan Procedure? Hear Lung Circ 2015;24(8):753–68.

75. Cordina R, D'Udekem Y. Long-lasting benefits of exercise for those living with a Fontan circulation. Curr Opin Cardiol 2019;34(1):79–86.

76. Rhodes J, Curran TJ, Camil L, et al. Impact of cardiac rehabilitation on the exercise function of children with serious congenital heart disease. Pediatrics 2005; 116(6):1339–45.

77. McCrindle BW, Rowley AH, Newburger JW, et al. Diagnosis, Treatment, and Long-Term Management of Kawasaki Disease: A Scientific Statement for Health Professionals from the American Heart Association 2017;135.

78. Thompson PD, Myerburg RJ, Levine BD, et al. Eligibility and Disqualification Recommendations for Competitive Athletes with Cardiovascular Abnormalities: Task Force 8: Coronary Artery Disease: A Scientific Statement from the American Heart Association and American College of Cardiology. Circulation 2015;132(22): e310–4.

79. Aggarwal V, Sexson-Tejtal K, Lam W, et al. The incidence of arrhythmias during exercise stress tests among children with Kawasaki disease: A single-center case series. Congenit Heart Dis 2019;14(6):1032–6.

80. Gravel H, Curnier D, Dallaire F, et al. Cardiovascular Response to Exercise Testing in Children and Adolescents Late After Kawasaki Disease According to Coronary Condition Upon Onset. Pediatr Cardiol 2015;36(7):1458–64.
81. Banks L, Lin YT, Chahal N, et al. Factors associated with low moderate-to-vigorous physical activity levels in pediatric patients with kawasaki disease. Clin Pediatr (Phila) 2012;51(9):828–34.
82. Yang TH, Lee YY, Wang LY, et al. Patients with Kawasaki disease have significantly low aerobic metabolism capacity and peak exercise load capacity during adolescence. Int J Environ Res Public Health 2020;17(22):1–11.
83. Brothers JA, Frommelt MA, Jaquiss RDB, et al. Expert consensus guidelines: Anomalous aortic origin of a coronary artery. J Thorac Cardiovasc Surg 2017; 153(6):1440–57.
84. Cheezum MK, Liberthson RR, Shah NR, et al. Anomalous Aortic Origin of a Coronary Artery From the Inappropriate Sinus of Valsalva. J Am Coll Cardiol 2017; 69(12):1592–608.
85. Basso C, Maron BJ, Corrado D, et al. Clinical profile of congenital coronary artery anomalies with origin from the wrong aortic sinus leading to sudden death in young competitive athletes. J Am Coll Cardiol 2000;35(6):1493–501.

Printed and bound by CPI Group (UK) Ltd, Croydon, CR0 4YY

08/05/2025

01864704-0006